The Stigma of Mental Illness

Strategies Against Social Exclusion and Discrimination

The Stigma of Mental Illness

Strategies Against Social Exclusion and Discrimination

Nicolas Rüsch
Professor of Public Mental Health and Consultant Psychiatrist
Department of Psychiatry II and BKH Günzburg
University of Ulm
Germany

Adaptation Author
Shoshana Lauter
Department of Health Policy
London School of Economics and Political Science

With contributions from Yukti Ballani, Janine Berg-Peer, Anish V. Cherian, Petra C. Gronholm, Martina Heland-Graef, Santosh Loganathan, Gurucharan Bhaskar Mendon and Graham Thornicroft

ELSEVIER

The right of Nicolas Rüsch to be identified as author of this work has been asserted by him in accordance with the Copyright, Designs and Patents Act 1988.

First published in Germany under the title:
Rüsch, *Das Stigma psychischer Erkrankung*, 1st edition 2020 © Elsevier GmbH, Munich
ISBN 978-3-437-23520-7

Elsevier GmbH, Urban & Fischer Verlag
Bernhard-Wicki-Str. 5
80636 Munich
Germany

This adaptation of *Das Stigma psychischer Erkrankung* by Nicolas Rüsch was undertaken by Elsevier Limited and is published by arrangement with Elsevier GmbH.

Notices

The adaptation has been undertaken by Elsevier Limited at its sole responsibility. Practitioners and researchers must always rely on their own experience and knowledge in evaluating and using any information, methods, compounds or experiments described herein. Because of rapid advances in the medical sciences, in particular, independent verification of diagnoses and drug dosages should be made. To the fullest extent of the law, no responsibility is assumed by Elsevier, authors, editors or contributors for any injury and/or damage to persons or property as a matter of products liability, negligence or otherwise, or from any use or operation of any methods, products, instructions, or ideas contained in the material herein.

ISBN: 978-0-323-83429-2

Content Strategist: Robert Edwards
Content Project Manager: Tapajyoti Chaudhuri
Design: Ryan Cook
Marketing Manager: Deborah Watkins

Printed in Poland
Last digit is the print number: 9 8 7 6 5 4 3 2 1

Working together
to grow libraries in
developing countries

www.elsevier.com • www.bookaid.org

To my father Alfred Rüsch (1938–1983)

The neighbours of the Nasamones are the Psylli, but they no longer exist. There is a story which I repeat as the Libyans tell it: that the south wind dried up the water in their storage tanks, so that they were left with none whatever, as their territory lies wholly within the Syrtis. Upon this they held a council, and having unanimously decided to declare war on the south wind, they marched out to the desert, where the wind blew and buried them all in sand.

—HERODOTUS, *HISTORIES*, BOOK 4, 137

CONTENTS

I am delighted to see this important book by my dear friend and colleague, Nicolas Rüsch, is translated into English. Mental illness strikes with a two-edged sword. On one hand, people must cope with the symptoms and disabilities wrought by mental health challenges. On the other, the individual must deal with the public and self-stigma that come with mental health labels. Its consequences are vast and harmful. Stigma robs people of rightful life opportunities, for example, the employer who won't hire people or landlords who won't rent to those with labels. It leads to self-stigma and what has been called the *profound irony* of stigma and mental illness. Dealing with the sadness and self-doubt of symptoms like depression and anxiety are already hard enough. In addition, people are made to feel ashamed of themselves. Stigma also dissuades people from engaging in beneficial services. They avoid evidence-based mental health services in order to escape hurtful labels. 'That's Harry coming out of the psychiatrist's office; he must be nuts.'

The pain of stigma is classic. Nicolas uses his deep roots in ancient literature to frame stigma in terms of long-standing metaphor. Consider the sea god Proteus: with his many vagaries and slipperiness, he is an excellent metaphor for stigma. And consider the Greek hero Ajax: driven insane by Athena, he throws himself on his sword in shame. As archetype, the tragedy of stigma permeates the human conditions; stereotypes, prejudice and bigotry are at our core. Hence, we need to be aware of stigma's pernicious impact in order to change its course.

Stigma change is no easy task. In fact, we are often fooled by simple answers which actually exacerbate stigma. Nicolas notes the unintentional effects of stigma change strategies gone awry. Prominent among these is the inaccurate idea of changing stigma by framing mental illness as disease, typically genetic and inescapable. Yes, research shows mental illness as brain disorder may be effective in decreasing blame: 'It's not Harry's fault he has schizophrenia. It's inherited in his genes.' But mental illness as a brain disorder challenges notions of recovery, and this is what leads to discrimination. 'I'm not going to hire Harry. He looks good now, but his schizophrenic brain is a ticking time bomb. He could flip out and be violent any moment.' The research base highlighted by Nicolas is essential to figure out what does and does not lead to meaningful impact.

If there is any agreed-upon direction for beating stigma, it lies in the first-person efforts of people with lived experience. Research seems to suggest stories of recovery by people with lived experience replace stigma with notions of hope and aspiration. That is why I am pleased to see Martina Heland-Graef and Janine Berg-Peer joining Nicolas as coauthors from the perspective of persons with lived experience and family members. Together, the authors have produced a scholarly text that unpacks the complex challenges of stigma and ways forward to overcome. But I am reminded of Ajax because the authors of this book are heroes, seeking to defeat a major dragon in the lives of those with mental illness.

Pat Corrigan
Chicago, USA
16 January 2022

PREFACE

The stigma of mental illness is a complex burden for people with mental illness and for society. This book attempts to link research and practice on this topic. It aims to draw attention to stigma as a burden and injustice and to provide a basis for discussing antistigma initiatives. This text does not claim to be complete with regard to coverage of research literature or antistigma projects. It is primarily about clarifying the concepts and promising approaches of antistigma work. Apologies to all those whose initiatives or publications are not mentioned.

How might one read the book? The subsequent chapters build on each other. Those who have the time can read the book from beginning to end. Do not get distracted by the cross references (to other chapters). They only serve to make it easier for readers in a hurry to find references to other parts of the book, such that they can look up a specific topic or example (e.g. basic concepts in the first chapters or examples of antistigma programmes nearing the end). If you don't understand a particular idea or term, it is worth taking a look at the book's 'Glossary'.

This book is not a scientific reference book on methodological details or specific findings in research. Although I always refer to the underlying research literature, in the interest of readability I tend to focus more on recent systematic reviews than on individual studies (Sect. 1.5). When I quote from a review that brings together texts from various studies, I cite the review as evidence for the quote and not the original source. This may be considered philologically sloppy, but it shortens the bibliography and makes the book more readable. Quotes from non-English original sources are translated by me, if not indicated otherwise, and the translations are not authorised.

In some places, my irritation may be evident. This happens when dealing with issues such as discrimination and social injustice. Righteous anger is a term used in stigma research; it can motivate people and contribute to social change. At my age, I could pass as an angry old man.

Writing this book has taught me gratitude. I would first of all like to thank those who have made my work on mental illness stigma possible and who have accompanied me on my journey for many years. In chronological order, they are Pat Corrigan, stigma researcher from Chicago, who has been my mentor and friend for over 20 years; Mathias Berger in Freiburg, Germany, who gave me the freedom to devote myself to stigma in addition to brain research; and Wulf Rössler in Zurich, Switzerland, and his colleagues with whom I worked on stigma as part of a local project. For years I have had the good fortune to work with Thomas Becker at Günzburg and Ulm in Germany. We both deal with social aspects of mental illness, and I owe a lot to my exchanges with him and his support. I would like to thank the Bezirkskliniken Schwaben, to which the Günzburg psychiatric hospital belongs, and their CEO Thomas Düll, who has encouraged my work over the years. Finally, I am grateful to my fabulous colleagues at the Günzburg Home Treatment Team and to all of my patients for bringing me joy in clinical work.

For the last few years, my work at Ulm University and the Section of Public Mental Health there would not have been possible without my colleagues: Nathalie Oexle, who deals with, amongst other issues, stigma and suicidality (Sect. 5.2); Ziyan Xu, who contributed a rich East–West perspective in addition to her studies (Sect. 10.3); Moritz Wigand, with his interest in culture and stigma; and Nadja Puschner, who calmly helped me to get on top of the vast amount of literature. I am grateful for the exchange with my research colleagues in Günzburg: Reinhold Kilian, Markus Kösters, Silvia Krumm and Bernd Puschner. My observations on stigma would not be possible without my constant and long-standing exchanges with Sara Evans-Lacko and Graham Thornicroft in London, in addition to Pat Corrigan. Special thanks go to my friend Roland Zahn and our conversations, without which this book would not exist.

I am very grateful to the authors of three chapters that contribute key perspectives: Martina Heland-Graef and her view as person with lived experience of psychosis; Janine Berg-Peer on her experience as relative and carer; and Gurucharan Mendon, Yukti Ballani, Anish Cherian, Petra Gronholm, Graham Thornicroft and Santosh Loganathan, my colleagues from India and the UK, and their text on mental illness stigma in low- and middle-income countries.

Many of my relatives, friends and colleagues gave important comments on an earlier version of this manuscript that led to changes in content. My sincere thanks go to them all: Reinhold Aschenberg, Cornelia and Thomas Becker, Alexander Gallus, Joachim Hein, Rainer Höflacher, Andreas Jung, Johannes Keller, Florian Rüsch, Hans Joachim Salize, Georg Schomerus and Roland Zahn. I would like to thank other readers for finding various oversights and ambiguities. All remaining errors are mine. Many thanks to my colleagues at Elsevier, Uschi Jahn, Christine Kosel, Robert Edwards and Tapajyoti Chaudhuri, as well as to the editor Karin Beifuss and illustrator Heike Hübner. My special thanks go to Shoshana Lauter, who vastly improved the text's clarity, language and style; the process of translation and cultural adaptation for an international audience only worked due to her care and acuity, and it was a true pleasure to work with her.

While working on this book, I immersed myself again and again in reading and writing. This was necessary for the book, but was a burden on my family. I therefore thank not only my wife for her important advice on all parts of this book but also her and our children for their patience with me during this time.

If you as a reader of this book encounter gaps or ambiguities or simply have a different opinion, I would be pleased to receive constructive feedback at nicolas.ruesch@uni-ulm.de.

Nicolas Rüsch

Studied classics in Munich and Tübingen, with a master's degree at University of Oxford, UK. Medical school and training in psychiatry and psychotherapy in Freiburg, Germany, and two years of neurology in Rome, Italy. Postdoctoral work in the field of brain research (MRI). Two years of research on mental illness stigma at the Illinois Institute of Technology, Chicago, USA, with Prof. P.W. Corrigan; three years at the Zurich Psychiatric University Hospital, Switzerland, in clinical work and stigma research. Since 2013, Professor of Public Mental Health and consultant psychiatrist in a home treatment team at the Department of Psychiatry II, Ulm University and BKH Günzburg, in southern Germany. Visiting researcher with Sir Graham Thornicroft and colleagues at the Institute of Psychiatry, Psychology and Neuroscience, King's College London, UK, for more than 10 years.

Shoshana Lauter

Doctoral candidate in health policy at the London School of Economics and Political Science, UK. Is currently conducting an ethnographic study on the use of trauma-related diagnoses and concepts in urban social care services. Studentship is funded by the UK's National Institute for Health Research School for Social Care. Received her BA in sociology at Barnard College from Columbia University (2018) and MPhil in sociology from the University of Cambridge (2019). She has done both clinical counselling and academic research in psychiatric, reproductive and emergency healthcare settings and intends to work as an academic–practitioner in the field of psychotherapy. Her interests lie at the intersection of mental illness, urban poverty, social welfare and psychosocial studies.

Yukti Ballani has completed a master's degree in psychology and a postgraduate fellowship in mental health education. During her fellowship, she worked on projects about mental illness stigma in India. She has started her own practice as a psychotherapist and mental health educator in Gurugram, India, and currently manages a variety of social media platforms with the aim of raising awareness about different mental health concerns.

Janine Berg-Peer

Author, coach and blogger. Daughter of a mother with bipolar disorder and mother of a daughter with schizoaffective disorder. Four children, three grandchildren, one great-grandchild. Studied sociology in Berlin and Cairo, worked in research at an international business school and as a management consultant, and since 2013 as a consultant and coach for relatives of people with mental illness, giving lectures and readings to relatives in Germany and abroad. Author of several books.

Anish V. Cherian is Associate Professor of Psychiatric Social Work at National Institute of Mental Health and Neurosciences (NIMHANS), Bengaluru, India. He holds a PhD from NIMHANS and a Fogarty Postdoctoral Fellowship from the University of Florida, USA. His research interests include public mental health, suicide prevention, stigma and obsessive-compulsive disorder. He won a Public Health Research Initiative Fellowship from the Public Health Foundation of India (PHFI) to carry out public mental health research. He is part of the International Study of Discrimination and Stigma Outcomes (INDIGO) partnership and its Medical Research Council (MRC)-funded multicountry study on stigma.

Petra C. Gronholm is a Postdoctoral Research Fellow at the Centre for Global Mental Health at the Institute of Psychiatry, Psychology and Neuroscience of King's College London, UK. She has a background in health services research (PhD), mental health (MSc) and psychology (BSc). Her work is focused on understanding and reducing stigma and discrimination experienced by people with mental illness, particularly in relation to children and young people and global mental health. She is the Scientific Coordinator of the INDIGO Partnership research programme, a landmark global study to reduce mental illness stigma in low- and middle-income countries funded by the MRC.

Martina Heland-Graef

Psychiatric nurse, 57 years old, married. Active in peer support and as mental health advocate to speak for people who are unconfident or cannot represent themselves: 'I speak loudly for those who are too quiet.' Works mainly politically and organises self-help events in Bavaria. Board member of the Bavarian Association of Service Users. She likes knitting and crocheting, and she sews a lot of her own clothing. Her motto on good and bad days is 'Nothing is impossible! Psychosis does not mean you are dead. Psychosis means you live more intensely.'

Santosh Loganathan is Professor of Psychiatry at the NIMHANS, Bengaluru, India. His interests include social and cultural aspects related to stigma and mental health, mental health literacy, qualitative research, psychotherapy, adult and geriatric psychiatry, and family therapy. He is part of the INDIGO research programme with its cross-cultural study to reduce stigma and discrimination.

Gurucharan Bhaskar Mendon is a Senior Research Fellow in the ongoing INDIGO

research project at the Department of Psychiatry at NIMHANS, Bengaluru, India. His interests include the implementation of stigma reduction strategies in the community and mental health literacy trainings for teachers. He has experience in dealing with mental illness stigma among primary care workers as part of INDIGO project. At NIMHANS he was trained in skills-based training for psychosocial aspects of persons with mental health problems and their families. He is pursuing a PhD on strategies to reduce mental illness stigma with the long-term goal to contribute to culture-based interventions and programmes.

Sir Graham Thornicroft is Professor of Community Psychiatry in the Centre for Global Mental Health at the Institute of Psychiatry, Psychology and Neuroscience of King's College London, UK. He worked with colleagues to establish the Movement for Global Mental Health, a network of 200 institutions and 10,000 people to improve services for people with mental health problems and psychosocial disabilities worldwide, especially in low- and middle-income countries. He is cofounder of the INDIGO Network, a collaboration in over 40 countries worldwide working to reduce discrimination against people with mental illness. He has published over 575 scientific papers and 30 books. He chairs the Guideline Development Group for the World Health Organization (WHO) guidelines on work and mental health, and he is a Trustee of United for Global Mental Health. Graham was made a Knight Bachelor in the 2017 Queen's Birthday Honours for services to mental health.

CHAPTER 1

Introduction

People with mental illness face compounding challenges. They not only deal with the symptoms of their illness—be it deep sadness, hearing voices, loss of energy, suicidality—but they also face the consequences of being *labelled* mentally ill. Stigma is often aptly named *the second illness:* its social consequences can have just as, if not more of, a negative effect on those living with mental illness than the actual symptoms [1]. Discrimination by others (public stigma) can be augmented by self-stigma and shame about the illness, as well as structural discrimination in legal or organisational procedures.

Support and treatment options of all kinds, from mutual help groups and peer support to psychiatry, are better known and more frequently used than just a few decades ago. But not enough is being done to counteract stigma. This is a serious shortcoming and in itself a sign of discrimination against a large population group. Our society would never accept such pronounced social exclusion of and discrimination against people with physical illnesses. Stigma is not a trivial problem or a small hiccup in social interaction. The consequences are numerous and brutal: exclusion from family, friends and community; isolation, desperation and suicidality; poverty and need due to employment and housing discrimination; avoidance of seeking help; discrimination in the healthcare system; a much lower life expectancy; distorted images in the media; and disenfranchisement and discrimination in the legal system (such as the German federal electoral law upheld until 2019). Stigma is ultimately a barrier to recovery, managing illness, social justice and a fulfilling, equitable life.

1.1 Aims and Content of the Book

This book has two aims: to present the various aspects and effects of mental illness stigma and then to discuss ways of reducing it.

The consequences of stigma are often underestimated or hidden; only individual aspects are seen, if at all. But stigma can take many forms in different contexts and has numerous effects. Only by knowing about stigma's multidimensionality can we develop antistigma programmes that realistically and helpfully reduce it. The goal of reducing stigma is not simple, and even the most well-intentioned approaches can misjudge or reinforce the issues at hand (Sect. 1.3).

Stigma is like the sea god Proteus of Greek mythology, who takes on many forms and is difficult to capture (Homer, *Odyssey*; 4, 349 ff.). But once seized, Proteus can predict the future. Likewise, once we have grasped the different types and consequences of stigma, we can discuss future ways of reducing it and the social exclusion of people with mental illness. This is the second aim of the book. We know a lot about what helps, but good antistigma programmes are used far too rarely—even though hundreds of millions of people are affected across the world. It's time to act.

The book is divided into the following parts. Following this first chapter, the concepts of mental illness and stigma are introduced with a focus on their history, social contexts, and issues of burden and social inclusion (Ch. 2). This is followed by a description, based on sociological and social psychology studies, of what stigma is and what function it fulfills for individuals and groups (Ch. 3). Chapter 4 deals with the consequences of stigma for those who are stigmatised as well as for the general public. In these chapters, we lay down the foundations critical to understanding the stigma not only of mental illness but of related experiences and characteristics, for example, the case of long-term unemployment.

Chapter 5 addresses the topic of stigma for people with mental illness in general (Sect. 5.1), followed by certain groups who, due to the nature of their illness, their specific troubles (e.g. suicidality) or their role in society, have to deal with stigma in a particular way (Sects. 5.2–5.8). This is followed by personal perspectives on stigma from the viewpoint of a service user (Martina Heland-Graef, Sect. 6.1) and a service user's family member (Janine Berg-Peer, Sect. 6.2).

Stigma operates in specific social contexts. Its manifestation in different areas of society, namely, work, housing, healthcare, media and the legal system, are therefore discussed (Sects. 7.1–7.5). Chapter 7 includes a discussion of antistigma interventions targeted specifically towards each of these spheres of society. The basics, effectiveness and examples of successful antistigma work beyond these specific areas are dealt with in Chapters 8 to 12. Chapter 13, written by Gurucharan Bhaskar Mendon and his colleagues, deals with sociocultural aspects of stigma and discrimination in low- and middle-income countries. The final chapter summarises key points and provides an outlook to the future (Ch. 14).

To orient and facilitate reading, the following are available: an alphabetical list of terms (a combined glossary and list of abbreviations), bibliographical references and an index at the end of the book. Throughout the text, there are references to other chapters or sections to establish links, for example, between stigma concepts at the beginning and antistigma interventions towards the end. Websites where further information can be found are occasionally mentioned. Translations of non-English quotations are mine (except the English Standard Version of the Bible), but they are not authorised. References for the original quotations are given for those interested.

1.2 Language

Our actions are influenced by the words we use to speak and think about ourselves and others. If I as a doctor treat *a schizophrenic*, I will treat him (and he will treat me) differently than if I address Mr Jones, who has a profession, children, a dog and schizophrenia. Each of us hold many identities, roles and characteristics; no one *is* his or her illness. The resulting principle of addressing or naming the person first (Mr Jones), instead of the illness, is called *person-first language*. For some people, the emphasis on politically correct language these days may seem too drawn-out. But to name the person first and to deal with him or her in this way is both logical and sensible—in this book, we therefore do not talk about *the mentally ill* but about *people with mental illness*.

Language can become a battlefield: words such as stigma and discrimination often connote issues of social injustice and can elicit anger and contention. The term *stigma* can also be rejected when perceived to lay blame on the person himself (Sect. 3.1.2). The conversation about stigma falters when we get wrapped up in choosing the correct words. I remember a conference where I sat on the podium next to a man with a history of mental illness. The aim of the meeting was to talk about common approaches and initiatives of service users, relatives and healthcare professionals in antistigma work. The conversation broke down, however, before it had begun. This panelist said first that there were no *mental illnesses*, and as such there could be no programmes against the *stigma of mental illness*. End of discussion.

Of course, every person is free to choose a preferred expression for his or her own experience of mental crisis, emotional upheaval, etc. However, the refusal of an exchange on the stigma of mental illness because of the words used to describe it seems to me to be a fallacy for three reasons:

- A woman released from a psychiatric hospital may experience discrimination on returning to work because, in the view of her colleagues, she was in a 'the looney bin' and is now *crazy* or a *psycho*. The term chosen in a panel discussion to describe the stigmatised characteristic is irrelevant to the situation of the woman.

- The adversity faced by those with mental illness is far too pressing for us to get bogged down in linguistic disputes. I ask myself: do we really want to fight about words? Isn't the ongoing discrimination suffered by people with mental illness too important for that?
- There will be no choice of words that satisfies everyone (nor is this even desirable in a pluralistic society that respects different perspectives). American stigma researcher Pat Corrigan once reported that service users had advised him to use the term *mental health challenges* in future lectures on stigma; the term *mental illness* appeared too negative, too psychiatric. Pat followed the advice in his next presentation. Thereupon an angry listener came up to him and said: 'Mental health "challenge"! What's that? I have a mental illness. "Challenge" waters down the whole thing. Call it what it is: mental ILLNESS' ([2], p. 105).

My conclusion is to strive for language and actions that do not devalue people. Linguistic sensitivity is important—words can be painful and denigrating. But in this book I will not lean into the wishes of thought police who dictate how we should speak and who get stuck on terms instead of focusing on meaningful antistigma work.

1.3 Aims of Antistigma Work

Reducing stigma as a manifestation of social injustice is of course an honourable goal. But does antistigma work always result in *good*? Not quite. A well-meant initiative can actually aggravate the matter, for example, by focusing on biological or medical models of mental illness (Sect. 5.1.2). Additionally, antistigma work often overlooks and fails to prioritise certain key objectives. There are three overarching objectives or agendas of antistigma work [3], namely, the reduction of stigma aimed to improve:

1. use of available services (services agenda),
2. rights and equality (rights agenda) and
3. self-esteem of people with mental illness (self-worth agenda).

First, stigma leads to people not seeking help and treatment because of their fear of public stigma, self-stigma and shame (Sect. 5.1.7). An antistigma programme would aim to reduce this avoidance of treatment such that more people with mental illness could seek assistance (services agenda). The people behind programmes with this objective are often people with mental illness and positive treatment experiences themselves, as well as relatives and mental healthcare professionals.

Second, stigma often leads to limitations and restrictions on social participation in important areas of life, such as education, work and independent living (Ch. 7). Antistigma initiatives can thereby support a second objective—strengthening the rights of people with mental illness and reducing discrimination against them—in line with the UN Convention on the Rights of Persons with Disabilities (UN-CRPD; Sect. 7.5.2, rights agenda).

Finally, self-stigma and shame can lead to one's loss of self-esteem (Sect. 5.1.3). Antistigma work can thereby maintain a third objective of removing self-stigma and instead promoting and building self-determination, empowerment, hope and self-confidence (self-worth agenda). Important to this goal are self-help groups, peer support (Sect. 7.3.4) and programmes that help service users make confident decisions regarding disclosure (Sect. 9.2).

Why is it important to differentiate between the objectives? First and foremost, no antistigma programme can achieve all three objectives equally well. Resources such as money, social commitment and attention are limited, and it is therefore critical to consider where a programme's focus should be placed. Additionally, unintended side effects are possible. Let us assume that an antistigma programme has the goal of increasing treatment participation. It will provide a picture of mental illness with a focus on symptoms, risks of untreated illness and functional limitations which can be improved with treatment. Such a programme could facilitate treatment participation while reinforcing prejudice by emphasising the deficits and differences of people with mental illness. Research on the side effects of different agendas such as these is rare. However, service users who are free of self-stigma seem to prioritise antistigma work aimed at rights and equality over other approaches [3].

Finally, a possible misconception should be pointed out. When psychiatrists or other mental healthcare professionals engage in antistigma work, it is sometimes suspected that they would like to 'psychiatrise' people. In these instances, they are said to be more concerned with expanding their area of treatment and power than with the goal of reducing stigma. I cannot evaluate the motives of others. But from my point of view, good antistigma work for increased treatment participation (Ch. 10) has a simple goal: to encourage people who would otherwise be deterred by fear of stigma, shame or lack of good support to seek and maintain help (Sect. 5.1.7). Sources of help should be understood in a broader sense (rather than restricted to psychiatry) and include not only professionals but family, friends, self-help and peer support as well ('Glossary'). If people refuse support for other reasons (e.g. because they don't think it will help), then that is their right. But antistigma programmes with a services agenda are not about psychiatrisation; they are about enabling free decisions that are not restricted by fear of stigma, self-stigma or shame.

1.4 Dismissing Concerns?

After one of my lectures on this topic, I spoke to relatives of people with mental illness about stigma. One young woman came up to me and reported that she was sometimes afraid of her father when he was tense during an acute psychosis. She asked about her fear: 'Am I stigmatising?' The quick answer: no. People (with and without psychosis) can be aggressive, and fear is an obvious reaction. Stigma is a tendency to judge and react to someone on the basis of the qualities attributed to the group he is labelled a part of, rather than to him as an individual ('All psychotics are dangerous and frighten me, even if they seem calm at times.'). To fight stigma, one does not have to dismiss or override all fears and concerns in certain situations.

This young woman's question shows us that we cannot ignore real problems when dealing with the stigma of mental illness. Glossing over her fear may sound positive, but it doesn't really do any justice to the suffering that is (also) associated with mental illness. *Schizophrenia Sucks, Mum!*, a book by Janine Berg-Peer (Sect. 6.2), ultimately takes its title from something her daughter said about her own illness. Service users often point out that antistigma work should not minimise real problems. It should not be denied that people with severe mental illness may be less able to cope in certain situations (e.g. with stress at work). Regardless, they should be enabled to participate despite their limitations or disability.

In this context, it is helpful to distinguish between being socially labelled as *mentally ill* on the one hand and actual functional impairment or disability due to the illness on the other (label versus disability). If someone has an alcohol addiction and continues to drink, they are not allowed to work as a pilot or truck driver. This is not discrimination, but simply the consequence of illness-related impairments. However, depriving someone of the right to vote just because they are labelled as *mentally ill* could very well be a case of discrimination (Sect. 7.5.4).

1.5 Studies and Evidence
1.5.1 CHATTING ABOUT WEATHER, FOOTBALL ... AND THE BRAIN

There are many vying opinions and approaches as to what should be done about the stigma of mental illness—it's almost like when we discuss football or the weather. The amount of interest in this topic is unsurprising. Mental illness is incredibly common; everyone has to deal with it to a certain extent either in themselves or in their private or professional environments. The problem is, however, that some opinions and approaches are nonsensical—and unlike the weather or football, they can have serious repercussions. During my time in Zurich, I was once invited to another region of Switzerland to consult a foundation that wanted to start an antistigma initiative. A decision had already been taken on the strategy: first, in order to remove stigma, the general public should learn that mental illness is a brain disease. Nobody has prejudices against metabolic disorders such as diabetes, they figured. Would people still have anything against schizophrenia if they understood that it was a metabolic brain disorder? A marketing company was commissioned to design fancy logos, pictures, balloon promotions and the like. When I heard this, I remarked that the focus on the brain was likely to aggravate, not improve, stigma (Sect. 5.1.2). I suggested giving the money not to the marketing company but instead to initiatives of service users, so that they could control the programme and carry it out themselves (e.g. through contact-based anti-stigma work; Sect. 8.4). None of this stirred the interest of the foundation. Service users and relatives withdrew from the collaboration, as did I. The moral of the story: well-meaning work is not the same as good work.

1.5.2 TYPES OF STUDIES, INFORMATION, CAUSALITY

So how do we separate the strong approaches in antistigma work from those merely well intentioned? Good research helps in this regard; there are certain studies that provide evidence on which types of antistigma work are effective or not—as well as for whom, how much effort is needed, long-term sustainability, etc. The basic structures of these studies and methodologies are explained in this section. However, it is important to note that researchers themselves can be biased. Even researchers are blinkered, stick to certain procedures and can have pet projects. Studies can be perceived, interpreted or conducted in skewed ways. Rarely are one's motivations made explicit; goals for antistigma work (Sect. 1.3) often remain vague. Self-marketing is not uncommon. On the whole, this book does not intend to simply express opinions but rather to present points of view which can be substantiated by sound research whenever possible. Readers should be able to understand what kind of information these points of view are based on.

First up are the *first-person accounts* of those with mental illness, which are pivotal in demonstrating how stigma is experienced in the daily lives of those most affected. Second, one must distinguish between quantitative and qualitative research. *Quantitative studies* ultimately collect numbers and measure something: I can measure the increase in heart rate when someone experiences stigma; I can use a questionnaire to measure the degree of self-stigma or shame experienced on a scale of 1 (not at all) to 7 (extremely high). Qualitative studies, on the other hand, collect the views of different people in the form of individual or group interviews, for example, on their experiences with stigma. The resulting reports and perspectives are rich in content but not in numbers. Quantitative and qualitative studies thus provide different types of information that complement each other. Both are indispensable for stigma research; in this book, therefore, in addition to quantitative findings, statements by people from qualitative studies are cited.

Next, it is important to distinguish between longitudinal and cross-sectional studies. *Cross-sectional studies* ask people with depression, for example, about their symptoms and self-stigma at a certain point in time. In a *longitudinal study*, questions are asked and data is collected repeatedly over the course of a longer timeline.

There are also *observational studies* regarding process: 'How do people who are unemployed and have mental health problems fare over the course of a year?' These are different from *intervention studies*, wherein those unemployed subjects may, for instance, participate in a group programme with an intended goal of some kind of change. Intervention studies may simply investigate how participants feel before and after the intervention. These 'pre–post' studies are common but limited; they cannot prove the effectiveness of an intervention. For example, if I administer medication for fever and the fever drops, I don't know if it was due to the aspirin (intervention) or if the fever would have dropped in any case. Similarly, I don't know whether self-stigma diminished because of the group programme or because things improved for the participants with time, regardless of the intervention.

Controlled studies therefore examine the effectiveness of an intervention by comparing participants who receive the intervention with a control group (without the intervention). The most sophisticated form of controlled trials is the *randomised controlled trial* (RCT; see 'Glossary'). In it, study participants are randomly assigned to receive the intervention or control. This type of random placement is critical. Examiners could otherwise place particularly motivated study participants into the programme and unmotivated ones into the control group, resulting in a misleading impression that the intervention is effective. In the course of an RCT, a comparison is made between how participants fare with or without intervention. If, for example, self-stigma is only reduced amongst those participants receiving the intervention, this is a strong indication of its causal effectiveness.

CAUSALITY

Beyond RCTs and related research methods, the question of causality in the case of stigma is important to consider: can stigma itself worsen someone's mental health and well-being? Can self-stigma contribute to suicidality?

A statistical correlation alone does not imply causality. A well-known example is that of the storks and birth rates: the decline in the number of the storks in the second half of the 20th century shows a clear statistical correlation with the decline in the number of births in the same period. So do storks deliver babies after all? Who knows. It is more likely, however, that both processes could be due to social changes that have led to families having fewer children, as well as a decline in frog-friendly environments—these two facts put together are therefore known as a spurious correlation.

The topic of causality is important because the role of stigma should not be exaggerated. Not every correlation between stigma and the poor status of people with mental illness or with social grievances alarmingly points to stigma as a *cause*. If in a cross-sectional study of people with mental illness more self-stigma is correlated with more suicidality, this could just be a spurious correlation—higher levels of depression can increase both. However, a study of this nature could provide a strong indication of self-stigma as a (co)cause of suicidality if it is first performed as a longitudinal study (i.e. investigates self-stigma at the beginning of the study and suicidality months later) and if the role of psychological symptoms is statistically taken into account [4].

1.5.3 HOW CAN THE RESEARCH STATUS BE SUMMARISED?

Every year, thousands of scientific papers on the subject of stigma are published worldwide; not even specialists can keep track of them all. These studies employ all of the research methods mentioned above and countless others. The situation is made more difficult by the fact that research follows trends. Important issues are not investigated if they are not in vogue. The relatively few studies on psychosocial interventions and their implementation (Sect. 7.3.3) is one such example. Within this reality and amongst piles of individual studies, how can a data-based summary be obtained? There is an international research network focused on the collection and summary of evidence from many separate studies: the international *Cochrane Collaboration* (https://cochrane.org) systematically reviews the effectiveness of a wide range of healthcare and policy interventions.

I will now outline a number of ways to summarise the available evidence because I refer to the underlying research that produces it throughout this book. Sometimes there is a complete lack of (good) studies or evidence on a specific topic. This does not mean that an intervention is not effective: the absence of evidence is not the evidence of absence. But mere opinions and ideations do not provide certain ground.

Individual studies provide useful, detailed evidence that enriches our understanding of specific cases and concepts; this book occasionally presents these studies to illustrate how they are conducted (method) and what information they provide (results). But for a comprehensive overview, reviews or summaries of a large number of these individual studies are preferable. In systematic reviews, available studies are searched for in electronic databases in a traceable and verifiable manner and then selected and summarised according to previously defined criteria.

Many systematic reviews contain, if possible, meta-analyses. These are analyses that calculate and average the effectiveness of an intervention across various individual studies. However, several issues arise from this kind of approach:

- The boundary conditions and contexts of interventions are often not taken into account, which is why average values often need to be taken with a grain of salt. Let us assume that a meta-analysis finds that a programme used in various studies has a weak average effect in reducing public stigma. This average may hide the fact that the programme does not work at all for GPs but is in fact very effective for employers.
- The scaling of intervention strength in the field of antistigma interventions and social psychology is not well defined. A meta-analysis of the effect of aspirin may show that 500 mg reduces fever by an average of 0.5 °C. However, in the case of antistigma interventions, the 'dose' used in various programmes is uncertain—there is no milligram scale. Some meta-analyses therefore group together individual antistigma interventions for which the length, type of implementation and medium are all completely different. Such summaries can lead to half-baked information.
- Information from meta-analyses can only ever be as good as the individual studies on which it draws. If individual studies are not available or methodologically flawed, even the best meta-analysis will not help. We cannot possibly examine and measure everything, and this is one of the limits of so-called evidence-based medicine. For example, one review published in the respected *British Medical Journal* wrote up evidence on the life-saving effectiveness of parachutes. Lo and behold, there was not even evidence to exhibit—there had never been an RCT conducted on the use of parachutes [5].

When one digs through mountains of literature (as when working on this book), one *experiences* the peculiarities of today's scientific world first-hand. Quantity is preferred over quality. Complete nonsense can be published, and editors and reviewers of journals often fail to do their jobs. Even strong research groups publish fragments of their overall studies in multiple separate papers, such that a huge number of articles end up on these colleagues' publication lists, but the knowledge gained from the overall study remains hidden. It is astonishing that, in tax-financed research, this concealment of knowledge due to a craving for recognition is tolerated. All of this has to do with the Sovietisation of our scientific system (Plaggenborg, FAZ, 3 Jul. 2019): target figures for research grants and publications are set, diligently fulfilled and recorded. But really new ideas hardly ever emerge in this way, as they are perceived as too challenging to measure.

The data presented in the book contain many gaps and deficiencies. First, I have undoubtedly overlooked or been biased while choosing and reproducing some of the literature. Second, I mostly limit the studies I engage with to those in Western countries. The issue of stigma in low- and middle-income countries is therefore dealt with in a separate chapter by my colleagues (Ch. 13; see also https://indigo-group.org and the work of Vikram Patel and Graham Thornicroft [6]). Third, I have decided to summarise the findings from various Western countries into one account. I recognise there are differences between these countries that affect the stigma of mental illness and its consequences. However, data from only the EU or even only from German-speaking countries would be too sparse, and a great deal of information would be lost. And the results of Western studies on stigma, for example, from the United States or Europe, are not so different that a summary would be harmful. Nevertheless, a (regional) fuzziness remains. To make this clear, the countries of origin for individual studies are occasionally mentioned.

And so while this book offers a rough summary, the goal is to make the evidence easier to read. While the details, contradictions and gaps in knowledge of available literature are typically discussed in depth in a singular research article, in this book I summarise—intentionally and despite the weaknesses of the procedure mentioned above—whole meta-analyses that are dozens or hundreds of pages long in just one or two sentences. This gives a better overview, albeit with less detail. The literature references offer suggestions for further reading.

1.6 Diagnoses and Continuum

Diagnosis is a controversial topic for various reasons, particularly in the field of stigma research. First of all, there are several advantages and disadvantages to obtaining and having a psychiatric diagnosis that depend on the person, the point of view and the context [7].

Among the possible *advantages* of a diagnosis are access to treatment and reimbursement of treatment costs, rehabilitation and other support services; possibility of temporary sick leave; and labour law protection, for example, in the context of an illness-related disability. Some people with mental illness are relieved that the diagnosis finally gives their condition a name and makes it more tangible—in this respect, diagnostic labelling of symptoms or behaviour (not the person) is helpful. With a diagnosis, service users can often find better support in the form of literature, mutual-support groups, therapists, etc. Diagnoses also facilitate communication with and between healthcare practitioners. Finally, a diagnosis can protect people from punishment if they have committed a crime while in a state of illness-related incapacity.

On the other hand, diagnoses can mean considerable *disadvantages*, as they often lead to being labelled as *mentally ill* and subsequently to public stigma, self-stigma and/or structural discrimination. Either way, people with severe mental illness in particular report that their initial diagnosis represented a profound turning point in their lives, after which little was as it had been before.

Does the *type of diagnosis* play a role in the stigma associated with it? This is a complex issue. There is stigma attached to mental illness in general, regardless of an individual's diagnosis. When someone has been in a psychiatric hospital and their neighbour stops being friendly, that neighbour may not know what their diagnosis is (or may be indifferent to it). The label and association of them *being crazy* or *bonkers*, however, could drive that neighbour's change in behaviour. But the characteristics of some specific psychiatric diagnoses, and the social attitudes towards people with these illnesses, do in fact lead to particular aspects of stigma (Sect. 5.4). One example is the accusation that service users are responsible for their illness, particularly pronounced in the case of addictions (Sect. 5.4.7).

Despite certain undeniable differences in individual diagnoses, progress in stigma research and the development of antistigma interventions should be possible through a transdiagnostic view (i.e. by looking beyond the often artificial boundaries of the diagnosis). There are three key reasons for this: first, many of the effects of stigma are not diagnosis specific. The example of the neighbour mentioned in the previous paragraph applies to other areas of life. The experience of being different (socially attributed or self-experienced) is more important than differences in symptoms. Second, there is more to lose than gain when stigma research is broken up into countless diagnosis-related subareas, and there is a strong methodological case for a uniform, *transdiagnostic approach* [8, 9].

A third reason is the limited plausibility and temporal stability of psychiatric diagnoses, both in practice and conceptually amongst patients and practitioners alike. In practice, people with serious illnesses regularly receive many different diagnoses over the decades: schizophrenia, schizoaffective disorder, bipolar disorder with psychotic symptoms, in addition to perhaps an anxiety, addiction or personality disorder. A random sample of letters from psychiatric hospitals regarding one person often reveals a mixed bag of labels. Stigma is therefore a transdiagnostic problem because after each treatment episode, neither the employer nor the neighbour will react differently according to the new diagnosis. They will simply say: 'Mr Jones was in the loony bin again!'

Conceptually, the issue is much more difficult. Even though certain psychiatric classification systems provide and continuously update hundreds of diagnoses, they do not define what a mental illness actually is. This problem has long been a point of contention in psychiatry [10]. Mental illness is often pragmatically referred to as a combination of subjective suffering, disrupted social participation or functioning, and some core symptoms of the particular illness that have been present for a certain amount of time. When considering social functioning, however, it should be noted that this is not (only) determined by the person's deficiencies but also by the social environment—in the latter case, stigma and discrimination play a role.

So what about a man who hears voices, thinks he is the Roman emperor Caligula, thereby makes his horse a senator, and otherwise lives a very solitary but not unhappy life on his farm? Is he *mentally ill*? From which external perspective should this be assessed, and who would have the right to do so? Historians too find this question tricky the other way round [11]: was Caligula a case of 'Caesar madness' or rather a healthy cynic who made fun of the Roman senatorial aristocracy with his horse? Examples such as this one show that the definition of mental illness is always influenced by social norms. The topic is well known because of long-standing debates within the field, such as criticism from the antipsychiatry movement in the 1960s: psychiatry establishes boundaries around 'normal' social behaviour, classifies certain behaviour arbitrarily as disordered and thereby contributes to the suppression of people with deviancies (Sect. 2.1.3).

Two further, related reasons for doubting the meaningfulness of psychiatric diagnoses should be mentioned, and both have to do with the fact that diagnoses imply a distinction between a *normal* and an *ill* state. First, it can be unclear as to whether a commonly defined mental illness is in fact a 'normal' reaction to a cruel environment. Second, there is undoubtedly a continuum that exists between a completely healthy mental state on one end and the most severe mental illness on the other. According to the *continuum model*, there is no dividing line between being *ill* and *healthy* (Sect. 3.1.4). In contrast to many physical illnesses, determining a mental illness is not made any easier by the fact that there are no definitive biological measurements available to it: no blood test, no genetic test, no MRI image of the brain that can prove or exclude the presence of depression or schizophrenia, anxiety or an obsessive-compulsive disorder.

Do the problems in defining mental illness thereby suggest that mental illness is made-up (possibly by psychiatrists)? I don't think so (although I am of course biased). Madness or insanity, as it was once called, has been fundamental to the human experience for thousands of years (Sect. 2.1.1). To make a simple comparison: falling is a problem. People can fall when it is slippery, when their blood pressure drops, or when they are drunk or have some genetic defect. They can sink to the ground in despair and die there (Sect. 2.3.1, 'Deaths of Despair'); they can throw themselves off a bridge. All of these falls can be dangerous or even fatal. Yet no one would say that falling is a *singular* problem or disease—obviously there are countless different ways of falling, varying in cause, course, treatment and consequences. Assessing a fall is relatively straightforward: low blood pressure can be measured and treated. Even epilepsy, which used to be called falling sickness, is no longer a 'sacred disease' (Lat. *morbus sacer*) but has been demystified by measuring brain waves and can be assessed and treated.

Mental illnesses, on the other hand, are much more complex. This is due to the biological intricacies of the brain, with its many billions of neurons and neuronal connections. And the brain is also a deeply social, *mediating organ* [12]; understanding it cannot be reduced to neuronal (mis)function alone. To stick with the comparison of falling: like a cluster of *falling illnesses*, there are many different, and very real, kinds of mental illnesses with a variety of causes, courses and consequences—from enriching to threatening. They are simply difficult to define. But this rather lofty and academic challenge does not alter the fact that we need to remove the stigma associated with these illnesses. Choosing a term for the illness is secondary. Disputes over this issue distract from the task (Sect. 1.2).

To summarise, psychiatric diagnoses in this book are regarded as a way of communication. They can be useful or harmful, and they are not devoid of content. On the contrary, Karl Leonhard's *Classification of Endogenous Psychoses and Their Differentiated Etiology* [13] contains a wealth of insight on psychoses. Leonhard claimed the ability to distinguish between many different subtypes of psychoses according to their course and cause. But the question of what a mental illness is remained unanswered for him as well. With our current level of knowledge, many in the field acknowledge that psychiatric diagnoses cannot perfectly delineate naturally distinct realities in terms of exact causes, courses, symptoms and treatments.

Pragmatically, there is much to be said for a model that identifies different stages of symptoms and illness course (Fig. 1.1) and thereby serves as a compromise between a diagnostic model (illness: yes or no) and the continuum model mentioned above. This model with different stages includes (as described in Fig. 1.1 from top to bottom) mental well-being, unspecified mental stress (e.g. worries), significant impairment from symptoms that fall below the threshold of a diagnosis or are temporary (e.g. exhaustion, anxiety), and fully defined syndromes (mainly an anxiety or affective/mood or psychosis syndrome). Not shown in the figure but important in the course of the illness are persistent symptoms or symptoms that recur in the event of relapse. The term 'aberrant salience' in Fig. 1.1 refers to the fact that in psychoses, everyday issues can take on a special meaning.

What is considered to be a *mental illness* in the general public can also be empirically investigated. In a Finnish study, more than 3200 people were interviewed: politicians, nurses, doctors and the general public [14]. There was general agreement (>75% in each of the four groups) only insofar as schizophrenia and autism were considered mental illnesses, but not grief and homosexuality. There was more widespread disagreement as to whether one should refer to mental illness when speaking of conditions such as eating disorders, anxiety and personality disorders, ADHD, depression, addictions, work-related exhaustion and transsexuality. In an English survey,

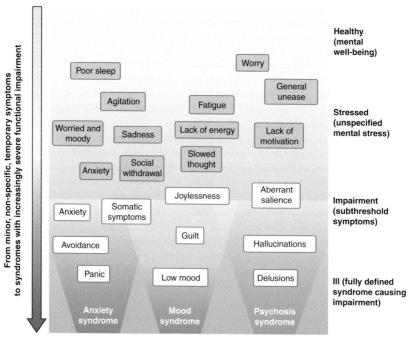

Fig. 1.1 Different stages of mental health/illness. (Based on Patel V, et al. The Lancet Commission on global mental health and sustainable development. *Lancet.* 2018;392:1553–1598.)

people who regarded bipolar disorder or schizophrenia as mental illnesses had more positive attitudes towards people with mental illness. Respondents who endorsed a broader concept of mental illness, such that stress and grief were also seen as illnesses, had increased negative attitudes but felt that disclosure to employers would be easier [15]. It is therefore worth clarifying what precisely is being talked about in the field of antistigma interventions. Focusing on individual diagnoses is probably less helpful than separating between severe mental illnesses and common mental disorders (e.g. anxiety or nonsevere depressive disorders). Even more important than such distinctions, however, is the context: only context-based campaigns can also address structural discrimination, for example, in work settings (Sect. 7.1), the healthcare system (Sect. 7.3), the media (Sect. 7.4) or the legal system (Sect. 7.5). Before examining those campaigns, it is worth looking at particular disorders or age groups that uniquely deal with stigma (Sects. 5.2–5.4).

1.7 Stigma in Times of Social Upheaval

Mental illness has social causes as well as consequences. Stigma is an expression of social attitudes. In this respect, issues in society and the stigma of mental illness are intrinsically linked. Ulrich Beck once pointed out that the terms 'change' and 'transition' no longer suffice to describe our world; transition implies that some things change, but others remain the same. In our world, however, nothing seems to stay as it is. A fundamental transformation—a metamorphosis—is taking place: 'The world is unhinged' ([16], p. xi). Like Gregor Samsa in Franz Kafka's story *The Metamorphosis*, we may suddenly find ourselves lying on our backs like a beetle. Gregor in his new form faces the disgust of his environment and ultimately dies, while his family no longer speak of him as a person but as a thing: 'It must go away ... just to try to get rid of the thought that it is Gregor.' The resonance of Kafka's 1912 story today suggests that the metamorphosis taking place all over the modern world finds countless people in weak positions, estranged from others, experiencing exclusion, dehumanisation and death.

The *metamorphosis* of our world comprises strands and processes that can no longer be separated. Global phenomena such as climate change, obesity and malnutrition are so intertwined that they are referred to as a *syndemic*, meaning a synergy, an interaction, of epidemics [17]. The impact of this syndemic on mental health is diverse: climate change, poverty, hunger, conflict, habitat loss, migration, viral pandemics and the fear of all of these threats combined are likely to increase the incidence of mental illness [18, 19]. The existential crisis will not only contribute to physical and psychological illnesses. In a vicious cycle, people in a crisis situation will also have dwindling resources to maintain or recover their health. And in a digitally connected world with large population migrations (Sect. 5.8), this will be felt everywhere.

Physical and mental health follow a *social gradient* [20]. This means that poverty, low professional qualifications and low social status are strongly associated with illness. People of low income are more often physically and mentally ill. This can also be observed at a societal level: in societies with greater social inequality, poor mental health is more common [20, 21]. A societal approach to addressing mental illness thereby remains crucial—treating individual people is not enough (Sect. 2.3). This is not a new insight. In 1848 Rudolf Virchow investigated a typhoid epidemic in Upper Silesia, which had claimed around 16,000 victims after a famine [22]. He saw that societal changes were necessary to solve the problem. He drew the famous conclusion: 'Medicine [is] a social science (...) and politics is nothing but medicine on a large scale' ([22], p. 287). For Virchow, doctors were therefore the natural advocates of the poor. One can hardly claim that, in our time, this social perspective has truly been internalised by the healthcare system and psychiatry.

1.8 What Is Missing in This Book?

Many topics important to the stigma of mental illness are not discussed in this book or are only touched upon briefly. These include people with mental illness who are placed in forensic psychiatry clinics following a criminal offence [23]; prison inmates, many of whom have mental illness [24]; and the stigma of mental illness amongst marginalised social groups such as sex workers [25]. None of these have been left out because they are unimportant, but because a book of this size cannot cover all topics. It is important to note that these examples also demonstrate how the stigma of mental illness is even more challenging for people who suffer from multiple other stigmas (Sect. 5.5). I have also omitted rather technical information (e.g. on effect sizes for interventions) in order to keep the book readable.

My knowledge is limited: I am not a sociologist, anthropologist, social psychologist, epidemiologist, historian, philosopher or lawyer. As a young man I studied Classics, which comes up now and then in the book. Apart from that, work from other disciplines is often only briefly referred to. To facilitate further reading, literature is cited. This is a compromise between too much information and detail on the one hand and too much simplification and neglect of those on whom this book has depended on the other. As with every compromise, not everyone will be wholly satisfied.

1.9 Perspective of This Book

Objectivity is difficult to achieve. This is known to be true in the natural sciences but especially so for the subject of this book. Every observation or seemingly objective measurement is done following a specifically crafted method or comes from a particular perspective, and observation changes that which is observed (as well as the observer). This book therefore cannot be objective, nor does it want to be. In the great Macedonian film *Before the Rain*, it is said (in another context): 'You have to take sides.' As stigma often carries devasting consequences and reflects social injustice for people with mental illness, I choose to take sides in a fact-based fashion.

I would like to clarify my points of view and perspectives: I wrote this book as a researcher, as a doctor, as a peer and as an antistigma worker. I came into contact with stigma research on a cold winter morning in early 2000, when I entered Professor Pat Corrigan's Chicago office towards the end of my time in medical school. This developed into a friendship and collaboration on the topic of stigma that has stretched over 20 years. As a researcher, I strive to test my hypotheses and present complex findings in a fact-based and straightforward manner (Sect. 1.5). I also work as a psychiatrist at the psychiatric hospital of Günzburg with wonderful colleagues in a Home Treatment Team (Sect. 7.3.4). We visit and treat people with severe mental illness at home. Through my clinical work, I have gained deep respect for all those who manage their illness and learn to live with it. I am a peer insofar as I had an anxiety disorder as a young man and have known times when my world seemed grey and the day was hard to get through. I have therefore made my own decisions about help-seeking and disclosure. Finally, I am an antistigma worker trying to not only investigate interventions that reduce stigma and its consequences but also communicate about them and make them available to those in need.

The perspective from which mental illness is written about is traditionally that of the doctors or scientists who write about their patients. Fortunately, in recent decades, awareness has grown such that people with lived experience of mental illness (i.e. service users) are increasingly involved in research and presentations on this topic. Keywords are participatory research (i.e. the participation of people with mental illness) or 'survivor research' (i.e. not research *on*, but *by* survivors of psychiatry [26]). In this book, the perspectives of service users are represented by multiple quotations throughout the text; Martina Heland-Graef (Sect. 6.1) and Janine Berg-Peer (Sect. 6.2) also describe their personal perspectives as a service user and family member, respectively. Jasna Russo has pointed out that researchers and practitioners often decide on the nature and interpretation of studies and narratives in this field due to their position of power. She criticises this trend as an *epistemic injustice* [27]. This book offers only one approach among many; I bear this power imbalance in mind as I acknowledge my limitations and aim to incorporate diverse voices and perspectives into the final text.

CHAPTER 2

Historical and Social Contexts

'Stigma is more than just an injury to an individual, but an indicator of the health of the social environment' ([9], p. 3). How well people with mental illness can live in our society is a sign of social (in)justice (Sect. 7.5.1). In this chapter, the topics of stigma and mental health/illness are embedded in three broader discussions: first regarding their historical development, since these topics have occupied our society for centuries (Sect. 2.1); next in a conversation on the prevalence and burden of mental illness for individuals and society (Sect. 2.2); and finally in a discussion on social factors and policies (Sect. 2.3). Using this background, Chapter 3 will follow with a presentation of models and aspects of stigma (for a short explanation of the term *stigma*, see 'Glossary').

2.1 Historical Examples

How a society and its people come to think about mental illness does not develop overnight. Three points in history that bring us to the present moment are here briefly outlined. First, we look to the ancient Greeks, because they stood at the beginning of what we now (using the name given in the Greek myths) call Europe. Their thinking about mental illness or madness, as it is often called in ancient texts, influences us fundamentally today (Sect. 2.1.1). Next, we examine the exclusion and murder of people with mental illness (and other disabilities) during the Nazi regime (Sect. 2.1.2). It is an example of what discrimination can lead to if implemented with great brutality, significantly by doctors. Finally, we discuss the 1975 West German Psychiatry Enquete and other psychiatric reforms (Sect. 2.1.3).

2.1.1 MADNESS IN GREEK ANTIQUITY

It's human nature that we tend not only to think about ourselves, the past and the future, but to dwell on them and despair from time to time. Since antiquity, written texts have described mental illness. In the Old Testament, King Saul of the Israelites became ill (1. Book of Samuel). Nebuchadnezzar II, the New Babylonian king around 600 BC, similarly went mad. He lived apart from other humans for seven years, like an animal in the fields (Book of Daniel). Both of these instances are described in the text as punishment from God. Likewise, in ancient Greek mythology, the superman of Greek myths, Heracles, was punished for offending a goddess and killed his wife and children in a fit of madness. These examples show that from the very beginning, narratives of mental illness were linked to questions of causality and experiences of social exclusion, guilt and punishment.

The following is not an attempt at a historical outline. The topic is too complex for that, and comprehensive presentations are available elsewhere [28]. Rather, two examples will be highlighted: (1) Ajax as hero of the Trojan War in Sophocles' tragedy *Ajax* around 440 BC and (2) the concept of melancholy in the fourth century BC.

Ajax

Ajax was, after Achilles, the greatest hero of the Greeks in the 10-year fight for Troy (Fig. 2.1; Aias is his Greek name, Ajax the Latin version). When Achilles fell, Ajax rescued Achilles' body from the battle (Fig. 2.2).

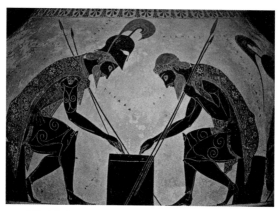

Fig. 2.1 Exekias, approx. 540 BC; Ajax and Achilles playing a board game. (From World History Archive, Alamy stock photos.)

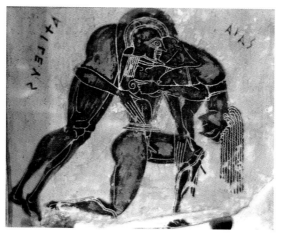

Fig. 2.2 Kleitias, 565 BC; Ajax carries Achilles' body from the battlefield. (From ART Collection, Alamy stock photos.)

Nonetheless, the Greek leaders did not award him with Achilles' armour, instead awarding it to Odysseus. Ajax's honour was insulted: he wanted to kill Odysseus, but the goddess Athena instead made him go insane ('by throwing unbearable delusions upon his eyes'; *Ajax*, 51 f.). In his delusions, Ajax killed a flock of sheep, thinking he was killing Odysseus. When he awakened from his delusion (Greek nósos, manía) and realised what he had done, Ajax despaired. Getting his revenge on Odysseus would have been fine, but killing sheep was a disgrace incompatible with his identity as a hero. He saw himself not only robbed of his honour but exposed to the shame and hatred of both gods and men. In this state, he felt he could not appear before his father after returning from the war (*Ajax*, 364 ff.), and so he threw himself on his sword (Fig. 2.3).

The tragedy is a moving reflection on how difficult it can be to go on living after an episode of serious mental illness, especially when the person fears social exclusion as Ajax did. There is not much difference between Ajax's suicide and the suicide of a hero today, be it an athlete, soldier or celebrity. The timelessness of Sophocles' portrayal of this kind of pain is demonstrated by modern readings of his play in front of American soldiers who recognise themselves in Ajax: 'I've

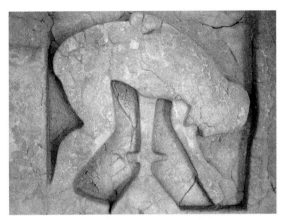

Fig. 2.3 Ajax throws himself on his sword—Metope, Hera sanctuary near Paestum, 6th century BC. (From PRISMA ARCHIVO, Alamy stock photos.)

been Ajax, I've spoken to Ajax' (*Theater of war*, *New York Times*, 11 Nov. 2009). As seen in the examples of famed mythological heroes, tragedy deals with themes that are deeply human and universal. The danger of despair about mental illness and the threat of social exclusion concerns everyone.

The Greeks would not be the Greeks if they had not also thought through an alternative ending and transformed it into poetry: surviving madness is possible with social support. Euripides described this around 415 BC in his play *Heracles*: Heracles is made to go insane by a goddess and in his delusion kills his wife and children, mistaking them for others. Afterwards he too thinks of suicide. But his old friend Theseus comes to him and says: 'Nobody mortal and nobody immortal is unaffected by fate ... now you need friends' (*Heracles*, 1313 ff.). Theseus not only abstractly points to the omnipresence of suffering and guilt, classifying Heracles' situation as human, but offers Heracles his friendship. On this basis, Heracles can continue to live.

Melancholy

Albrecht Dürer's copper engraving from 1514, *Melencolia I,* shows a dark, winged female figure who rests her head on her hand and looks into the distance while surrounded by strange objects (Fig. 2.4). In order to explain the picture, the art historians Raymond Klibansky, Erwin Panofsky and Fritz Saxl investigated the motif of melancholy and its history [29]. The foundation for their inquiry is a short text, the so-called *Problem XXX, 1*; it likely comes from the fourth century BC and was written by Aristotle's disciple Theophrast. The text begins with the question of why all exceptional men are melancholic and ends with the statement that all melancholic men are exceptional—not through illness, but through their natural disposition (phýsis). The text takes up the motif that connects heroic greatness and genius with madness (as with Ajax and Heracles in Greek tragedy) through Hippocrates' theory of the four humours (an early biological model of mental illness; Sect. 5.1.2). According to this doctrine, melancholy is caused by an excess of black bile (mélaina cholé) in the body's mixture of humours. The author of *Problem XXX, 1,* differentiates between a temporary excess or overheating of this black bile, which causes pathological depression (melancholia), and the constitution and personality traits determined by it that characterise great (melancholic) men. Sometimes there is only a fine line between the two, which is evident from the fact that great heroes are often threatened by madness. *Problem XXX, 1,* takes up the motif of genius and madness that originated in Greek tragedy. The text is important for our theme, as it is an example of how a melancholic character, even if predisposed to mental illness, can be seen positively as a sign of greatness.

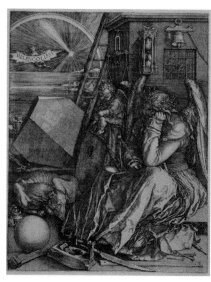

Fig. 2.4   Albrecht Dürer: *Melencolia I*, 1514. (Courtesy Metropolitan Museum, New York City.)

2.1.2 FORCED STERILISATION AND MURDERS DURING THE NAZI ERA

A social group defined as *different* or *ill* can be excluded to such an extent that the group members are denied the right to life. Their lives can be declared worthless, and such dehumanisation (Sect. 3.1.4) can lead to their systematic killing, a most extreme form of discrimination. That this was even possible in a modern, Western country not too long ago is demonstrated by the mass murders of psychiatric patients during the Nazi regime [30]. The ideologies driving these actions date back to the 19th century, when the eugenics movement began to spread internationally. During the Nazi era, however, they were enforced with unique brutality. According to the eugenicist idea of racial hygiene, the 'ethnic body' would be strengthened and preserved by preventing those with 'hereditary diseases' from reproducing. This can be seen as a perversion of Virchow's approach to medicine as a social science (Sect. 1.7): when he went to Silesia in 1848, Virchow took the social circumstances of those facing famine and disease into account in order to help them; in the Nazi era, vulnerable individuals were sacrificed for the supposed welfare of the 'ethnic body'.

Among those with 'hereditary disease' were people with mental illness as well as many others, such as those who were deaf or had epilepsy. After the Law for the Prevention of Hereditarily Diseased Offspring came to pass in Germany in early 1934, at least 360,000 people were forcibly sterilised. The law was formulated with the active participation of high-ranking psychiatrists. Among them was Ernst Rüdin (1874–1952), a Swiss–German psychiatrist, internationally leading psychiatric geneticist and director of the German Research Institute of Psychiatry in Munich (predecessor to today's Max Planck Institute of Psychiatry).

As stated, the foundation for this kind of brutality against psychiatric patients was laid out long before the Nazi era. The lawyer Karl Binding and the psychiatrist Alfred Hoche, director of the newly opened psychiatric hospital in Freiburg since 1902, published the book *Allowing the Destruction of Life Unworthy of Life: Its Measure and Form* in 1920. The language used in it presented people with mental illness or other disabilities as being 'mentally dead', 'empty human shells' and 'dead weight'. The beginning of World War II nearly 20 years later would bring on radicalisation and use these ideas to justify their systematic murder. In October 1939, backdated to the beginning of the war on 1st September, Hitler wrote: 'Reichsleiter Bouhler and Dr Brandt

MD have been commissioned as responsible for extending the powers of designated physicians to grant incurably ill patients a merciful death after critical appraisal of their condition' ([30], p. 114). The act of killing was euphemistically called an act of compassion, a 'merciful death' or 'euthanasia' (Greek for 'good death').

Aktion T4, named after the administrative centre Tiergartenstraße 4 in Berlin (https://gedenkort-t4.eu; https://t4-denkmal.de), was the major Nazi campaign for the mass murder of the mentally ill. Psychiatric hospitals would report on their patients, and 40 T4 medical assessors, among them psychiatry professors, would then determine whether said patients should be killed. More important than the diagnosis was the economic question as to whether these individuals were able to work and could, for instance, be useful in agricultural areas of the psychiatric institutions. The patients selected for killing were taken in grey buses to one of six killing centres, often using other clinics as intermediate stops as a cover-up. The killings took place in gas chambers, and by August 1941, at least 70,000 people had been murdered. The experience gained here with industrialised killing was applied, partly by the same personnel, to the construction of the extermination camps in Eastern Europe.

Despite best efforts, the murders that took place in the territory of the Reich could not be completely concealed. Protests were driven by victims' relatives and church representatives [30]. And although Aktion T4 formally ended in the summer of 1941, the murders continued on a decentralised basis: around 100,000 patients were killed in their hospitals through targeted starvation or injections of medication over the course of World War II. Experiments on patients in psychiatric institutions by microbiologists were conducted. Psychiatrists, nursing and administrative staff actively participated. Mentally ill, forced labourers who were no longer able to work were killed in hospitals. Psychiatric patients were also murdered in occupied parts of Poland and, from the summer of 1941, in the Soviet Union as well.

The murdering of patients was committed by my grandfathers' generation. The horror of it echoed for a long time. My colleague Iris Zimmermann told me about a patient from Günzburg who, as an elderly lady around 1990, was still panic-stricken to step out from the hospital building in which she had lived since the 1930s: 'Outside, the grey buses are coming. Those who got into them never returned.' The German Association for Psychiatry, Psychotherapy and Psychosomatics (DGPPN) remained silent for decades on its professional association with this part of history. The false but digestible myth that the murders were forced upon psychiatry from the outside, by a few fanatical Nazi perpetrators, was cultivated in part by the DGPPN until the end of the 20th century. Volker Roelcke has contradicted this myth with good reason: Aktion T4 took place with active participation, including as frontline T4 assessors, from numerous leading academic representatives in German psychiatry [31]. The psychiatrist Paul Nitsche, temporary leader of Aktion T4, expressed himself euphorically: 'It is certainly marvelous if we can get rid of the dead weight in the hospitals and practice proper therapy' ([30], p. 225).

Given the scale of these crimes, memorial sites and local commemoration work have given us an idea of the names and fates of many lost individuals. In 2019, for example, a memorial was opened in Ulm on the site of the former Hereditary Health Court, which ruled on forced sterilisations of people with mental illness or other disabilities. At the psychiatric hospital in Günzburg, Thomas Düll and Thomas Becker had the rose garden reinstated as a place of remembrance. The site commemorates the lives of approximately 400 patients who were taken from Günzburg to killing sites in Grafeneck in the Swabian Alb and in Hartheim near Linz in Upper Austria. And at the Grafeneck Memorial, there is a preserved biscuit on display marked with the words 'All Murderers'. It was an inscription made by one patient with schizophrenia, Theodor Kynast, before he was murdered there on 25 November 1940. That the victims were 'mentally dead' and did not understand their situation is one of the deepest prejudices with which their murders were justified after 1945. Ernst Klee gave numerous proofs contradicting this, including a report from a nun at the Bavarian Irsee psychiatric hospital: 'She was also gassed ... she guessed what was happening. "Murderers" she called us, as they got her onto the bus, "You are murderers, you are killing us'" ([30], p. 168).

2.1.3 REFORMS IN PSYCHIATRY

In 1975 a commission of experts appointed by the German Bundestag in Bonn published a report on the state of psychiatry in the Federal Republic of Germany entitled *Psychiatrie-Enquete* (enquête, French for investigation [32]). How did it come about? After the murders of patients during the Nazi era (Sect. 2.1.2), the psychiatric institutions had filled up again. Many had been built in the 19th and early 20th centuries, typically far away and isolated from urban life (Sect. 7.3.3, 'Architecture'). The conditions were inhumane and the dormitories overcrowded. Inmates were detained without privacy and often neglected in what sociologist Erving Goffman would refer to as a total institution [33].

The environment changed in the 1960s: in Germany, the student movement was concerned with social inequality as well as Nazi crimes, which were both intrinsically linked to psychiatric care. The welfare state in Germany was also expanding, and the conditions of institutions were increasingly criticised in psychiatric circles as they were unable to keep up with the advancements of other Western countries [34]. There were numerous attempts at mental healthcare reform in the United States and other European countries, led by deinstitutionalisation and community mental health advocates. It was also the height of the antipsychiatry movement, which criticised psychiatry as a discipline and an institution.

Criticism of the practice of psychiatry at this point was nothing new: as early as 1900, unjustified incapacitation, internment and coercive measures by psychiatrists were heavily criticised in some spheres of the German Reich [35]. Antipsychiatry of the mid-20th century, however, not only called for change in malfunctioning institutions but also questioned attitudes and concepts that were seemingly fundamental to psychiatric care. This meant that prominent representatives of the antipsychiatry movement found an audience far beyond in-field experts. For the US psychiatrist Thomas Szasz, mental illness had proven to be a myth. His writing argued that society, with psychiatrists at the helm, merely labelled conspicuous or unpleasant behaviour with psychiatric diagnoses (Sect. 3.2.4, 'Behaviour or Label' [36]). The French psychologist, philosopher and social historian Michel Foucault was a similarly prolific, widespread influence on these issues. His analyses, many of which first appeared in his 1961 book *Madness and Civilization,* focused on the exercise of power and control in modern psychiatry. Foucault went on to engage, write and speak about psychiatry for decades. His lectures of the early 1970s, published as *Psychiatric Power* [37], describe the architecture of prisons and psychiatric institutions that gave wardens complete control over their inmates. In England, philosopher Jeremy Bentham had developed a design principle called the panopticon, in which radially arranged cells or blocks could be easily viewed and controlled from a central office. For Foucault, this type of architecture was an 'intensifier of power' and psychiatry an 'institutional enterprise of discipline' ([37], pp. 74 and 85). Foucault also dealt with the interactional processes and roles in psychiatry that mark the power dynamics between doctor and patient: the 'questioning [of the patient by the psychiatrist] is precisely this: Give me some symptoms, make some symptoms from your life for me, and you will make me a doctor' ([37], p. 276). Even though many of the views of antipsychiatry did not prevail, and psychiatry was by no means abolished, antipsychiatry provided crucial momentum for psychiatric reforms. And the issues of social labelling, architecture and power held by doctors and institutions which were raised by critics such as Szasz and Foucault remain central to the critical approaches of stigma and mental illness researchers today (power, Sect. 3.1.4; labelling, Sect. 3.2.4; patient–professional interaction, Sect. 7.3.1; 'Architecture', Sect. 7.3.3).

In 1963, in the German Democratic Republic (GDR), the Rodewisch Theses were formulated during a congressional session in Rodewisch, Saxony. These reforms were social-psychiatrically oriented; they focused on rehabilitation and social integration; they discussed prevention and deconstruction of broader 'intolerance towards the mentally ill'. There was some subsequent progress in, but no structural reform of, GDR psychiatry [38]. Besides economic difficulties, the challenges of operating under the communist regime should not be underestimated: reform and development of good care in the field of psychiatry only succeed if patients can trust their doctors. But in the 1970s (if not earlier), the Stasi, or Ministry for State Security—the East German secret police—had placed its own doctors in probably every hospital and outpatient clinic as unofficial employees. These physicians reported to the Stasi not only about their colleagues but also about their patients, breaching medical confidentiality [39].

By 1975, the West German Enquete made the following proposals to remedy the inhumane conditions in institutions and improve care: reductions in the size of the hospitals; the establishment of psychiatric departments in general hospitals; a wide expansion of outpatient psychiatric care; a stronger network of psychotherapy and social work in the in- and outpatient sectors; equality for people with physical and mental illness in health and social systems; and improved cooperation between various care and support systems. For decades, the Enquete acted as a driver of change. Its original objectives have not been fully achieved. But this is less the fault of the Enquete and more a task for us as their successors. One challenge remains the fragmented care system (Sect. 7.3.3) and the often-precarious social conditions of people with serious mental illness.

The Enquete was also about breaking down prejudices—and not only in the sphere of psychiatric and psychotherapeutic treatment. In his contribution to the Enquete, Asmus Finzen discussed topics that remain important for antistigma work [40]: limits of educational approaches, the continuum between illness and health (Sect. 1.6), advantages of local projects and contact as an antistigma strategy (Sect. 8.4), involvement of service users and media (Sect. 7.4.7) and the importance of perseverance in creating sustainable programmes (Sect. 8.4.4).

2.2 The Prevalence and Burden of Mental Illness

2.2.1 PREVALENCE

Given their widespread stigma, it may seem odd that mental illnesses are quite common. Given their frequency, one might even call them 'normal'. Frequency refers to the proportion of the population that has an illness or a group of illnesses; this rate is also called prevalence. The period for which a frequency is specified is important: the prevalence at a certain point in time (point prevalence) is lower than the prevalence estimated for one year, or for a lifetime. A one-year prevalence is most frequently used in research (and, unless otherwise stated, in this book as well). A *one-year prevalence* of 10% for an illness means that 10% of the general population will have that illness within one year. Prevalence numbers can appear low depending on the sample population being used; for example, the prevalence of dementia across all age groups is only 1% but is much higher among older people (Sect. 5.4.4).

Which illnesses have a high one-year prevalence? Those that occur frequently and early in life and that are more likely to have a recurring or long-lasting course. All of this applies to mental disorders, which, apart from dementia, typically begin in adolescence and young adulthood. In 2011, about one-third of the European Union's total population, approximately 150 million citizens, had a mental illness (including dementia and addictions [41]). These numbers were proportionally similar for Germany [42]. The prevalence stayed consistent between 2005 and 2011. Most common were anxiety disorders (14%), sleep disorders and depression (about 7% each). Prevalence rates for some other disorders can be found in Section 5.4.

How can one understand such figures, and are they plausible? The numbers are based on methodical, thorough studies and a broad database and follow diagnostic criteria. Those who do not think the figures are credible can consider two issues. First, not all 150 million are severely ill; some disorders are mild and temporary, with or without treatment. Second, some of the strongest studies in this field are those that examine large random samples of the general population regardless of a formal diagnosis. They systematically survey everybody—including those who have never reported alcohol abuse, depressed mood or anxiety to a family doctor or colleague and likely never would. These studies report on people and conditions that, because of the widespread stigma and taboo associated with mental illness, typically go unnoticed.

2.2.2 WHY IS THE PREVALENCE NOT DECREASING?

The prevalence of mental disorders has stayed relatively constant over the last few decades (Sect. 2.2.1). At the same time, more and more people with mental illness are being treated: in recent years, the use of psychopharmacotherapy and psychotherapy has increased. The number of psychotherapists in private practice in Germany has risen sharply since 2000. The number of beds in psychosomatic hospitals has also risen sharply—often under the control of profit-oriented private hospital companies that do not participate in providing mental health service coverage for people with mental illness in defined geographical areas [42]. An increased uptake of treatment was accompanied by a sharp rise in the number of sick days and early retirement and disability pensions due to mental illness—both in absolute figures and in relative terms compared with physical illness [42]. This raises a question: if there's been an increase in treatment, why has the prevalence of mental disorders not decreased? More frequent and available treatment of mental health problems should theoretically result in their being detected and treated completely (i.e. cured) at an early stage, or at least before full development (secondary prevention). Both would reduce the prevalence.

There are three possible explanations that may simultaneously contribute to the paradox of stable prevalence and increased service use [42]:

1. inadequate care,
2. increased prevalence masked by increased service use and
3. the psychologisation of our world, such that misfortune and suffering are increasingly understood as illness.

For the first explanation, there is abundant proof (Sects. 7.3.1 and 7.3.3): primary prevention for the general public (e.g. in schools) hardly ever takes place. And the vast majority of people with mental illness do not take advantage of existing treatment options. Help or treatment is typically not sought until many years after the onset of the illness, if at all; treatment programmes are often discontinued prematurely. This *treatment gap* arises from, among other things, fear of public stigma, and from self-stigma and shame (Sect. 5.1.7). When people make contact with their healthcare system, they often do not receive effective help. In many cases, GPs do not recognise depression or do not treat it adequately. Outpatient psychiatric and psychotherapeutic care in Germany is completely insufficient, which leads to long waiting times and unnecessary hospital stays (Sect. 7.3.3). Poor care does not reduce the prevalence of mental illness.

The second explanation is based on a gloomy assessment of our modern world, which has become increasingly global, confusing, fast and stressful—rapidly leading to higher rates of mental disorders. From this perspective, it would appear that new cases and types of diagnoses are emerging but concealed by more frequent treatment. And researchers are increasingly aware that social issues also play a significant role below the surface: 'Something central to recovery appears to be missing in the social fabric of developed countries. It seems likely that factors such as income inequality, discrimination, prejudice, unemployment and strongly materialistic and competitive values may contribute to increased mental stress' ([43], p. 1176). All of this sounds plausible, but diffuse; where the burden of stress precisely arises from is ill-defined. We are also often dealing with contradictory social trends: over the last 15 years, unemployment in Germany has fallen sharply, while the number of people living alone has increased. The first trend would be expected to reduce the prevalence of mental disorders (Sect. 7.1) and the second to increase it—the overall impact of these and other influences, however, remains unclear. There is also much to suggest that, at least for members of vulnerable social groups, the disintegration of previously reliable social networks can increase rates of mental disorders, including suicidality (Sect. 2.3.1, 'Deaths of Despair').

Disability arises from the interaction between the person and his environment. It is not easy to interpret the link between societal changes towards a more demanding work environment and the prevalence of mental health problems [42]. When I was young, it seemed like every building entrance, even auxiliary buildings at hospitals and universities, was staffed with a porter or two. I wasn't always clear on what their jobs were—they were just there, with low-pressure work. These are the employment niches in which employees with mental or physical disability might thrive. But it seems today that those jobs have virtually disappeared. The reintegration of people with mental illness into the labour market (Sect. 7.1.2) is not only about training and working with the deficits of participants but also about constructing and safeguarding niches for them—a kind of ecology of work for people with psychiatric disabilities. This is not charity, but their right (Art. 27, UN-CRPD; Sect. 7.5.2).

The third explanation also assumes a cultural trend; namely, the popularisation of psychologising certain human experiences. Stress and burnout are on everyone's lips, and differentiating them from mental illness is not always easy—for the public and experts alike (Sect. 1.6). Exhaustion is considered to be a modern-day diagnosis and an explanation for the prevalence of depression in our time [44]. This can lead to an exaggerated assessment of the general stresses of life as illness. Studies worldwide show that the frequency of anxiety and depression disorders is not increasing, but at the same time more and more people feel 'stressed' [45]. This phenomenon presents a slippery slope for educational programmes that aim to improve knowledge about mental health (mental health literacy; Sect. 3.1.7) and normalise help-seeking behaviour (Sect. 8.1.5): when raising awareness about mental illness, there is the risk of prematurely regarding any suffering or grief as an illness. This could have the paradoxical effect whereby more knowledge leads to subjectively worse mental health [46]. If *stress* is to equal *illness*, we also risk trivialising the experiences of those with severe mental illness (who are undoubtedly dealing with more than *stress*).

2.2.3 BURDEN ASSOCIATED WITH MENTAL ILLNESS

Because the above-mentioned prevalence figures summarise very different diagnoses and degrees of severity, the question arises as to what burden is caused by mental illness. A good measure of illness burden is how many years of 'healthy' life are lost through an illness in an overall population. For this purpose, the disability-adjusted life year (DALY; 'Glossary') was developed by the World Health Organization (WHO) in the 1990s. A DALY is a healthy life year lost due to early death or due to living with illness-related impairments or disability. The quantified loss of years varies depending on the disabilities themselves. DALYs are not measurements that simply classify people according to their usefulness or ability to work; rather they focus on impaired quality of life and social functioning, including among children and the elderly (who are, however, outside the working age and thus assigned less weight). Traditionally, assessments of illness burden would focus on whether illnesses led to early death. However, as life expectancy has increased worldwide, and as rates of all kinds of chronic illnesses have risen, the impairments of living with illnesses have become a more pertinent subject for study. The DALYs have helped to raise awareness of the enormous loss of healthy life years due to mental illness. However, the DALY concept also has weaknesses and has been criticised in multiple ways: DALYs are based on expert estimates and definitions of impairments rather than on how they may truly manifest for those affected. They also underestimate the role of social context, because the disability caused by an illness is not simply due to the illness itself but depends on available help and support options.

The proportion of all healthy life years (DALYs) lost due to mental illnesses in the EU is 20.2% [41]. In other words, one-fifth of the burden presented by all illnesses, including cancer, cardiovascular diseases, diabetes and so forth, is attributable to mental disorders. Depression leads with the highest contribution of 7.2% of DALYs, ahead of dementia and alcohol addiction, and thus carries a higher burden of disease than any other illness, including physical illness, in the EU. The proportion of DALYs due to mental illness is slightly higher among women than among men. The burden of disease due to mental illness is rising sharply worldwide, but this is not due to increasing prevalence. Instead, it is because of rising life expectancy: more people are living longer with their illness [47].

Although this one-fifth statistic indicates an enormously high burden of disease, it still underestimates its true extent [48]. Suicides, which are typically associated at least in part with mental illness, are not included. Nor does the measurement take into account the reduction in life expectancy by around 15 years for people with severe mental illness due to comorbid physical illnesses (Sect. 7.3). If a man with schizophrenia develops obesity, high blood pressure and diabetes as side effects of his psychiatric medication and therefore dies of a heart attack at the age of 50, the 30 years of his life that are lost (DALYs) are attributed solely to heart disease in this calculation. Due to these and other misattributions, the burden of disease from mental illness is considerably underestimated [48].

2.2.4 COSTS OF MENTAL ILLNESS

There are several issues at play in the relationship between economics and mental illness. For one, these illnesses hold enormous societal costs: direct costs in the form of treatment and the much higher indirect costs (including those due to loss of working capacity and early retirement). There are additional costs in the social environment as well, including those that affect families (e.g. relatives who are less able to work due to caregiving) and social and educational systems (e.g. those unable to graduate or complete training due to mental illness). Mental disorders are expected to account for more than half of all follow-up costs of noncommunicable illnesses worldwide by 2030 [49]. To further complicate matters, those living in poverty are often more susceptible to mental illness, leading many into a vicious circle of financial hardship and psychological distress.

As the London health economist Martin Knapp (whose name is quite apt; 'knapp' means scarce in German) is wont to say: the resources that can be distributed politically are always scarce [49]. Therefore an economic perspective on mental health can inform decision-makers and society as to the sensible allocation of resources. From this point of view, the significance of an intervention's cost should be weighed alongside that of its effectivity. This ultimately aids in the allocation of limited financial resources. Let's say we're considering two interventions to reduce self-stigma with the goal of a better quality of life and recovery for people with mental illness, and that we're safe to assume they are equally effective. If the first intervention costs 1000 euros per participant and the other 3000 euros, the first is undoubtedly more cost-effective. Another test might determine the cost of two interventions that aim to improve the healthcare system in order to gain an average of 10 years of good quality of life for people with different illnesses. The costs (sum per year for quality of life gained) allow comparisons for investment decisions on different subareas of medicine (e.g. between cancer and mental illness). These factors are not the be-all and end-all, but they enrich decision-making when resources are scarce: 'Economic evidence cannot make decisions, but it can make decisions better "informed"' ([49], p. 10).

Level of Costs

The Organisation for Economic Co-operation and Development (OECD) estimated the costs of mental illness for European countries in 2015 [50]. The total cost in Germany was just under

150 billion euros and about 106 billion euros in the UK. Of this, about a third was accounted for by direct costs in the treatment system (e.g. visits to doctors, clinics and medication), under a third by social expenditure (e.g. sickness benefit, disability benefit, unemployment benefit) and more than 40% by the labour market through loss of income and productivity. That 40% increases when people are more absent from work (absenteeism) or when they are physically present but work less efficiently (presenteeism). Total costs in Germany correspond to 4.8% of the gross national product and are higher than in the EU on average (4.1%), in Austria (4.3%), Switzerland (3.5%) or the United Kingdom (4.1%). The cost of mental illness can also be estimated by looking at how much people would be willing to pay to reduce their risk of having a mental illness. That estimated cost is slightly higher than that of cardiovascular diseases and more than three times that of cancer [51].

Outlook and Political Response

The costs of mental illness are expected to rise sharply in the coming decades, especially in wealthier Western countries, which have an ageing population and risk a loss of overall productivity and wealth. All of this should be a wake-up call for politicians. What is their reaction? None that comes even close to meeting the challenge. On average, mental healthcare accounts for 13% of health expenditure in EU countries. In relation to the 20% of DALYs due to mental illness (Sect. 2.2.3), this represents a massive financing gap of one-third—not to mention the increased discrepancy that will emerge in the coming decades as well as the economic follow-up costs. The lack of political response is illogical; providing more resources for better care of anxiety and depression, for example, is not only an ethical imperative but economically worthwhile. The *return on investment* in the form of increased labour productivity is two to three times the cost of treatment [52]. Investment in prevention would also pay off but hardly ever takes place [53]. Not only is this economically foolish but it also signals politicians' complicity in broader, structural discrimination against a large population group whose suffering could be avoided or greatly reduced (Sect. 5.1.8).

Why is there no adequate political response? One explanation is that political decisions are usually made in the short term with a myopic view to the next few years, determined by election cycles and term limits. These decisions are also typically made within one department (e.g. health or social affairs), and cross-sectoral relationships and effects are neglected. Martin Knapp calls it the problem of *diagonal accounting* [49]. The treatment and prevention of mental illness is usually funded from the health budget, and most of the costs are upfront. But the economic benefits of, say, preventing mental disorders among youth only reveal themselves decades later. Moreover, these savings mostly manifest in other areas: education, employment, social welfare, housing, justice and pensions. It is thereby a challenge to convince current policymakers to see the long game and invest in prevention and treatment. This problem is also called 'silo budgeting disincentive' (deterrence through silo/separate sector budgeting [49]). And yet it remains critical that there be increased acknowledgement and prioritisation of the far-reaching social consequences of mental illness across all policy areas (mental health in all policies; Sect. 2.3.3).

Mothers and Young People

Two examples illustrate the economic value of investing in prevention: mothers with pre-natal and postnatal mental illness (usually depression) and children and adolescents with mental illness.

1. Screening for depressive symptoms, and the treatment of mothers at an early stage of natal care, if necessary, is incredibly worthwhile from an economic point of view. The short-term cost of healthcare (e.g. a hospital stay for the mother) should be taken into account, but the long-term savings are undoubtedly greater: while close to one-tenth of the follow-up costs of maternal depression land in the health and social care sector, almost three-quarters of the follow-up costs are incurred by the child later in their life [49]. These costs are

generated in education, justice and penal systems, and in lost quality of life (if financially estimated). Effective prevention programs are often straightforward and adaptable, such as training midwives to pay attention to mothers' depressive symptoms and to refer mothers to help services if necessary.

2. Therapy for depression in children and adolescents is cost-effective—psychotherapy even more so than pharmacotherapy in the long term [49]. Consistent education on and prevention of bullying in schools [54] is also economically worthwhile; peer violence leads to higher demands for mental healthcare down the road (not to mention care costs for victims of it [55]; Sect. 7.3.4, 'Prevention'). These and other investments are worthwhile from a societal perspective, not least early intervention for psychoses [56].

Recovery and Economy

Recovery essentially consists of achieving self-defined life goals and lifestyles (Sect. 5.1.6). Because the path of recovery is unique and different for each person, it is difficult to evaluate recovery economically. Are there nevertheless clues that investing in recovery could be economically worthwhile? A number of programmes, which range from peer support (Sect. 7.3.4) to psychosocial interventions (Sect. 7.3.3) and recovery colleges (Sect. 5.1.6), promote recovery. While the longitudinal data is still incomplete, what is available indicates that most of these approaches are also good investments; they do not increase costs but are more efficient uses of resources than traditional approaches [57].

Conclusion

Data in this field routinely demonstrate the enormous societal costs of mental illness well beyond the healthcare system. Interventions have the capacity to save society as a whole far more than they cost. Nevertheless, they are rarely used (Sect. 7.3.3 and Sect. 7.3.4, 'Prevention'). Foresighted and cross-sectoral policy reforms are needed. An appeal to state or federal officials for social affairs and for education could simply be: 'Please co-finance better prevention and treatment efforts for mothers with postnatal depression, and for children/adolescents with mental health problems, in equal measures. The effects will benefit your budgets for decades!'

2.3 Mental Health as a Social Task

2.3.1 SOCIAL CAUSES

The conditions under which people live have multiple effects on their physical and mental health, including their life expectancy [20]. Social factors that influence health include those that are external or mutable (e.g. poverty, education, social isolation or support, work, housing, trauma and violence), and those that are usually stable or inherent (e.g. gender and ethnicity). Some modifiable social factors can be summarised as social or socio-economic status, which is essentially determined by education, work and income. The influence of social factors on health follows a social gradient. The lower a person's social status is, the worse their health is on average [20].

Three things are important in this context (Fig. 2.5). First, the effects of social factors add up over the course of one's life, from womb to old age. Second, seemingly impenetrable and long-lasting cycles are typical: a boy from a poor family has a much higher risk of demonstrating developmental challenges at school, which in turn limits his educational opportunities, leads to increased risk of mental illness and diminishes his chances at socio-economic mobility. Finally, social factors are often incorrectly presented as defects or weaknesses of individuals; they are in fact products of social inequality, and only this view of the problem will lead to social answers.

What is the evidence for the link between unfavourable social living conditions and mental health? The more unequal and disparate the living conditions of a society, the more common are

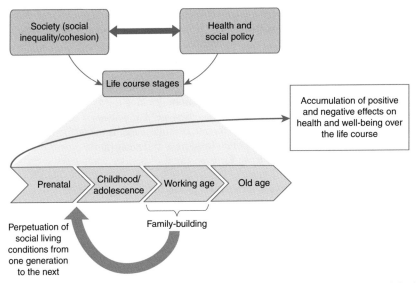

Fig. 2.5 **Model of the effects of social living conditions over the course of life.** (Based on WHO Regional Office for Europe. Review of social determinants and the health divide in the WHO European region: Final report. Copenhagen: WHO; 2014. fig. ES3. Courtesy of Heike Hübner, Berlin.)

mental disorders, especially depression, amongst its population [21]. People with lower relative social status have a much higher risk of mental illness over their life course [58]. This applies to the general public as well as to disadvantaged groups, including immigrants (Sect. 5.8), the unemployed (Sect. 7.1.2) and the homeless (Sect. 7.2). To mention just one example, psychoses are much more common among people who have experienced violence, bullying or discrimination in their childhood and youth (Sect. 5.3).

DEATHS OF DESPAIR

The link between social factors and mental illness mentioned so far may sound abstract. However, the consequences of adverse living conditions can create emotional distress and despair, leading so far as to fatality. Anne Case and Angus Deaton have investigated this in an unsettling study [59]. Their starting point was that in Western countries the average mortality rate of people aged 50 years has fallen sharply for decades—with one exception. In the United States, the number of 'deaths of despair' among (non-Hispanic) whites with a low level of education has risen dramatically since about 2000. Included are deaths from suicide, drugs, alcohol or cirrhosis of the liver. The increase was found only in this group—not among blacks, Hispanics or higher-educated whites. Case and Deaton interpret these death rates in the anomic tradition of Émile Durkheim (Sect. 5.2.1 [60]) as a product of social disintegration and chronic strain for people of this class and generation. They argue that continuity and reliability in work, family, marriage and church had dissolved for this demographic of society. Older members of this population had not been as burdened by social disintegration as those in midlife, and for younger people such challenges lay ahead. Many people with lower levels of education struggle to cope with their social and economic surroundings, and despair.

The study is important for our topic for several reasons: economic inequality, political upheaval and social disintegration only continue to increase (Sect. 1.7), and vulnerable groups will be particularly at risk. People with fewer resources need support. The stigma of mental illness will likely contribute to deaths of despair amongst vulnerable people. Finally, it would be misleading to understand and treat these deaths as though they are the results of individuals' isolated problems.

2.3.2 INCLUSION OF SOCIAL FACTORS

Causes of illnesses may be obvious and proximate, or more distant [61]. Let us assume that there is a group of people who live by a river and fall ill from drinking the water because it has been contaminated some kilometres upstream by factory sewage. The proximate cause of their illness is that they drink from the river. The more distant, or distal, cause is the factory upstream. Our conception of a cause determines what we do to address it: if we focus on proximate causes, we could give the people water filters; if we focus on distal causes, we could reroute the factory's sewage.

It is useful to distinguish between three causal factors influencing health:
1. very proximate (i.e. when seeking help, treatment and individual behaviour for particular issues, like smoking),
2. intermediate (i.e. the living and working conditions of an urban district),
3. distant (i.e. the social and economic conditions of a society, such as social inequality).

Psychiatry and the healthcare system tend to focus on proximate causes. We diligently hand out our water filters, with varying success, and neglect 'upstream' social factors—often because we do not know or recognise them. Yet distant causal factors are fundamental to the many ways that the damage can take shape (as can easily be imagined in the factory wastewater scenario)—they are therefore also referred to as 'causes of the causes'. Good school education, for example, leads to better mental health in many ways: greater knowledge (Sect. 3.1.7), better work and income, and larger and stronger social networks [61].

Greater incorporation of social factors into both clinical and policy understandings of mental illness is long overdue (i.e. looking at the social causes, intervention options and consequences of an illness [62]). A biological (and biopharmaceutical) paradigm currently dominates psychiatry. It has been of limited usefulness. If psychiatry as a medical science has the overriding goal of curing and preventing mental illness, then this approach has proven unsatisfactory [63]. Instead of limiting ourselves to biological factors, it is worth taking a step back and looking upstream—to the social causes of the causes. This is ultimately a more progressive approach and engages fundamental critical and conceptual ideas [62]: what is considered a mental illness is socially defined (Sect. 1.6); social adversity causes mental illness, which in turn has social consequences (not least social isolation); stigma as a social consequence of mental illness is the *second illness*; and finally, treatment can be seen as a social process (not only in a psychotherapist's office).

The inclusion of social factors in no way excludes the import of considering biological processes; they are vital, for example, to the study of generational transmission of social disadvantage. Take Germany, where pregnant women within a low socio-economic status are 13 times more likely to smoke than those within a higher status ([64], p. 309). This habit greatly increases the risk of foetal damage, which in turn can impair a child's psychological development and future mental health needs.

If psychiatry does not succeed in incorporating social factors more comprehensively into its medical practice, it is likely to wither away as an academic subject into a subdomain of applied neuroscience. Society, health policy and psychiatry are thus faced with the challenge of thinking about mental health in social terms. This has already been the subject of reforms such as the Psychiatry Enquete (Sect. 2.1.3), but many of the questions it addressed are now being asked again. This is in part due to the way our world changes (Sect. 1.7): social interactions are increasingly taking place, for example, in the digital realm—redefining our forms of support and carrying unknown consequences for mental health. We must also recognise that it is a tremendous challenge to incorporate diffuse social factors more comprehensively into the field of mental health when up against a reductionist zeitgeist. For example, even in sophisticated media reports, the essence of a mental illness seems to be decoded only after its genetics have been examined or colourful images of the brain have been presented—however scanty these findings may be (for an example, see Sect. 5.4.5).

The deficiency of one-sided views has long been known. The psychiatrist and philosopher Karl Jaspers (1883–1969) pointed out in his *General Psychopathology* that only *one* perspective or method cannot do justice to the complexity of mental illness. He spoke of a *somatic prejudice*, where only the physical (somatic) aspect counts: 'Tacit assumptions are made that, like everything else biological, the actual reality of human existence is a somatic event. One can only be comprehensible when one is understood in somatic terms' ([65], vol. 1, p. 18). Jaspers also critiqued the belief that all psychological processes can be explained in terms of the organic structure of the brain as '*brain mythology*'. Of course, these biological–somatic prejudices are by no means the only ones that exist. Moralising, psychologising or other theoretical assumptions also lead to distorted images of mental illness—not least among psychotherapists (for examples, see Sect. 6.2). Matthias Bormuth, a scholar who works on Jaspers, spoke in this context of 'reductive relief': by limiting oneself to one point of view ('schizophrenia is a genetic illness'), one no longer needs to take its limits into consideration or take note of other approaches. It certainly is not wrong to have a point of view, but to make it absolute is myopic and ineffectual.

In a broader sense, a social paradigm shows that how we deal with diversity and the *otherness* of other people affects the mental health of everyone as well as the fabric of our society. Extending far beyond the field of psychiatry, this is a discussion of societal inclusion and equality as fundamental rights (Sect. 7.5.2). It will not suffice to solely remove stigma or exclusion; a social paradigm for understanding mental illness relays the need for an altered social attitude, in which the acceptance and support of those who are different is a natural goal.

2.3.3 SOCIAL ANSWERS

Social interventions can sustainably improve the situation of people with mental illness [66, 67]. These include programmes for the unemployed (Sect. 7.1.2, IPS), the homeless (Sect. 7.2.6) and the impoverished [68]. Other interventions promote the development of social networks and reduce social isolation [69]. Support schemes can help people with various disorders find solutions to social problems, from finance to loneliness; this approach is also called *social prescribing* and seems to help many [70]. Collectively, these are approaches that pave ways back into society for people who withdraw out of fear of public stigma, out of self-stigma or shame, or because they've reached a sense of deep despair.

Inge Schöck used to tell me about her decades of work in the Stuttgart *Bürgerhilfe* (Citizen Support Group) for and with people with mental illness. A few dozen people, members of the general public and active service users alike, would meet there once a week. Mutual support and exchange of all kinds were created without any therapeutic aspirations. The communally planned programme would facilitate discussion about and participation in the everyday social and cultural life of the city, and there would be occasional group activities outside of weekly meetings. One participant described his experiences like this: 'This is the only place where I can say: "I am what I am." Here I do not need to keep watch over my soul ... I am very proud to be able to say: "I am what I am, which is all I need to live"' ([71], p. 213). Such support from others builds bridges into society and has a destigmatising effect. The opening of the Trialogue, to be discussed in Section 7.3.4, to the Tetralogue—an exchange between service users, relatives, professionals and citizens—is a step in this direction.

Programmes that support the healthy development of young people also promote mental health. One example of this is the *Communities That Care* (CTC) project in Germany, which focuses on a reduction in drug use and violence among young people through primary prevention at a local level. The effects of the programme are seen and maintained for years, and its cost is vastly lower than potential long-term costs to the health, social and justice systems that would occur without the programme [72].

Mental health interventions that reduce social inequalities can be divided into different levels [73]: interventions for individuals and families, such as programmes that support families at risk; programmes and campaigns for cities and municipalities; and, most broadly, national and international policy measures. The larger the target group, the more difficult it becomes to prove the effects of such measures; interventions with multiple components and layers become increasingly complex, and outcomes become harder to study. Nonhealth policy measures, which tend to start 'upstream', seem to be effective in the areas of the labour market, social care and welfare, and housing [73]. This approach is also known as *Mental Health in All Policies* and argues for the improvement of mental health in multiple integrated sectors. In a certain sense, this is a broader policy equivalent of the attempt to overcome fragmentation within the healthcare system (Sect. 7.3.3). The causes and consequences of mental illness are so complex that only an integrated approach could prove effective.

CHAPTER 3

What Is Stigma?

Section 3.1 gives an overview of stigma—the origins of the term as well as common models and forms of it. Section 3.2 discusses categorisation and stereotyping as fundamental aspects of stigma. Section 3.3 deals with the function of stigma for individuals, groups and society and thus with reasons why stigma is so common. Chapter 4 describes the consequences of stigma and stigmatised individuals' ways of coping.

3.1 Terms, Models and Forms of Stigma

3.1.1 ORIGIN OF THE WORD

Stigma comes from the ancient Greek verb στίζειν (stízein). It is related to the English verb 'stick' and the German words 'stechen' and 'sticken'; the root means to sting, to mark, to tattoo or to brand. Stigma is the corresponding noun and denotes the marking or the mark. In ancient Greek it is used as a sign of ownership (e.g. of horses or land), or as a sign of shame and social ostracism (e.g. of criminals or runaway slaves). The Greek historian Herodotus (*Histories* 7: 35) describes an entertaining scene from the year 480 BC: King Xerxes of Persia was angry after his Pontoon Bridges across the Hellespont Strait were torn apart by the stormy seas. The Hellespont is the strait south of the Bosporus between Asia Minor and Europe; Xerxes and his army had wanted to cross it to subjugate the Greeks. Not only did Xerxes angrily lash out and have chains thrown into the Hellespont, insulting the sea, but it is said that he even sent his men to brand it (stíxontas tòn Hellésponton). The Hellespont's reaction is unknown, but with subtle irony Herodotus calls its punishment a thankless honour for Xerxes' underlings. One can see that there are no limits to the imagination of people, especially the powerful, when it comes to whom and how to stigmatise.

A completely different context in which the term stigma is used regards those who bear the wounds (stigmata) of Jesus. Jesus was executed on the cross as a convicted criminal, and the ensuing stigmata remind us of his fate of fatal exclusion. Especially in the Catholic faith, these stigmata are an expression of mystical closeness to God, as in the case of Francis of Assisi and based on the Epistles of Paul, who said he bore the wounds of Jesus on his body (Galatians 6:17). Contrary to an illness-related stigma today, such marks represent something positive. Even the mark of Cain, which is often used as a biblical reference to stigma, is not simply a sign of ostracism: God marked Cain upon his killing his brother Abel, but God did so to protect him against others' retaliation (Genesis, chapter 4). The mark of Cain, unlike a stigma in the sense of this book, is therefore not a purely negative term.

3.1.2 STIGMA AS A GENERIC TERM

In *Stigma: Notes on the Management of Spoiled Identity* (1963), American sociologist Erving Goffman describes stigma as a characteristic of a person 'that makes him different from others in the category of persons available for him to be, and of a less desirable kind—in the extreme, a person who is quite thoroughly bad, or dangerous, or weak. He is thus reduced in our minds from a whole and usual person to a tainted, discounted one' ([8], p. 3). Much of modern research on stigma and mental illness follows in Goffman's tradition.

Stigma as a term has been criticised [74]. Some people say that the term places blame on the stigmatised person, when in reality the problem lies in structural injustice. Others similarly criticise it by arguing that we should concern ourselves with what truly matters: behaviours and issues of discrimination in society. These criticisms are valuable—nobody should be blamed for being stigmatised, and discrimination is often the most important aspect of stigma. However, in this book I will continue to use the term stigma for two main reasons: as indicated by the Greek origin of the word, stigma implies a social attribution or marking by others. And stigma as an umbrella term explicitly includes discrimination.

Next, two leading models of stigma will be briefly outlined. These models are compatible but use different frameworks: one is social-cognitive and the other sociological. These are followed by an overview of the different types and expressions of stigma. Aspects such as categorisation and stereotypes that appear here in Section 3.1.3 are explained in more detail in Section 3.2.

3.1.3 SOCIAL-COGNITIVE MODEL OF STIGMA

The social-cognitive model has three components: stereotypes, prejudice and discrimination (Table 3.1).

- *Stereotypes* are general statements about social groups, such as 'Scots are stingy' or 'women are bad at maths' [75]. Stereotypes generalise: they carry assumptions about people who hold specific identities regardless of whether they are true, and they usually reflect widespread, societal opinions. They persist because they are helpful and effective when it comes to referencing and associating others in one's own mind (however wrong or distorted they may be). When you meet a Scotsman, it is easier to be guided by a stereotype than to find out whether he is in fact stingy or generous. Stereotypes facilitate rapid cognitive orientation in complex social environments. Common elements of stereotypes about people with mental illness are that they are dangerous, incompetent, weak and responsible for their illness.

TABLE 3.1 ■ Two-Factor Theory of Stigma: Stigma Focus (Public/Self) and Social-Cognitive Components—Stereotypes, Prejudices, Discrimination

	Public Stigma		Self-Stigma
Stereotypes	Negative opinions about people with mental illness* (dangerous, incompetent, responsible for illness)	Self-stereotypes	Negative opinions about your own group (dangerous, incompetent, guilty)
Prejudices	Agreement with the stereotype and emotional reaction (anger, fear)	Self-prejudice	Acceptance of the stereotype and emotional reaction (reduced self-esteem/self-efficacy, shame, guilt)
Discrimination	Behaviour as a result of the prejudice (e.g. discrimination in work settings, withholding of assistance)	Self-discrimination	Behaviour as a result of self-prejudice/why try (e.g. giving up looking for work or housing)

*After Corrigan PW, Watson AC. The paradox of self-stigma and mental illness. *Clin Psychol Sci Pract.* 2002;9:35–53.

- *Prejudice* occurs when someone not only knows a stereotype but also agrees with it and reacts emotionally (Table 3.1). The stereotype that a mentally ill person is dangerous evolves into a prejudice when accompanied by fear: 'Yes, it's true, all mentally ill people are dangerous and frighten me!' Gordon Allport defined a prejudice as 'a hostile attitude towards a person who belongs to a group, simply because he belongs to that group, and is therefore presumed to have the objectionable qualities ascribed to the group' ([76], p. 8).

- While prejudice refers to thinking and feeling as a result of the stereotype, *discrimination* refers to the way one behaves as a result of prejudice. Discrimination therefore consists of how someone acts towards a stigmatised person. Depending on the nature of the prejudice and its emotional component, discrimination can take different forms: a prejudice of fear might lead to avoidance, a prejudice of anger to hostility or punishment. *Self-stigma* is when a person with mental illness, for example, agrees with the negative stereotypes attached to their condition, internalises them and thereby puts them upon themself (more on self-stigma in Sect. 5.1.3).

3.1.4 SOCIOLOGICAL MODEL OF STIGMA

American sociologists Bruce Link and Jo Phelan developed a model that engages with and complements the social-cognitive approach. In their model, stigma is defined as the culmination of four processes that occur within a power discrepancy [77]: distinguishing and labelling of differences, the association of human differences with negative attributes, separating *us* from *them*, and status loss and discrimination (Table 3.2).

The first step, *distinguishing between groups and labelling,* is the most fundamental. Differences in human characteristics considered important are socially defined and delineated. Consider, for example, eye colour: hardly anyone would consider eye colour so significant that they would say: 'My neighbour is a brown-eyed man!' The same cannot be said, however, of skin colour. Group classifications tend to be oversimplifications; characteristics do not tend to fall along clear dividing lines such as *white* or *black*, *healthy* or *sick*, and *heterosexual* or *homosexual* (Sect. 1.6). The separation into *them* and *us* has a clarifying and even calming effect on those who see themselves as *normal* (Sect. 7.4.6, 'Cultural Knowledge and Self-Assurance').

The second step, the *association of differences with negative characteristics,* corresponds to stereotyping in the social-cognitive model. In Section 3.2 we will deal with stereotypes, their content and functions in more detail. What is important to note about stereotypes in Link and Phelan's model is that they are often applied automatically and involuntarily, without conscious control or reflection. Like in the social-cognitive model, stereotypes here are generalisations, such that members of a stigmatised group are not judged by their personal characteristics but by their group membership.

TABLE 3.2 ■ **Core Elements of Stigma**

1. Distinguishing and labelling of human characteristics	
2. Cultural beliefs link labelled individuals with negative stereotypes	Social, political, cultural and economic power differences to the disadvantage of the stigmatised group
3. Labelled people are categorised (us ↔ them)	
4. Labelled people experience loss of status and discrimination	

Based on Link BG, Phelan JC. Conceptualizing stigma. *Annu Rev Sociol*. 2001;27:363–385.

The third step, the *separation between us and them*, is an expression of desire for social distance based on perceived difference. In extreme cases, this can lead to the dehumanisation of stigmatised people and can be misused as justification for any kind of discrimination, even genocide (Sect. 2.1.2).

The fourth step, *status loss and discrimination*, is, as in the previous model, the significant final stage. Status loss is a key aspect of the overall model for two reasons. First, stigmatised people suffer from loss of status in society regardless of blatant discrimination. Second, loss of status has a concrete effect on social performance. This connection was investigated in studies on status and expectations [78], which demonstrated that assumed characteristics of a lower-status group are associated with expectations about how a person in that group will behave. In turn, these expectations strongly influence behaviour and performance (Sect. 4.2.3). Take for example the prevailing negative stereotype that women are weaker in maths than men. In a maths class group project, internalised insecurity due to this expectation may result in girl students withdrawing, while the boys dominate the meeting. Differences in status thereby risk becoming self-fulfilling prophecies: later in life, in the professional world, men tend to hold more positions of power (e.g. hierarchically, in universities or companies). Concepts of status are effective because everyone, men and women, whites and blacks, know them.

In the Link and Phelan model, discrimination appears in both individual and structural forms. *Individual discrimination* refers to a single person's discrimination of another. A classic example of this is when an employer disregards an application from a woman, a foreigner or a person with a mental illness despite their being highly qualified. While this example is clear and common, it underestimates the various harmful dynamics and complexities of stigma; stigmatised people often experience discrimination from many sides and in many areas. Discrimination as a practice or corporate culture of businesses or government bodies can also have an impact without individuals behaving in a discriminatory manner. This is dealt with later under the topic of structural discrimination (Sect. 5.1.8).

Link and Phelan pointed out that stigma can only develop when there is a *power difference* between those who discriminate and those who are discriminated against [77]. One example is the relationship between psychiatrists and their patients. Patients can associate psychiatrists with negative stereotypes—that they lack empathy or are fixated on medication management. But even if patients have this view and behave accordingly towards psychiatrists, psychiatrists do not become a stigmatised group [77]. Patients do not have the social, cultural, economic or political power to turn psychiatrists or other healthcare professionals into a stigmatised group.

Situating stigma within a power dynamic is critical for three reasons:

- If stigma can only occur when certain social groups have and exercise their power, these groups (e.g. employers or professionals in the healthcare system) should be considered key targets of antistigma programmes (Sects. 7.1.1 and 7.3.2).
- There is a conceptual misunderstanding when certain groups, such as psychiatrists, think of themselves as stigmatised. Prejudices may of course be circulated against them, but they do not face any known systematic discrimination. On the contrary, they are often in a position of power, at least with regard to their patients (Sect. 7.3.1, 'Are Psychiatrists Stigmatised?').
- The concept of stigma should not be used in a vague or excessive way, otherwise it loses its significance for marginalised groups. If everyone was 'stigmatised' because of existing stereotypes about their group, politicians and investment bankers would also be stigmatised. 'Stigma' would appear to be a harmless process that everyone is confronted with—but none of this is true.

3.1.5 FORMS OF STIGMA: PUBLIC, SELF, STRUCTURAL

Three major forms of stigma are outlined here. *Public stigma* is when members of the general public have prejudices against a stigmatised group and discriminate against those in it. This does not suggest that the behaviour has to take place in the public realm; it more so connotes the behaviour of, for example, a neighbour, doctor, teacher, police officer, landlord or employer. This stigma is part of the public domain insofar as employers, for instance, act on widely known prejudices as part of the nonstigmatised 'normal' public ('Glossary': general public).

Self-stigma occurs when a stigmatised person is not only aware of prejudices against her group but also agrees with and applies them to herself. A woman may say, 'Yes, I am a woman, so I must be bad at mathematics', or a person with mental illness may think, 'Because I am mentally ill, I must be incompetent and to blame for my illness.' This internalisation of prejudice damages one's self-esteem and self-efficacy—the judgment of ability to achieve one's own goals. This can lead to a state of demoralisation, known as the 'why try' effect: 'Why should I try to achieve my goals? I'm not worth it or am not able to do it.' Goals in the areas of living and working, relationships or even the search for good treatment can be affected (Sect. 5.1.3 [79]). It is important, especially for those working in psychiatry, to realise that self-stigma is not the fault or a defect of the service user; rather, it is a reaction to the existence of public prejudice.

Structural discrimination manifests in the form of rules, policies and procedures in the political, cultural, legal or social sphere; this tends to be a systematic hindrance or endangerment of a group of people without regard to the individual. Internal processes in companies, public authorities or universities can also be affected, for example in the realm of human resources or in dealing with disability or compensation for disadvantage. Structural discrimination can occur even without explicit discriminatory behaviour from individuals (e.g. administrative staff who simply follow the rules [80]). While the term structural discrimination is used in this book, other authors may refer to it as systemic or institutional discrimination or, in regards to companies and organisations, as organisational stigma. (These distinctions are not clearly defined and will therefore not be pursued in this text.)

Structural discrimination can be either intentional or unintentional. One example of deliberate structural discrimination is the prohibition of same-sex marriage in many countries around the world. Unintentional structural discrimination can be found, for example, in the US university admissions system. The standardised achievement tests (SATs) required for acceptance are considered to be 'objective' but in fact highlight underlying societal problems and discriminatory realities: students of colour from underresourced and low-income schools in the United States have historically performed worse on these entrance tests. Coming from a disadvantaged school means you are less likely to be accepted at elite universities. Educational (mis)opportunities are intertwined with discriminatory practices in housing and employment as well; this has been the matrix of racial discrimination in the United States since the end of slavery in the 19th century. To make matters worse, individuals most affected also face stereotype threat (Sect. 4.2.3). Forms and consequences of structural discrimination for people with mental illness are discussed in Section 5.1.8.

3.1.6 DEGREES AND TYPES OF EXPRESSION OF STIGMA

A Matter of Degree

Stigma is not a case of all or nothing; it contains nuances and can vary in intensity. The distinction between groups (*mentally ill* or *mentally healthy*) often exists on a continuum between the extremes of complete health and most serious illness (Sect. 1.6). Similarly, the stereotypes, discrimination and extent of status loss associated with this distinction may vary in strength. For this reason, antistigma initiatives tend to be less focused on eliminating stigma altogether and rather aim to gradually reduce its manifestations and consequences (Ch. 8 ff.).

Explicit and Implicit Attitudes

People can make their prejudices explicit. There's a Mr Smith sitting at a pub somewhere blatantly saying: 'I don't want to have anything to do with mentally ill people!' But even if he does not explicitly express himself in this way, prejudice can still influence Mr Smith's behaviour. He may automatically associate people with mental illness with certain character profiles, feel uncomfortable or tense, and thereby keep his distance. This unintended prejudice and discomfort is also known as an implicit attitude. The explicit–implicit distinction is a much-studied phenomenon regarding how people process, judge and react to their environments (dual process theories [81]). Both explicit and implicit prejudice can influence behaviour. People with mental illness can also express these kinds of prejudices against themselves (Sect. 5.1.3); both processes seem to have an effect on their quality of life [82].

An impressive US study of more than two million members of the general public looked at the link between racist attitudes and the incidence of black people being killed by police in certain areas [83]. Implicit attitudes were recorded by measuring participants' reaction times when assigning word pairs that represented the connection between black people and negative characteristics; namely, 'black–bad' and 'black–danger'. The results showed that the stronger the implicit prejudices in an area, the higher the incidence of black people being shot by the police in that area. Given the high proliferation of firearms in the United States, police officers on duty often decide within fractions of a second whether to shoot; the result can be unarmed blacks being severely injured or killed. This study emphasises the seriousness of implicit prejudices for making automatic and fast decisions (and is applicable to far less dramatic or grave scenarios). And because the study subjects consisted of the general population rather than police officers alone, the results illustrate just how much the broader social climate can influence individual behaviour.

Open and Indirect Discrimination

There is much to be said for the fact that we are living in an era when open discrimination against minorities and the marginalised is less tolerated; this is generally good news. But it unfortunately does not mean that discrimination has disappeared. Discrimination also occurs indirectly, and subtle discrimination puts those affected by it in a difficult position—they might be less able to recognise and give it a name (Sect. 4.2.5). The following experiment is about the expression of prejudice taking place openly or in a subtle and indirect way.

EXPERIMENT

An instructive study was conducted about discrimination against homosexual job seekers [84]. In addition to its careful design, the study had four strengths that are important for our topic:
1. investigation into the stigma of homosexuality which, like mental illness, is usually invisible,
2. the observation of behaviour towards stigmatised people in the everyday world rather than in the laboratory,
3. the distinction between open and subtle discriminatory behaviour and
4. the recording of all subjects' reactions, including those who are stigmatised.
As part of the study, students in a city in Texas were recruited to walk into large businesses, inquire about job opportunities and ask the person in charge if they could apply. Students were given a tape recorder and wore a hat on which either the words Gay and Proud or Texan and Proud were clearly visible. As per the study design, the students did not know which hat they were wearing. Using the tape recordings, two types of discrimination were evaluated by the researchers (who also did not know which hat was worn at the time): was there obvious discrimination (e.g. was the student denied an application)? Or did the employer demonstrate a more subtle discrimination, in the form of a shorter, taciturn conversation or negative attitude (in terms of choice of words and language)? As expected, there was no evidence of overt discrimination; no student was sent away immediately. But the conversations with the students wearing hats with Gay and Proud turned out to be much shorter and colder. This was not only the result of the evaluation of the tape recordings, but also of the students' assessments—even though they did not know which hat they had worn. The students wearing Gay and Proud hats reported, for example, that employers had avoided eye contact with them. The more negative an employer's behaviour, the less likely he'd mention vacancies, offer a job application or call the applicants back afterwards.

Microaggression

As exemplified earlier, indirect discrimination can be administered in smaller doses, so to speak. But its poison can nevertheless cause damage. The term microaggression has been used for this purpose since the 1970s but was only popularised at the beginning of this century [85]. Microaggression was the word of the year in 2015, according to the Global Language Monitor; American universities now offer training programmes aimed at reducing them. Microaggressions are described as instances in everyday life when hostile or pejorative attitudes are intentionally or unintentionally expressed towards a minority. One example might be of a white professor who compliments a black student: 'That's a particularly good answer!' From the point of view of many microaggression researchers, this is a pejorative-aggressive statement because it tacitly implies that a good answer should not be expected from black people.

There is no question that discrimination today, including against people with mental illness, is often very subtle. Nevertheless, the concept of microaggressions, and especially the guidelines, interventions and training programmes derived from it, has been criticised [86]. The research field on microaggressions faces many problems. For starters, microaggression is not clearly or universally defined, neither as a concept nor in the questionnaires used to study it. The statement from the professor in the previous paragraph could not only be well-intentioned but could also be received by the black student in a variety of ways—as unreservedly positive or as subtly racist and aggressive. This is a dilemma for researchers who seek to prove the alleged spread and negative consequences of microaggressions for members of the stigmatised minority (Sect. 4.2.5). The above example also presents a dilemma of the white professor: both ignoring the black student and praising her might be labelled a microaggression [86]. The impact of stigma on the nonstigmatised is further discussed in Section 4.1 [87].

3.1.7 STIGMA AND KNOWLEDGE: MENTAL HEALTH LITERACY

Stigma is more than ignorance. But distorted, generalised or simply false convictions that lead to negative stereotypes and prejudices (Sects. 3.1.3 and 3.2) demonstrate how little people know about mental health and illness. This is why Australian researcher Tony Jorm coined the term 'mental health literacy' [88]: knowledge that is helpful for the recognition, management and prevention of mental disorders. Jorm's starting point was that although much is being done to educate people about heart disease, HIV and so on, the issue of mental illness receives little attention. According to his approach, the general public should be able to recognise common mental disorders such as depression, panic disorder and suicidality, and to identify the symptoms and acute crises associated with them. We should know about resources that can help and be able to point them out to those in need. And we should also know about prevention and ways to strengthen one's mental health. Jorm uses a broad definition of help when describing said resources, ranging from the help of one's friends and family, to self-help and counselling centres, to psychiatric-psychotherapeutic treatment. Ideally, people should learn which type of assistance or support is appropriate depending on the degree of severity of the illness. Studies have shown that having more knowledge in this regard better facilitates the search for help [89].

In this book I refer to overgeneralised statements and distorted opinions as stereotypes, as this term facilitates the link to a wealth of social psychological research on the broader topic of stigma (Sect. 3.2). Graham Thornicroft cites ignorance as one of three core elements of the stigma of mental illness [90], which is consistent with Tony Jorm's approach to fighting stigma by providing information. Jorm developed a training programme for the general public which bears the catchy name *Mental Health First Aid* and is discussed in more detail in Sections 8.1.5 and 8.1.6 [88]. Fighting ignorance with education is clearly important. However, due to the many aspects of stigma—its functions, emotional reactions and cultural characteristics (Sect. 3.3)—the provision of information alone is unlikely to suffice.

3.1.8 MORE THAN ONE STIGMA: INTERSECTIONALITY

Everyone carries with them multiple social roles and identities. I am a husband, psychiatrist, father, brother, son, colleague, neighbour and so on. But what happens when several of those held by one person are stigmatised? Let us suppose that someone with mental illness is also a black man who is homeless and formerly incarcerated: he is exposed to various types of prejudice and discrimination that stem from these coexisting identities.

The concept of intersectionality refers to the intersection and co-occurrence of several characteristics or attributes [91]. The term was first introduced by American lawyer and critical race theorist Kimberlé Crenshaw in the late 1980s, who from her own experiences as a black woman had grown well-acquainted with discrimination [92]. Crenshaw argued that when one holds multiple identities, she does not singularly experience, say, sexism *or* racism. Rather, the combination of one *and* the other leads to a new quality of discrimination. Crenshaw was amongst the first to point out that feminists of that time concerned themselves with the fate of white women, and antiracists with that of black men, but that the plight of black women was too often overlooked.

As an example, Crenshaw cited the futile struggle of black women in a court case against the American car manufacturer General Motors over discriminatory termination practices. General Motors had never hired a black woman before 1964, and during a recession after 1970 they were all laid off. The district court rejected the black women's claim: discrimination for being women was not apparent, as white women had been able to keep their jobs. The claim of racial discrimination was also rejected, as black men had not been dismissed. The court rejected the notion that the two identities could be combined into a new minority worthy of protection; it argued this would open Pandora's box and the floodgates for all kinds of 'subgroups' to sue. But intersectionality is not about creating endless new minority categories; rather we need to open our eyes to the particular and unique challenges of experiencing multiple forms of discrimination in everyday life [93].

The concept of *intersectionality* is closely related to structural discrimination (Sects. 3.1.5 and 5.1.8). Some social groups are structurally disadvantaged (e.g. women and black people). Being a woman *and* a black person thus makes one vulnerable to the *structural discrimination* of both groups. There are many intersections: poverty, illness, unemployment and so forth. People with mental illness often hold multiple stigmatised characteristics as well, and they are therefore similarly affected by structural discrimination and challenges of intersectionality (Sect. 5.5).

3.2 Categorisation and Stereotypes as Basic Elements of Stigma

3.2.1 WHAT IS CATEGORISATION?

Human beings are social creatures for whom cooperation is essential for survival. This has been a feature of human life throughout evolution (Sect. 3.3.4). Cooperation works well when the support is mutual, and it is best achieved within an in-group that is clearly distinct from its social environment and out-groups. Human ability to categorise quickly allows us to assign each other to our own or other social groups [94]. In a more complex social environment, this allocation is usually made 'by itself'—automatically, or outside conscious awareness. This relieves the burden on the perceiver so that we can simultaneously perform other tasks. In this sense, *categorisation* is a highly efficient process. Yet it can come at the expense of precision in our perceptions of others. Categorisation as well as the lack of precision in doing so is evident even in the first year of life [95].

People form impressions of others in two ways (*dual process models* [81]; Sect. 3.1.6, 'Explicit and Implicit Attitudes'):

1. cognitive processing of social information that is detailed and elaborate, originating (bottom up) from the individuals whom we meet,
2. cognitive processing based on categorisation, using the general (the social category or group) to judge the individual (top down); this is often automatic, fast and efficient.

Categorisation leads to members of one social group being perceived as more similar to each other than they really are; at the same time, the differences between the in-group and the out-group are overestimated. This results in the often artificial distinction between *us* and *them* mentioned in Section 3.1.4 as the basis of stigma. The categorisation of people as *mentally healthy* or *mentally ill* automatically leads to the assumption of two distinct groups, even if in reality all people are on the same continuum (Sect. 1.6).

Categorisation, and thus the distinction between *us* and *them*, can increase under various conditions [94]. There are external conditions, such as real-world conflicts for limited resources (e.g. food and water), that may force the divide. There are also internal conditions, such as the process of developing one's own self-concept and determining the groups to which he or she belongs. The latter deals with the much-studied *self-categorisation theory*, which assumes that people define their identity personally and socially [96]. In the case of personal identity, personal characteristics and motives determine how we think and act. Social identity evolves from when people see themselves less as individuals and more as members of a group, such that their own actions are determined by the collective's goals and values. The two identities are not mutually exclusive but can be more or less in the foreground depending on the person and situation. Most people have the need to both belong to a group (social identity) and be their own distinguishable person (personal identity). Other factors that promote categorisation are the threat of losing one's own self-esteem (Sect. 3.3.1) or the need for system justification (Sect. 3.3.3).

3.2.2 CATEGORISATION AND REDUCTION OF PREJUDICE

Contact with members of an out-group can, under certain conditions, reduce prejudice. The necessary conditions broadly include equal status and cooperation between the groups, common goals, support from the institution or those in authority, and the opportunity for personal meetings and friendly exchange [97]. We will discuss this in more detail later on in the context of antistigma interventions (Sect. 8.4). The question now is how contact reduces prejudice and the role of categorisation in doing so. We all belong to different groups, but our self-assignment to these groups is often in a state of flux. For example, depending on the context, I can feel like a citizen of and associate myself more closely with a neighbourhood, a city, a country, Europe or the earth. These categorisations include others to a greater or lesser extent.

Three approaches to the reduction of prejudice center on categorisation: decategorisation, group differentiation and recategorisation [94]. In programmes that use *decategorisation*, people are encouraged to see and describe themselves primarily as individuals and not so much as group members. This also means that when they come into contact with members of the out-group, they share personal details about themselves and become recognisable as individuals. This approach reduces prejudice by minimising the significance of social identities and group boundaries.

The *group differentiation* approach assumes that the distinction between the in-group and out-groups does serve an important function (including for one's own identity) and should not be downplayed. The approach supports the idea of continuing to differentiate between groups while establishing good, cooperative contact between them. The contact works if members of the out-group are typical representatives of it and remain recognisable as such.

The approach for finding a common, overarching identity that is inclusive of both groups is known as *recategorisation*. Let us assume that there is a conflict between two football teams in a school, from two different classes. Through recategorisation, one would try to remind both teams that they belong to the same school and thus emphasise their common identity. Prejudice diminishes because those who were previously *others* now belong to the new in-group (and this in-group is usually viewed positively).

EXPERIMENT

Social psychologist Jason Nier investigated recategorisation in an elegant study [98]: when it comes to the relationships between black and white people, can recategorisation change everyday behaviour? The study was conducted at a football match between two rival university teams on the American East Coast. Researchers, both black and white, wore the hat of either of the two teams. They would ask arriving fans, who were also recognisable as fans of one of the teams by their clothing, for a short interview. The percentage of white fans who agreed to be interviewed was recorded according to whether their interviewer was black or white and whether the interviewer was a fan of their own or the opposing team. The results showed that when it came to white interviewers, white fans did not care which team they affiliated with. But black interviewers were much more likely to obtain interviews from white fans with whom they shared team clothing. What does this demonstrate? White fans let themselves be interviewed by white interviewers, regardless of team affiliation, because they felt they belonged to the same group (i.e. shared skin colour). With black interviewers, it was only the higher-level identity of shared fandom that led to a decrease in rejection and an increased willingness to be interviewed among whites. This study showed that everyday behaviour is strongly influenced by categorisation processes.

These three approaches to how categorisation can be used to reduce prejudice between groups are not mutually exclusive; depending on the situation, they can complement and promote each other. For example, recategorisation, which is the formation of a common, overarching identity, can lead to members of other groups being perceived more as individuals and less as members of a group (decategorisation).

3.2.3 WHAT ARE STEREOTYPES?

Stereotypes are preconceived beliefs we hold about the characteristics and behaviour of certain social groups [75]. In social psychology, these are seen less as faulty thought patterns and more as efficient means of finding one's way around a very complex social world without much use of cognitive resources (thinking effort).

The question of why stereotypes are so widespread will be dealt with in more detail in Section 3.3 in connection with the functions of stigma. Briefly, they fulfil different functions depending on the person and context:

- They can make orientation easier, as people are judged quickly according to stereotypes that correspond with the group they belong to rather than cumbersomely, according to their individual personalities.
- They can constitute a reaction to an environment or event. When there is a conflict between groups, for example, there may be a negative stereotype created or perpetuated about those who belong to the competing group.
- They can also fulfil personal needs for social identity, for demarcation from others or for the legitimisation of social differences.

Five aspects of stereotypes will be described first: their content and whether they are based on truth (Sect. 3.2.4), how stereotypes arise (Sect. 3.2.5), how stereotypes are perpetuated (Sect. 3.2.6), how stereotypes are applied to individuals (Sect. 3.2.7) and finally, how stereotypes can be changed (Sect. 3.2.8).

3.2.4 CONTENT OF STEREOTYPES

Content Dimensions of Stereotypes

Social psychologist Susan T. Fiske defined two main dimensions of stereotypes: warmth (or friendliness) and competence. These can be found across cultures and are applicable to all different social groups (Fig. 3.1 [99]). Warmth and competence as a stereotype's main content dimensions closely relate to a stereotype's function: both of these axes assist in quickening and easing our orientations of others. When I meet strangers, I first have to assess whether they have good or bad intentions (warmth) and then whether they can act on those intentions (competence). Some groups are highly associated with both warmth and competence (such as the wealthy middle class; top right in Fig. 3.1), while other groups are associated with neither of these characteristics (such as the poor and homeless, Sect. 7.2; bottom left in Fig. 3.1).

Fiske's model explains why stereotypes are often ambiguous (i.e. not only good or bad). Some groups are considered both warm and incompetent (top left in Fig. 3.1), while others are seen as cold and competent (bottom right in Fig. 3.1). Among other examples, this chart explains the phenomenon of so-called benevolent sexism. It attributes warmth to women (e.g. in the area of child-rearing), yet declares them to be professionally incompetent. As we will see later, this form of benevolent stigma, accompanied by pity, also exists for people with mental illness (Sect. 5.1) or with intellectual disability (Sect. 5.4.6). It may also play a role in the efforts of psychiatrists to chair antistigma programmes (Sect. 12.4).

Do Stereotypes Contain a Kernel of Truth?

Whether stereotypes are rooted in truth is often discussed, especially in regard to those with mental illness. I once brought up in a lecture the stereotype that 'schizophrenics are dangerous', and afterwards I was approached by a well-known psychiatrist who said this was not a prejudice;

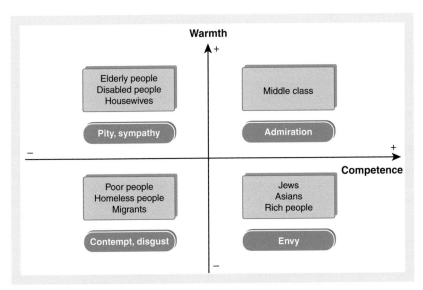

Fig. 3.1 Model of stereotype content; catchwords are used for the groups (e.g. disabled people instead of people with disabilities, etc.). (Based on Fiske ST, Cuddy AJC, Glick P, Xu J. A model of [often mixed] stereotype content: competence and warmth respectively follow from perceived status and competition. *J Pers Soc Psychol.* 2002;82:878–902. Courtesy of Heike Hübner, Berlin.)

he argued that 'schizophrenics' really were more dangerous than the general public. It is therefore worth taking a look at whether stereotypes are based on truth.

One can, broadly speaking, distinguish between stereotypes that reflect real group differences and those that do not. Examples of stereotypes that are plausibly related to reality include common notions such as 'basketball players are tall' or 'Chinese people like to eat rice'. A limitation is that such stereotypes are generalisations that only identify individual characteristics that emphasise group differences (and do not encapsulate the person): not all basketball players are tall; not all Chinese people like rice.

Whether negative stereotypes apply to people with mental illness is an important question. As with the above-mentioned psychiatrist, the stereotype that people with mental illness are dangerous is repeated time and again. Before we go further, it should be made clear that people with mental illness are much more likely to be victims of violence than those without mental illness [100]. This is particularly due to their higher chance of experiencing housing and employment discrimination as well as social isolation [90]. On the other hand, studies show that the risk of people with severe mental illness being violent is on average a bit higher than the general public [101]. But this risk of violence is just as closely related to other factors, including male gender, young age, and alcohol or drug consumption.

This discussion about whether there is an increased risk of harm from people with mental illness is problematic for two reasons and tends to reinforce rather than reduce prejudice. First, stereotypes are an overgeneralisation; individuals are not judged by who they are but by the group they are seen to belong to and the negative stereotypes associated with it. When it comes to stigma, the question of whether people with schizophrenia statistically have a slightly higher risk of violence is thereby no longer relevant. Stigma occurs when an employer does not hire Mr Smith, an applicant with a history of schizophrenia, because that employer believes the violent stereotype must apply to him—even though Mr Smith has never been violent.

Second, this discussion bears the risk of confirming prejudice. People who consider stereotypes to be true will feel confirmed by a slightly increased risk of violence amongst those with schizophrenia in large population studies, even if these figures say nothing about individuals. This is not to say that epidemiologists should not deal with such questions (of a relative increase in risk)—on the contrary, serious research has critical value, and it does not help anyone to conceal facts with good intentions (Sect. 1.4). But we should not promote conclusions from large samples about the behaviour of individuals. The risk of violence is increased in those with severe mental illness who do not seek treatment. Stigma itself is a reason why people remain untreated (Sect. 5.1.7). There is evidence here of a vicious cycle: negative stereotypes and stigma lead to avoidance of treatment, and avoidance of treatment leads to upsetting individual cases that seem to confirm those negative stereotypes (Sect. 3.2.5, 'Illusory Correlation').

Behaviour or Label: Stereotypes as a Normal Perception of Bizarre Behaviour?

Similar to the kernel of truth question is the argument that stereotypes are in fact based on the public's correct perception of people with mental illness. After one of my lectures, a social psychiatrist, of all people, said to me that if patients simply received sufficient treatment such that their behaviour returned to normal, stigma would no longer be a problem. Patients, in his opinion, only meet rejection if they behave in a bizarre, threatening or conspicuous manner.

These issues were first intensively discussed and conceptually and empirically clarified in the second half of the twentieth century. In the 1960s, Thomas Scheff formulated his provocative labelling theory [102]. According to this theory, socially deviant and conspicuous behaviour is labelled as mental illness, and in many cases this labelling leads to people becoming permanently mentally ill. In other words, stigmatic labelling is the cause of mental illness. Scheff's position was part of the antipsychiatry movement of that time (Sect. 2.1.3). His critics' response was that stigma does not play a significant role and has little effect on people with mental illness.

In response to the two extreme ends of this debate given by Scheff and his critics, Bruce Link developed a *modified labelling theory* [103]. He does not claim that labelling is the cause of mental illness, but he does argue that labelling and stigma have many negative effects, including psychological ones. The starting point is the well-documented fact that even children and adolescents are aware of negative stereotypes about people with mental illness [104]. These stereotypes tend to remain irrelevant for people as long as they do not fall ill themselves. But as soon as a person does fall ill and is labelled *mentally ill*, particularly when he seeks treatment, the stereotypes become personally relevant and threatening. He must now decide how to respond to public stigma and self-stigma. This leads to the matter of coping mechanisms (to which we will return later): choosing to keep the illness secret, socially withdraw or educate one's own environment (Sect. 4.3).

Link also investigated whether conspicuous behaviour or labelling led to greater social rejection of people with mental illness [105]. Some studies had previously shown that both conspicuous behaviour and the label of mental illness can lead to rejection, with behaviour often having a stronger effect than the label. But Link thoughtfully hypothesised that the effect of labelling can only be understood if existing prejudice is taken into account. For example, labelling someone as 'schizophrenic' will trigger a strong reaction in others if they are already of the opinion that schizophrenics are violent. This expectation was confirmed: in the experiment, being labelled as *mentally ill*, regardless of the extent of unusual behaviour, strongly influenced the desire of study participants for social distance if they already thought that people with that label were dangerous. This is consistent with the results of a German study by Matthias Angermeyer and Herbert Matschinger [106]: members of the general public were given descriptions of others showing symptoms of either schizophrenia or depression, though the descriptions did not explicitly refer to either diagnosis. Those study participants who identified and labelled the symptoms of the person being described as *mental illness* also indicated more fear and a stronger desire for social distance. This effect was only found for schizophrenia, not depression.

Conclusion

Bizarre behaviour does trigger negative reactions—everyone has borne witness or experienced this first-hand in public spaces. But being labelled as *mentally ill* independently triggers strong social rejection, even if a person does not show any conspicuous behaviour or signs of mental illness. This rejection has far-reaching consequences and leads to the long-term devaluation of the person.

3.2.5 ORIGINS OF STEREOTYPES

Broadly speaking, stereotypes originate in three distinguishable ways. The first are cognitive processes, reflective of the peculiarities of human thinking; three examples of this are explained below. There are also motivational processes (i.e. the emergence of stereotypes out of self-interest) which are discussed later in 'Functions of Stigma' (Sect. 3.3). Finally, the development of stereotypes is influenced by personality traits, such as a preference for authoritarianism and the social dominance of one's in-group (Sect. 3.3.3 [107]).

Unconscious Association

Stereotypes can arise when people unconsciously associate external features with characteristics. In one study, students were shown a few photos of professors [108]. The images showed people with long, narrow faces who were said to be fair examiners—conversely, those with short, broad faces were supposed to be unfair. In another group of students, the association of face shape with character trait (i.e. fair or unfair) was reversed. The results showed that the students, unaware of the arbitrary association between face shape and trait, had internalised and applied that association after being shown only a few photos.

In a second study, participants saw computer-generated face shapes with noses higher up or lower down than usual. As part of a learning phase, the participants were told that noses high up on a face belonged to personality type A and noses low down on a face belonged to personality type B. Again, the participants learned the connection quickly. Next, pictures with noses high up or low down were shown. The study participants were asked to say whether the face belonged to personality type A or B. Not only did they stick to the learnt association between face and personality, but the perceived connection became stronger and stronger over the course of being shown the series of pictures. Stereotypes can therefore be self-perpetuating (self-perpetuating bias; Sect. 3.2.6). This is important when understanding mental illness stigma: mental disorders are, for example, a common theme in the media (Sect. 7.4), which not only forms stereotypes but maintains them through the audience's self-exposure.

The *Others* Are All Alike

The formation of stereotypes is facilitated by the fact that, while we tend to judge members of our in-group as individuals with personal characteristics, we also tend to perceive members of out-groups as homogeneous, on the basis of the groups they belong to [109]. This is especially true when it comes to the negative behaviour of those who belong to other groups. The stronger the type of competition or threat which emanates from the out-group, the stronger this effect becomes (out-group homogeneity effect).

Illusory Correlation

Stereotypes about groups can arise even if there are no real group differences. Hamilton and Gifford investigated this issue in their experiment on the so-called illusory correlation [110]. This refers to a connection (correlation) between a group and characteristics that only appears to exist and is not actually real. In the experiment, study participants read sentences. Each sentence described a positive or negative behavioural characteristic of various people. Each sentence then stated whether it was representative of 'Group A' or 'Group B'. There were three key details to the set-up of this experiment:

1. Two-thirds of all of the sentences described positive behaviours, and one-third described negative behaviours.
2. Two-thirds of all of the sentences described behaviours of Group A, and one-third described behaviours of Group B.
3. Within both Group A and Group B, negative behaviour was less common (about 30%) than positive behaviour (about 70%).

The study participants were then asked which of the groups tended to behave positively or negatively, and how they might rate the groups. The participants correctly remembered that about one-third of all positive behaviour came from Group B. However, most of the negative behaviour was also attributed to Group B—even though only a third of the negative behaviour came from Group B. Group A was also rated much more positively than Group B.

How can such a distorted impression of a group arise after a simple experiment? It seems to be because significant incidents are easier for people to remember. In this case, the assumption of Group B's negative behaviour was significant because both variables (negative behaviour *and* Group B) were less frequent (compared to the frequency of positive behaviour and Group A). The combination of the two (negative and B) was therefore more conspicuous. More recent explanations of this phenomenon refer to attention processes through which people first form an opinion of the majority or 'normality', and minority impressions are then shaped by rare incidents [111].

This experiment on illusory correlation has often been replicated and is important for the stigma of mental illness for multiple reasons:

- First, the conditions of the experiment are very similar to those in everyday life. Members of the general public are less likely to meet people with mental illness than people who are deemed 'healthy'. And as in the general public, negative behaviour is less common than positive behaviour. Therefore illusory correlation can contribute to people with mental illness being associated with negative behaviour.

- Second, illusory correlation can help explain why media coverage of crimes committed by people with mental disorders has serious consequences: it reinforces negative stereotypes because a stigmatised minority is permanently associated with rare events (Sect. 7.4).

3.2.6 MAINTENANCE OF STEREOTYPES

Regardless of how stereotypes have been formed, they are maintained by various mechanisms. How we perceive, process and interpret new information or experiences is strongly influenced by our previous experiences. Established knowledge and thought structures control our perception and behaviour (biased processing). As a result, people tend to absorb and interpret information in a way that confirms stereotypes. Since social situations are often complex and up to interpretation, stereotypes strongly influence how people process and respond to what is occurring around them. In this way, stereotypes are unavoidable—but the damage they can cause is particularly serious.

EXAMPLE

Suppose someone believes in the stereotype that black men are both stupid and hostile [75]. If she then meets a black man who acts stupidly but friendly, she will think he is stupid. And if he behaves intelligently but in a hostile manner, she will consider him hostile. In both cases, she will feel confirmed in her beliefs.

We tend to overestimate how similar individuals are to their respective groups. This is especially true when it is not our own group but an out-group. So if someone thinks black people are aggressive, they will overestimate the aggressiveness of any black person. We also interpret situations in a way that confirms stereotypes. For example, we tend to attribute others' negative behaviours to persistent, long-lasting personality traits, while negative behaviours within our in-group are more likely to be interpreted as accidental or situational (and vice versa for positive behaviour). A person's memory supports the maintenance of stereotypes: people are more likely to remember information which conforms to their stereotypes. This is especially true in situations with high cognitive demands (as is the case in most social situations), as well as for people with strong prejudices [75].

Stereotypes can be maintained by *self-fulfilling prophecy*. If a teacher expects from the outset that a student belonging to a certain social group is outstanding, the teacher can behave in such a way that gradually strengthens that opinion within the student himself and results in his better academic performance. The opposite effect can occur with negative or demoralising stereotypes.

The use of *language* also helps to stabilise stereotypes (linguistic intergroup bias [112]). When people talk about social situations, they may describe observed behaviours of others more concretely ('He speaks loudly.') or abstractly ('He is aggressive.'). It has been shown that the behaviour of out-group members is more likely to be described in abstract and thereby inalterable terms. Conversely, negative behaviour of the in-group is described in specific, detailed terms, such that it appears more situation related and changeable. Thus our language contributes to the maintenance of stereotypes. Linguistic cues indicate differences in status and contribute to discrimination, not least in work settings, media, and healthcare and judiciary systems [112].

3.2.7 APPLICATION OF STEREOTYPES

Stereotypes only have a negative effect if they are applied to those who belong to stigmatised groups. So far, we have seen the content dimensions of stereotypes, how they are formed and how they are maintained. We will now briefly discuss when and how they are applied to people. Their application is important because it marks the transition from thinking to emotional reaction (prejudice) and behaviour (discrimination).

Usually, stereotypes are so culturally widespread that they can be automatically activated and applied to people belonging to a specific group. For example, a person who sees a skinhead could quickly apply common stereotypes to that person. Experimental studies show that although these stereotypes can be consciously suppressed temporarily, they recur all the more strongly afterwards [113]. This is especially true in situations where one's own self-esteem is threatened; this threat influences automatic processing and strengthens the motivation to devalue others (Sect. 3.3).

Most people do not want to give the impression that their behaviour is determined by stereotypes. If a situation were to clearly give the impression that a person holds certain prejudices, he or she would likely avoid it. A research study investigated this question with a hypothesis that negative stereotypes towards people with a physical disability lead to a desire for social distance [114].

EXPERIMENT

As part of the study, two research assistants were each placed in a corner of a room in front of a screen; one was able-bodied, and the other showed signs of a physical disability and had crutches. Participants in the experiment could choose to sit and watch a film together with either of the research workers. The key to the experiment was that on one occasion the same film was running on both screens; on a different occasion it was two different films. It turned out that more people chose to sit with the person with crutches if the same film was shown on both screens. But if different films were being shown, far more people sat down with the able-bodied person. Why is that? People do not want to appear prejudiced. When the same film is playing, the only plausible explanation why someone does not sit down with the disabled person is the desire for distance. However, if different films are being shown, one can say that the choice of where to sit is because of the film, not because of a desired distance from the person with a disability.

3.2.8 CHANGING STEREOTYPES

As stereotypes are the basis of stigma, how they might be changed is a key question for antistigma interventions (Ch. 8 ff.). Different models explain how stereotypes can be changed [75]. They can be changed incrementally, by continuously gaining new experiences (bookkeeping model). They may suddenly change if they have proven to be untrustworthy (conversion model). Encountering individual representatives from a group can change stereotypes (exemplary model). Finally, new information can lead to the creation of a new subtype (e.g. next to the stereotype 'Mentally ill people are incompetent' the new subtype 'Some mentally ill people are geniuses' can appear; subtyping model). This subtyping can have one of two results: it can lead to the stereotype being preserved and stabilised ('Apart from a few geniuses, the fact remains: mentally ill people are fools!'). Or it can lead to increasing differentiation such that the newly formed subgroups replace the parent group (in our example: people with mental illness) and the associated stereotype is reduced.

These models of reduction in stereotyping have consequences for antistigma work. For example, the above-mentioned stabilisation of stereotypes by subtyping shows the risk of deploying very unusual individual cases (i.e. 'exceptions to the rule') by antistigma campaigns. Campaign participants could respond: 'This celebrity with mental illness is a lovely person, but the others are dangerous fools' (Sect. 8.4.3).

In Sections 3.2.5 and 3.2.6 we saw that stereotypes have different functions and are created and maintained by different processes. On one hand, this helpfully opens up different starting points for the reduction of stereotypes (which will be dealt with later in Ch. 8 ff. in connection with antistigma interventions). On the other hand, this diversity of processes involved in making and maintaining stereotypes means that a singular intervention will likely have limited success. This is one reason why antistigma interventions should ideally have several components.

3.3 Functions of Stigma

Prejudice against different groups in society would not be as pervasive if it did not fulfil specific functions. In turn, these functions have allowed many prejudices to exist for centuries and across cultural lines. It is therefore worth taking a look at the functions of stigma. This is not meant to imply that stigma is an inevitable or unchangeable phenomenon. In order to discuss antistigma initiatives later on (Ch. 8 ff.), it is helpful to know that stigma is not only 'bad' but also serves a purpose for individuals and groups. This section therefore discusses four functional areas of stigma: for individuals, for one's own group, for the relationship between groups, and for society as a whole.

3.3.1 FUNCTION FOR INDIVIDUALS

This section deals with the function of stigma for nonstigmatised members of the general public [115]. First, devaluation of out-groups can increase one's own self-esteem—when I devalue others, it makes me feel relatively better about myself or makes me look good. This is a *downward comparison* [116]. This comparison through the devaluation of others tends to occur when one's own self-esteem is threatened after a failure [117]. This model has two limitations: it does not explain why components of stigma, for example the content of stereotypes, are broadly shared in a society. It also cannot account for why many stigmatised individuals in reality agree with the stereotypes put upon them.

A second function of stigma is to *stabilise a world view* by devaluing those who may endanger it. One of the assumptions of this model is that people are aware of their mortality. Knowing death is inevitable and unpredictable can be so frightening that human beings involuntarily seek a world view that reinforces their sense of order, meaning and security of life. This ultimately helps them cope and find a sense of stability (terror management theory).

EXPERIMENT

Abram Rosenblatt examined this model in a study using US court judiciaries [118]. He gave a cohort of judges documents about a woman who had been arrested for prostitution. Each judge then had to determine the amount of the bail he or she would give for the woman's release. However, right before making this determination, half of the judges received a questionnaire on how they might imagine and feel about their own deaths. This was intended to make the judges confront their own mortality. The result: the judges who had thought and written about their own death set a bail almost 10 times higher than those who had not.

These results indicate that after confronting their own mortality, people feel a stronger need to punish perceived rule violations by others. Devaluing and punishing those whose behaviours contradict and endanger one's own values helps stabilise the comforting view he or she has of the world.

The function of stigma in warding off fear of one's own vulnerability also has consequences for the way 'healthy' people tend to deal with those who have physical or mental disabilities and illnesses [119]. These people remind others of illness and death and can be socially shunned as a consequence. It poses an interesting problem for 'normal' people when the sick or disabled happen to manage their lives well and are happy and self-confident. This challenges certain stereotypical assumptions about the misery associated with illness and, as a result, negates 'normal' world views (Sect. 5.1.3, 'Empowerment and Stigma Resistance' [115]).

3.3.2 FUNCTION FOR THE IN-GROUP

Stigma can fulfil various functions for one's own group (in-group).

1. First, social cooperation often involves the dilemma of how far one should go to cooperate with others in a spirit of trust, without too much of a risk of being exploited by others (dilemma of trust). It is strategically risky to be the one person who cooperates and helps everyone else, because the favour might not be returned. Using categorisation to carefully draw one's own group boundaries thus has the signalling function of more likely cooperation and reciprocated support within the in-group.
2. Second, one function of valuing in-groups and devaluing out-groups is to develop a positive social identity (self-categorisation theory, Sect. 3.2.1). This corresponds at a group level to the process explained in Section 3.3.1, whereby individuals enhance their self-value by devaluing others.

The appreciation of the in-group and the devaluation of others is particularly common during intergroup conflict [115]. Again, this model struggles to explain why stereotypes are culturally shared and why stigmatised people often accept prejudice. This model is also insufficient when explaining the stigma of mental illness [120]. If the others (out-group) are *mentally ill*, my in-group is defined as 'normal' in a vague and negative way—by the absence of mental illness.

3.3.3 COMPREHENSIVE MODELS OF THE FUNCTIONS OF STIGMA

In this section we will discuss different functions of stigma that go beyond those for individuals and in-groups. Some of these models refer to concepts that cannot be discussed in detail here (and further literature is thus cited below).

Social Dominance

People differ in their attitudes as to whether resources should be equally distributed in society or not (Sect. 7.5.1). These debates tend to not only be about material things like money or land ownership but about education, influence, social status and access to social networks as well. When people object to equal distribution, they usually do so from a position of power where they themselves have access to resources. In other words, they prefer the dominance of their in-group (social dominance orientation [121]). Social dominance orientation has an overall societal function: it reduces conflict between those dominant groups who have access to resources on the one hand, and the disadvantaged groups on the other, by justifying group difference and maintaining the hierarchy. Negative stereotypes, prejudice and stigma towards disadvantaged groups are used to justify said dominance.

Belief in a Just World

The belief in a just world [122] has a related function. According to this model, people have the need to live in a just and therefore predictable world. Within this world view, people get what they deserve and deserve what they get. Here one must distinguish between the conviction of a just world for oneself ('I get what I deserve.') and for others ('Others get what they deserve.'). The belief in a just world for oneself is often associated with a sense of well-being. But the idea that others deserve what they get tends to be associated with a stronger sense of antipathy and prejudice.

The widespread need for a just world makes people want to correct injustice. There are two approaches to making this correction: first, you can help the victim such that injustice is eliminated. This often does not work if the injustice has taken place long ago, or if the power to make it right ultimately cannot land in the hands of the individual. In these instances, belief in a just world might otherwise lead to the second option of blaming the victim: one can blame the disadvantaged and explain away the injustice using stigma and prejudice (e.g. assuming someone who is mentally ill is unemployed because he is lazy and disinterested in employment [123]).

EXPERIMENTAL FINDINGS

A systematic review summarised the findings of experimental studies in which people were encouraged to believe in a just world [124]. The results found that study participants with low social status blamed themselves for their conditions and were worse off. Participants with higher social status were less inclined to help the disadvantaged, including in work and organisational contexts.

System Justification

The most comprehensive model for the function of stigma as a justification of the status quo is, arguably, the system justification theory [125]: an attempt at synthesising different approaches to social inequality as well as reactions of disadvantaged groups to that inequality. These include Marxist theories and the work of the social and Gestalt psychologist Kurt Lewin, who upon emigrating to the United States from Germany in 1933 studied issues such as Jewish self-hatred [126].

According to this theory, stereotypes function to justify the state of the system and maintain the status quo. (The term 'system' broadly refers to social or legal structures, such as institutions, groups or governments.) Why do people need justification of the system? Similar to the above-mentioned belief in a just world, members of both dominant *and* disadvantaged groups want to believe in a just social system that therein makes the status quo logical. Additionally, system justification leads to people being more satisfied with the state of society and their own situation, and less motivated to seek social change. Ultimately, it leads to less uncertainty about a world that is difficult to understand.

The theory, unlike models regarding the function of stereotypes for individuals or groups, can explain why stereotypes are culturally widespread. The theory cannot, and does not attempt to, explain all functions of stereotypes. But it does shed light on phenomena that are difficult to understand, including why members of disadvantaged groups might support a stereotype or discrimination despite it running counter to their personal interests. Women, for example, can agree with gender stereotypes that place them in a professionally passive role if and when this stereotype justifies the overall system. Of course, members of disadvantaged groups do not always accept the discrimination they face: they also follow their own legitimate interests, as well as those of their group, and strive for social change. But the system justification theory can explain why, even vis-à-vis disadvantaged people themselves, the status quo is often maintained.

This theory also points out a problem in research on stigma: when members of disadvantaged groups are asked whether they are treated unfairly, they might deny it because they consider the status quo to be legitimate (Sect. 5.1.1, 'Experience and Expectation of Stigma'; Sect. 5.1.3, 'Who Suffers From Self-Stigma?'). Now this does not necessarily mean that there isn't any discrimination from an external perspective. This is partly why the question of unfair treatment, which is often asked in research surveys, is likely to lead to an underestimation of everyday discrimination.

EXPERIMENT

Lee Ross conducted an illuminating experiment on how our perceptions of social roles serve to justify the status quo, even if these roles are completely random [127]. Students were given a quiz to play together. One played the questioner, one played the respondent, and others observed (and these roles were randomly assigned by playing cards). The questioner was then asked to think up 10 difficult questions on remote topics. It is important to note that the questioner and interviewee knew that their roles were randomly distributed and that the questioner could choose his difficult questions in such a way that only he would know the answers. During the quiz, the questioner asked his questions, the majority of which, as expected, the respondent was unable to answer. The questioner, respondent and observers then evaluated the participants' general knowledge. The researchers' hypothesis was that the participants did not take the random distribution of roles sufficiently into account while making their judgement. Therefore they would overestimate the knowledge of the questioner (who was able to formulate the questions) and underestimate the knowledge of the respondent (who was confronted with remote questions without having any influence over the formulation). In fact, both respondents and independent observers rated the knowledge of the questioners far higher than the knowledge of the respondents.

What does this experiment tell us? People underestimate the randomness and situational dependence of their social roles. We tend to infer long-term characteristics from what is right in front of us, even if there is no real justification for them. In this experiment, participants thought that they were clued in to each other's general knowledge from the quiz game arrangement, even though they were told exactly how randomly and unfairly the power to influence the game questions was distributed. Social roles therefore fundamentally shape our perception of people. Stereotypes or perceptions of characteristics confirm existing social roles. The role distribution in this experiment is easily transferable to many everyday situations, such as those in which an employer, teacher or examiner asks questions and thereby determines the conditions of the interview. In this regard, this experiment impressively demonstrates the status quo legitimation and maintenance explicated by system justification theory and signals an obstacle to social change: people from disadvantaged groups underestimate their competence.

The analysis derived from this experiment has implications for the stigma of mental illness. Historically, people with mental illness have been held in prisons, asylums or large institutions for long periods of time—and the number of people with mental illness living in institutions seems to be rising again across Europe after a period of deinstitutionalisation [128]. This history may have contributed to the emergence of stereotypes of dangerousness and incompetence amongst people with mental illness [120], as these stereotypes justify the status quo: 'If these people are in custody, it is probably because they are dangerous or cannot take care of themselves'.

Down, In or Away

Jo Phelan, Bruce Link and John Dovidio have described three main functions of stigma and prejudice in society under the concept of 'stigma power' [129]. The three functions are succinctly described as 'keeping people down, in, or away'. This means oppression and exploitation (down), enforcement of social norms (in) and avoidance of illness (away).

A historical example of the first function (down) is the oppression of and prejudice against black people in the United States, with slavery benefiting whites economically and prejudice legitimising slavery. Today, these researchers argue, prejudice against the poor or ethnic minorities serves a similar function. Examples of the second function, the enforcement of social norms (in), are negative stereotypes with regard to homosexuality, crime or substance abuse (Sect. 5.4.7). The function of stereotypes in these cases is twofold: people who are compliant with social norms are prevented from violating them, and those who have violated the social norms must be made to change their behaviour through sanctions in order to rejoin society. An example of the third function (away) is negative stereotypes about people with physical or mental illness and social avoidance of them. This function likely has evolutionary origins and is explained in Section 3.3.4. This model puts forward three plausible, basic functions of stigma that are useful to consider in antistigma programmes.

3.3.4 FUNCTION OF STIGMA FROM AN EVOLUTIONARY PERSPECTIVE

Humans have held onto the ability to adapt their behaviours to complex social environments over the millennia [130]. From an evolutionary standpoint, the most important goal of this *fitness* is the passing on of one's own genes (both by one's own descendants and those of close relatives). This does not only require the act of procreation but also the maintenance of good conditions for survival for oneself (including prevention of illness and higher social status) and within one's ingroup (including cooperation and exchange of resources). Evolutionary adaptations are very context specific. This explains why, for example, we humans are more afraid of snakes than of cars, despite the latter being far more dangerous in modern life. It is important to note that even though our social behaviours and mechanisms are contingent on evolution, this does not mean they are perfect. First, they are often not up to date or attuned to modern, current threats (see the snake and car example). Second, evolution does not function like the process of drawing up perfect plans on a drawing board and executing them; it is rather a process of selecting less-bad variants over long periods of time.

Third, evolutionary social mechanisms often operate on the principle that a stimulus or event should be quickly categorised and trigger a rapid response. In order to increase the probability of one's survival, such mechanisms must be fast and efficient. Of course, quick reactions are prone to result in errors. For example, if I were to consider a harmless peer dangerous, we might call this error a *false positive*—a danger is erroneously regarded as positive or present. Conversely, if I consider a dangerous peer harmless, this error is a *false negative*, as I have erroneously considered the danger as negative or nonexistent. Evolutionarily, these errors have very different consequences. If I meet someone in the woods and mistakenly consider them dangerous (false positive) and flee, not much happens, except that I may miss an opportunity for social contact or may abandon my hunt. But if I make a false negative error (i.e. do not recognise an enemy as such), the consequences for me and my descendants can be fatal. Therefore we humans are evolutionarily adjusted to react rather overcautiously (false positive). The number of false negative assessments of danger should ideally be close to zero—especially in complex situations, like social ones.

This problem, which is discussed in the context of signal detection theory, is also called the *smoke detector principle* [131]: in case of doubt, a good smoke detector should go off too many times rather than too few. If it goes off without there being a fire, it's just annoying. But if it does not go off when there is a fire, it can be fatal. 'In case of doubt' is important for the antistigma interventions discussed in later chapters: the more people learn and know, the better they can evaluate others. With regard to the stereotype of people with mental illness being dangerous, the more the general public knows, the better they can adjust their smoke detectors, so to speak, and avoid (false positive) overreactions. This is an example that evolutionary mechanisms are flexible and can be altered.

Two aspects of the evolutionary model are particularly important for the stigma of mental illness [132]: cooperation with others and prevention of illness. (A third aspect, the exploitation of others, is more significant for other forms of prejudice, such as that towards ethnic minorities, but is less so here regarding the stigma of mental illness.) In terms of cooperation and illness prevention, living in groups has certainly increased people's chances of survival. But it has also brought (and continues to bring) risks, including the risk that others will not reciprocate the help they are given or that we may become infected with communicable diseases. From an evolutionary perspective, the social exclusion of others serves to minimise both risks.

Cooperation is helpful when others support me as much as I support them. If someone's behaviour is unpredictable due to an illness or if he has few resources, he is unattractive as a cooperative partner and thereby faces the threat of social exclusion. This is all the more true when he accepts help but does not return it and does not follow social rules. People who show such behaviour are often punished by members of the in-group. This punishment is also called altruistic punishment, because it is in the public interest and caters to the observance of social norms that make the cooperation of the group possible.

As far as *illness prevention* is concerned, people have developed a highly sensitive warning system to avoid infection (smoke detector principle). Communicable diseases can often only be detected indirectly, for example through physical lesions or, in the case of infections of the central nervous system, through movement disorders or unpredictable behaviour. These signals suspect disease and therefore often lead to strict social distancing in order to avoid infection.

An evolutionary model leads to three functions of stigma that match the three functions mentioned at the end of Section 3.3.3 (down, in, away [129]):

1. oppression and exploitation of others (down),
2. punishment of behaviour that violates social norms (in) and
3. avoidance of people with diseases (away).

These functions correspond to Goffman's three types of stigmatised characteristics (Sect. 3.1.2 [8]): tribal stigma, blemishes of individual character and abominations of the body. Finally, the evolutionary model aides in our understanding of different emotional reactions—namely, anger and anxiety—as related to stigma: those who are perceived in violation of social norms or as unreliable co-operators (i.e. have blemished character) can spur anger, while those with bodily abominations, illness or infection risk can spur disgust or anxiety (as shown in studies about making contact with people with schizophrenia [133]).

The model is consistent with the results of a study in which around 13,000 members of the general public were questioned in 16 countries worldwide about their attitudes towards people with depression or schizophrenia [134]. Those whose attitudes were gauged expressed the strongest rejections (i.e. negative reactions) when it came to the description of an ill person having contact with children or marrying into one's own family. They also tended to believe that the ill person described would be unpredictable and a poor co-operator. Two-thirds of those asked about someone with schizophrenia, and about half of those asked regarding depression, agreed with these statements. From the perspective of the evolutionary model, these results make sense: stigma and stereotypes are closely linked to evolutionary concerns such as cooperation and reproductive fitness.

To avoid a misunderstanding: the discussion of this evolutionary model does not mean that such visceral reactions make sense today, that mental illness is contagious or that the desire for social distance from those who are ill is either good or justified. However, the evolutionary model contributes to understanding why the stigma of mental illness is stable and widespread across many different cultures (Sect. 7.6, Ch. 13). It also shows, as indicated above, which kinds of learning experiences might be necessary to overcome evolutionary reactions and thus reduce the stigma of mental illness.

CHAPTER 4

Consequences of Stigma

This chapter discusses the consequences of stigma for stigmatised and nonstigmatised people. Before Chapter 5 deals specifically with the consequences of stigma for people with mental disorders, four overarching aspects are discussed here; namely, the consequences of stigma for nonstigmatised 'normal' members of the general public (Sect. 4.1), for stigmatised individuals (Sect. 4.2), for the coping behaviour of the stigmatised (Sect. 4.3) and for the way stigmatised and nonstigmatised people deal with each other (Sect. 4.4).

4.1 Consequences for Nonstigmatised People

To fully understand the impact of stigma on minorities, it is valuable to understand how stigma affects nonstigmatised people. Four realities are discussed [115]: the widespread use of pejorative stereotypes aimed at certain groups (Sect. 4.1.1), the ambivalence (Sect. 4.1.2) and fear that 'normal' people feel when dealing with stigmatised people (Sect. 4.1.3) and the frequent contradiction between alleged attitudes and actual behaviour towards members of marginalised groups (Sect. 4.1.4).

4.1.1 WIDESPREAD STEREOTYPES

With regard to stigmatised groups in a society, negative stereotypes are generally consistent within the culture. This certainly does not come to be in adulthood; research shows that children from the age of three learn to devalue people who have black skin or who are disabled or overweight [95]. This presents a problematic reality whereby negative stereotypes are accepted as facts because they are both widespread and deeply entrenched. Even if stereotypes are explicitly and outwardly disapproved of, they can be automatically activated in many situations to thus influence behaviour (Sect. 3.1.6). While the influence stereotypes have can be consciously suppressed, it takes a significant energy expenditure and amount of attentiveness to do so (and therefore often does not work).

4.1.2 AMBIVALENCE

Many people in Western societies have an ambivalent attitude towards stigmatised people. This is probably due to two widespread, albeit oft-opposing, values: the first is the value of social justice and the notion that people who are ill or live in poverty should be able to live with dignity (Sect. 7.5.1). The other is individualism, a promotion of the idea that people are responsible for their own fates. The latter resembles the above-mentioned belief in a just world, according to which people deserve what they get and get what they deserve (Sect. 3.3.3). These value orientations tend to lead to different conclusions when dealing with disadvantaged groups: support and sympathy, or dismissal and resentment.

However, these reactions can occur simultaneously, be more or less pronounced at different times, and often lead to a deep ambivalence that shapes social interactions and reinforces the influence of prejudice on behaviour [135]. The idea that prejudice can consist of both positive and negative components is something we have encountered in Fiske's model of stereotype content (e.g. warmth and incompetence; Sect. 3.2.4, 'Content Dimensions'). When members of the general public behave ambivalently, stigmatised people are additionally challenged with identifying their contradictory or vague behaviours (Sect. 4.2.5).

4.1.3 FEAR AND INSECURITY

Members of the general public can feel fear or insecurity when dealing with members of stigmatised groups [136]. These feelings can have various causes:

- People who are strongly prejudiced have negative expectations and are therefore often tense when dealing with minority groups. For others, the ambivalence mentioned above can lead to uncertainty about how they should behave. Many people do not want to appear prejudiced, and it is exactly this effort that makes their behaviour seem artificial or strained.
- If members of the stigmatised group appear self-confident and competent, this contradiction of the cultural stereotypes affiliated with their identities (e.g. weakness) can also have a disconcerting effect on others.

For all these reasons, the behaviour of nonstigmatised people towards members of stigmatised groups can appear fearful, artificial or fraught. This applies in particular to nonverbal behaviour, such as avoiding eye contact. From the stigmatised person's point of view, it is very difficult to discern whether this behaviour is the result of prejudice or merely an effort to appear unprejudiced.

4.1.4 DISCREPANCY BETWEEN ATTITUDES AND BEHAVIOUR

What people say about their attitudes is one thing and how they behave is quite another; the two do not always go hand in hand.

Research on societal racism, for example, shows that explicitly expressed, or flagrant, prejudice has declined sharply since the 1950s. Nevertheless, the behaviour of white people, especially that which is nonverbal and/or takes place unconsciously, remains more negative towards black people. There are various explanations for the discrepancy between reported attitudes and behaviour [75, 115]: people may conceal their true attitudes in order to avoid appearing racist or prejudiced. A further explanation is that there are more subtle, conflictual attitudes towards minorities today: there is *aversive racism,* which is when white people consciously reject racism and stand for equality but react in an emotionally negative way to black people (e.g. with fear). This leads to ambivalent behaviour and has a detrimental effect on decision-making situations (e.g. of employers during job interviews). Attitudes whereby white people react emotionally and in a strongly negative way towards black people, combined with politically conservative views, are referred to as *symbolic* or *modern racism.* According to this mindset, discrimination should no longer be seen as a problem—if anything, black people should work harder, pull themselves up by the bootstraps and take responsibility for their own situations. A similar attitude is *ambivalent racism:* according to this, white people might welcome equal rights for black people but at the same time ideologically follow a Protestant work ethic, according to which people are responsible for their own destiny through hard work and discipline. This corresponds to certain ambivalent reactions towards black communities, particularly those living in poverty.

These more subtle and elusive attitudes towards discriminated groups also play a role in the stigma of mental illness. Open expressions of prejudice towards those with mental illness have decreased (Sect. 3.1.6), but it continues to have an effect. Attitudes of ambivalence and fear about this group can lead to tense and dismissive behaviour that thereby contradicts majority group members' self-evaluations as unbiased. People behave negatively towards the marginalised for various reasons, even if they report otherwise in surveys. For this reason, too, the extent of public stigma is often underestimated.

4.2 Consequences for Stigmatised People

Moving on from the consequences of stigma for the nonstigmatised, we now focus on the more serious consequences for those who *are* stigmatised. Five aspects are discussed [115]:

1. Experience with stigma
2. The awareness of one's own devalued social identity
3. Stereotype threat
4. Attributional ambiguity (in other words: is the negative behaviour of another person towards me really based on prejudice?)
5. Consequences of stigma for well-being and health

4.2.1 EXPERIENCES WITH STIGMA AND DISCRIMINATION

Stigmatised people come to expect that they will encounter prejudice and discrimination; this is the nature of stigma that is culturally pervasive. Many have had personal experiences of discrimination that vary greatly in form: aggressive or subtle, physical or verbal. Discrimination can threaten necessary access to important resources, such as employment or housing. It can also threaten personal self-esteem or how one values their own social group.

The situation for a victim of discrimination is made more difficult by the fact that the perpetrator may be genuinely convinced that they have not been discriminatory. As mentioned above, there is often a discrepancy between what people see as their attitude and their real behaviour. For the stigmatised, this means that in addition to the discrimination they have experienced, their perspective is regularly questioned. People who belong to a stigmatised group also tend to be aware of their societal devaluation (and the various forms and extent of it); they must always be on their guard because of it.

4.2.2 AWARENESS OF ONE'S OWN DEVALUED SOCIAL IDENTITY

Just as members of the general public become aware of prejudice against minority groups early in their lives (Sect. 3.2.4), so too do members of those minority groups learn negative stereotypes about their in-group in childhood and adolescence. People with mental illness are also aware of the widespread devaluation of their group in society, as studies by Bruce Link on his modified labelling theory have shown (Sect. 3.2.4 [103]). Such awareness of the devaluation of one's in-group can greatly impact self-esteem, though there are ways to combat and overcome this (Sect. 4.3).

4.2.3 STEREOTYPE THREAT

Stereotypes can be threatening for members of a minority group. The phenomenon of stereotype threat is when a stigmatised person comes to fear being judged negatively on the basis of a stereotype and ultimately is at risk of confirming it. Claude Steele has called this a 'threat in the air' [137]. Suppose a woman has to take an exam in mathematics. She is aware of the stereotype of women being bad in this subject and fears that her own, possibly weak, performance on the test will confirm it. This pressure effectively worsens her performance, and a self-fulfilling prophecy has thus been created. This effect can be seen in various minority groups in relation to various stereotypes. It explains many of the performance gaps we see in Western societies, for example in standardised math testing for women and in cognitive performance tests for members of certain ethnic minority groups [138].

The explanation for this threat is most likely that people in this situation have both a cognitively demanding task to solve (i.e. a test or performance) *and* a stereotype to contend with ('As a woman, will I do really badly now? Will it go wrong? No, don't think about that now! I must make a special effort...'). Such thoughts negatively affect one's working memory and performance. Stereotype threat is different from self-stigma; its results are independent of whether the person agrees with the stereotype. As per our previous example, a woman taking a mathematics test can adamantly reject the stereotype about her gender's inferiority in the subject, but the testing situation can make her so aware of this stereotype that her performance drops. And the more she is interested in a good performance, the more it will drop [115].

In contrast to what black people or women have to navigate, there is a question as to whether people with mental illness (which is often invisible) are also affected by stereotype threat. Diane Quinn examined this question using participants with a history of depression [139]. If the participants stated that they were mentally ill before taking an assigned test, their performance dropped significantly. If they did not have to state this before the test, their performance was no different from healthy subjects. Stereotype threat therefore affects people with mental illness if the stigma is disclosed (and may be even more of an issue in the real world, beyond the confines of a study). We will return to the subject of disclosure in Sections 5.1.4 and 9.2.

4.2.4 STIGMA AS STRESSOR

A consequence of stigma related to stereotype threat is that of stigma stress, or the effects of stigma as a stressor. The concept dates back to Richard Lazarus' work on stress and coping [140]. When it comes to feeling stressed, according to this model, people are not passive recipients. Rather, the ways people perceive a stressor influence its effects. There are two main appraisals we conduct: (1) How threatening do I find this stressor? and (2) What are my coping resources? Stigma stress thus occurs when the threat of stigma is assessed as high but when one's personal coping resources are perceived as low. If I had a mental illness, recognised prejudice against people with mental illness as a threat to me, and at the same time felt I could do little about it, I might very well suffer from stigma stress. Conversely, my stigma stress might be low if I assessed the threat of the stigma as low and had abundant coping resources.

This model can help explain why people who are stigmatised react differently to stigma and suffer differently from stress. The model also explicates different reactions to stigma stress, which are roughly divided into deliberate strategies (e.g. blaming discrimination for failure, Sect. 4.3.1) and involuntary reactions (e.g. anxiety or high blood pressure). There are many studies that demonstrate the negative consequences of stigma stress on people with mental illness (Sect. 5.1.5).

These models of stigma stress and stereotype threat can and should be considered jointly, as stigma is a threat to the integrity of a person (identity threat [141]). Incidentally, this applies to those nonstigmatised as well: not only can their self-image be threatened, as they run the risk of being characterised by prejudice (Sect. 4.1), but their idea of a just world can be shaken by stigma as well (Sect. 3.3.3). Taking a bird's-eye view here helps us understand how human the reactions of stigmatised people are—a key step in depathologising them [115]. Nonstigmatised people show similar reactions to those who are stigmatised when their self-esteem or social status is at risk. Our similar handlings of these types of social situations prove that this is not a clinical or pathological problem of the *mentally ill*.

4.2.5 ATTRIBUTIONAL AMBIGUITY

Everyone at some point or another finds themselves in an ambiguous and confusing social situation, with a sequence of events that prove challenging to cohere. For members of stigmatised groups, these types of situations are especially common and difficult. Imagine an overweight woman applying for a job: if she is rejected, she will wonder (like any rejected applicant) whether it was because of her poor preparation, a lack of qualifications or a weak presentation. But the overweight applicant might also wonder about the role of discrimination and whether the rejection was due to her weight and physical appearance. There is rarely a clear-cut answer to these questions; attributional ambiguity means that knowing the exact causes of certain outcomes is challenging for members of stigmatised groups. Successes and other positive developments can also feel ambiguous: if the applicant is hired, she may doubt whether this was due to her performance or whether she was given preferential treatment in order to avoid any impression of discrimination. In time, this can undermine her self-esteem.

EXPERIMENT

A study with 100 female students examined the question of whether they attributed negative feedback after a test to the sexism of the male examiners or to the poor quality of their own answers [142]. To this end, all participants took part in a written test. The participants were first told that one of eight male examiners would evaluate their test. They were also each given different information regarding the number of examiners (i.e. all of them, 75%, half, 25% or none of them) who were known to discriminate against women. In other words, the likelihood of discrimination perceived by the female students varied. After the written test, regardless of their answers, all of these subjects were told they had failed. They were then asked whether they thought they had failed because their performance was poor or because the examiner was sexist. There was a clear resulting divide: only those female students who were told that all examiners (100%) discriminated against women attributed their failure to discrimination. The remaining female students—even those who were expecting a 75% probability of discrimination amongst examiners—attributed their failure to their alleged poor performance over sexism. The broader conclusion: people in ambiguous situations tend to underestimate the extent of discrimination's role in their own lives.

Attributional ambiguity forces stigmatised individuals towards a number of specific challenges: first, since an evaluation can be performance related or not, it makes it more difficult for them evaluate their own performance. And struggling to self-evaluate makes it all the more challenging to realistically plan one's own goals. Also, similar to stereotype threat, persistent ambiguity can become an ongoing form of cognitive stress. The connection between effort and success (or failure) can become so dubious that one's own motivation can suffer. Finally, people can become suspicious of others' feedback, which in turn makes social exchange more difficult.

As previously discussed, prejudice tends to be expressed subtly in modern societies. This increases the ambiguity of social interactions, particularly for stigmatised minorities, and makes determinations of discrimination less clear. Today there is a paradox whereby despite a decrease in overt discrimination, the negative consequences of discrimination for those affected can increase [115].

4.2.6 STIGMA IS HARMFUL TO HEALTH

The effect of discrimination on physical and mental health has been extensively studied. Individual studies tend to focus on specific stigmatised characteristics, from sexism to racism to mental illness. But a meta-analysis involving 137 of such studies delivered two overarching findings [143]. First, there is a clear, albeit not very strong, correlation between perceived discrimination and worse mental and physical health. Second, the study explained this correlation (i.e. why does discrimination harm health?) by identifying two causative interim steps: *stress reactions* and *health behaviours*. The former includes stress effects on the cardiovascular system, such as high blood pressure, and on emotional reactions such as anger. Health behaviours refer to smoking, alcohol and drug consumption, eating habits and exercise. (Alcohol consumption as a health behaviour can also be understood as a risky or harmful coping behaviour.) These stress reactions and harmful health behaviours were found to be associated with an increased risk of physical and mental illness.

Stereotypes about certain social groups, like black people or those with mental illness, may also carry harmful attributions of incompetence or a lack of intelligence. Not only are members of these groups often excluded from social participation and advancement opportunities (e.g. in employment) because of these stereotypes, but they can also feel undue pressure to disconfirm them and prove particularly competent and efficient. As is asked in the 2019 film *Queen and Slim:* 'Why do black people always need to be excellent? Why can't we just be ourselves?' Ongoing pressure of this type often leads to health problems. The term *John Henryism* has described this phenomenon since the 1970s, when epidemiologists studied the plight of John Henry Martin, a black American who had worked his way up and out of sharecropper poverty yet suffered from high blood pressure and inflammatory diseases from an early age.

RELATED STUDIES

Discrimination causes concretely measurable and considerable damage even at the genetic level: the cells of people who experience discrimination more frequently show signs of pre-mature ageing at the end sections of their chromosomes (telomeres) [144]. A US study took two sets of data—one on 30 million recent births and one on trends of racism—and examined them together. Racism was recorded vis-à-vis online tests nationwide with almost two million participants [145]. The greater the implicit and explicit racism in an area, the more frequent the rate of premature births and underweight children amongst black women. This is an example of the inherited biological effects of social discrimination: being born prematurely and/or underweight increases various risks of illness throughout life, which in turn can lead to social disadvantage.

A Swedish study following about 28,000 members of the general public examined the connection between experiences of various forms of discrimination and mortality risk [146]. Participants were interviewed at the beginning of the study, and all deaths over the course of the next five years were recorded. It was found that the risk of mortality in participants re-peatedly experiencing discrimination was roughly twice as high. The effect was particularly pronounced among people who did not participate much in social activities, were poor or were psychologically stressed. Stigma can become a matter of life and death, especially for those on the margins of society or who face mental health problems.

4.3 How Can Stigmatised People Cope With Stigma?

Members of stigmatised minority groups are not passive targets; they react to what they face and try to handle stigma [115]. It is also not their fault if their attempts and strategies to cope are challenging or unsuccessful. The root causes of stigma do not lie with them but with society. Nevertheless, we here take a worthwhile look at certain coping mechanisms; they create a fuller picture of the reality of those stigmatised and can be helpful in identifying opportunities for the stigmatised to act.

4.3.1 BLAMING DISCRIMINATION FOR FAILURES

To face failure and social devaluation as a stigmatised minority can endanger one's self-esteem. Instead, one might protect his self-esteem by attributing that failure to discrimination rather than to his own shortcomings. This externalising attitude has two disadvantages. First, the feeling of capacity and control over one's own success decreases. Just as the failures are not his own fault, neither are any future wins. Second, his accusation of having experienced discrimination can lead to conflicts in the social environment, as others may feel they have been wrongly rebuked. This risk is high—members of the general public are not always aware of their negative or discriminatory behaviour (Sect. 3.1.6, 'Explicit and Implicit Attitudes'; Sect. 4.1.4).

4.3.2 SOCIAL COMPARISON WITHIN THE IN-GROUP

Who we compare ourselves to influences our self-esteem. Comparisons with people who have a higher social status (upward comparisons), for example, endanger it. Members of stigmatised groups have the opportunity, just like everyone else, to choose the reference points for their comparisons. A comparison with one's in-group can prove more helpful, since its members are often similar and comparisons with them are less threatening. The controllability of the characteristic(s) being compared also plays a role. For example, students who receive negative feedback on their essays but are told that they can improve the next time do not show evidence of a lower sense of self-esteem [147]. This is likely one reason why recovery programmes for people with mental illness are so often oriented towards taking control of their own lives (Sect. 5.1.3, 'Empowerment'). When I too have experienced failure, social comparisons with 'normal' people become less painful when I take back a sense of control.

There are, however, still risks if and when stigmatised individuals stop making external, upward comparisons and instead make them within their in-group. While it can stabilise their sense of self-esteem, avoiding comparisons with members of other, privileged groups can lead to underestimations of social inequality or discrimination. This can ultimately reduce motivation to strive for social change. Coping mechanisms help protect self-esteem and fight self-stigma but do make it difficult to look at broader structural problems. Additionally, only making comparisons with members of one's own disadvantaged group can lead to people setting lower goals for themselves and achieving less.

4.3.3 DISTANCING

Another way one might reduce the impact of failure or devaluation is to selectively distance herself from those areas which are impacted. A woman may know the stereotype that women are bad at mathematics; she may have failed a mathematics exam herself. Either way, her self-esteem would have suffered less had she decided that mathematics is not important to her, avoided it and placed her efforts for success elsewhere. This strategy of psychologically distancing can indeed stabilise one's self-esteem, but brings with it the long-term, unfortunate problem of undermining her motivation to engage, improve and participate in the subject. This might be seen by the woman herself and those in her environment as confirmation of the stereotype.

4.3.4 KEEPING THE STIGMATISED IDENTITY SECRET

A prerequisite for this coping strategy is that the stigmatised identity can be concealed, at least temporarily. This option is therefore not available to all stigmatised groups (e.g. women, overweight people or black people), though stories like Philip Roth's novel *The Human Stain* do examine the concept of passing [148]. The distinction between invisible stigmatised conditions and those where concealment is not possible is well-examined. Goffman (Sect. 3.1.2) makes this a central point in his thinking about stigma and its consequences. He distinguished between people for whom the stigma makes them 'discredited' or 'discreditable'. Both words are derived from the Latin verb 'credere' (believe) and mean that someone has either already lost their credibility and status (discredited) or that this would be a possibility as soon as their identity is revealed (discreditable).

Among the stigmatised conditions that can be and often are hidden are HIV, sexual orientation and mental illness. Studies show that a stigmatised condition that can be hidden often causes particular difficulties for those affected [149]. These people face complex decisions regarding whether and how to tell others, as well as who and what to tell. Keeping something hidden can protect against discrimination; disclosure always carries the risk of being labelled and discriminated against. On the other hand, keeping something hidden can lead to social isolation. Disclosure can also facilitate requests for help and social support, promote social contacts and increase authenticity: if you can talk to others openly, you can speak as yourself and be as you wish.

People with a hidden stigmatised condition are also burdened in other ways. If they keep it secret, others potentially finding out will not be on their terms. This risk is stressful and means that, in conjunction with all their other responsibilities and roles, they must always think about how they appear, what they say about themselves, what others might notice and so on. It is therefore not surprising that people in such situations have proven to perform worse in neuropsychological tests [149]. Keeping something hidden is emotionally stressful: studies show that secrecy is associated with increased fear, shame and depressive symptoms. This state of anguished secrecy is called a 'private hell'. One approach in order to bolster young people who suffer from secrecy and fear of stigma is to show that things get better later in life. One such project gives hope to young gay people who are discriminated against in school: adults who have overcome similar discrimination and have found more positive environments over time volunteer to relay their experiences (e.g. https://itgetsbetter.org).

STUDIES ON THE HEALTH CONSEQUENCES OF SECRECY

Regarding the emotional consequences of secrecy, social psychologist Brenda Major studied over 400 women who had chosen to have an abortion [150]. About half expected to be stigmatised because of their choice. About half also chose to keep it a secret from family or friends. Over the course of two years, secrecy amongst these participants led to mental health problems. Women who had chosen to keep it a secret were more preoccupied with the abortion and suppressing thoughts of it. The strength of this study is that it was an investigation over a long period of time and under everyday conditions. The results showed the dilemma for women: secrecy may have protected them from discrimination in their network, but it took its toll personally.

Keeping something hidden may also have a negative impact on physical health. In another study, gay men who were HIV-positive but otherwise healthy at the beginning of the study were examined over a period of nine years [151]. During that time, the HIV infection progressed more rapidly in those who kept their homosexuality a secret than in those who were open about their sexual orientation.

4.3.5 SECRECY AND STRUCTURAL DISCRIMINATION

The subject of secrecy does not only concern direct reactions from one's own network, or those from certain members of society (e.g. a discriminatory employer; Sect. 3.1.5 [152]). It also correlates to structural discrimination. Pachankis and Bränström investigated this relationship and evaluated data from 28 EU countries [153]. Around 85,000 adults from sexual minorities were asked whether they kept their sexual orientation secret, whether they experienced discrimination and how satisfied they were with their lives. At the same time, an index of structural discrimination against sexual minorities was compiled for each country. This index included both legal regulations (e.g. on marriage, partnership or adoption rights for members of sexual minorities) and public attitudes towards sexual minorities. There was a strong correlation between structural discrimination, reduced life satisfaction and increased secrecy. The differences between countries were significant: in countries with high levels of structural discrimination, such as Lithuania or Romania, 80% of individuals kept their sexual orientation secret, while in Holland or Denmark, less than

20% did. Furthermore, secrecy was associated with lower life satisfaction. None of this means, however, that secrecy is 'wrong' as a strategy. On the contrary, despite its impact on life satisfaction, secrecy can be a wise and protective choice in countries with high levels of structural discrimination. Disclosure decisions are complex and must be made individually (Sect. 5.1.4, Sect. 9.2).

4.3.6 SOCIAL WITHDRAWAL

A coping strategy related to secrecy is social withdrawal, when someone withdraws from others in order to escape labelling and discrimination. This concept can also be found in the work of Goffman (Sect. 3.1.2), who put it well: stigmatised people tend to limit their contact to 'the own' and 'the wise'. By this he meant those who belong to their own group (e.g. those who also have a mental illness) as well as those who understand the stigmatised condition, accept it, and are therefore people who can be trusted. Like secrecy, social withdrawal seems to be a double-edged sword. It can protect against discrimination but can also lead to social isolation or at least to being limited to one's in-group. These risks are similar to those linked with in-group comparison (Sect. 4.3.2). In a study by Bruce Link, social withdrawal among people with mental illness was associated with increased demoralisation and unemployment [154].

4.3.7 EDUCATING OTHERS AND CONTRADICTING PREJUDICES

The coping strategies discussed above regarding secrecy and social withdrawal into one's in-group or self are strategies of avoidance. This is not a negative assessment; both strategies can be helpful depending on the person and situation. These are rightful ways to avoid stigma such that one can try to appear 'normal' (pass as normal) or to submerge further into a group that feels similar and/or comfortable. Alternatively, there is the strategy of actively educating others about stigma, in the hopes that they will stop or reduce their discriminatory behaviour if they are made aware of it. A related approach is to directly call out and contradict prejudices when they are expressed. I have not found clear results on the success of these strategies for people with mental illness. The above-mentioned study by Link [154] suggests that informing or educating others does not have a positive effect on demoralisation or unemployment. This is not to say that these strategies cannot prove helpful in individual cases. However, they run the risk of irritating others (however prejudiced and unjustified their opinions may be) and stigmatised individuals experiencing even more discrimination following the critique.

4.4 Contact Between the Stigmatised and Nonstigmatised

In today's global world, not least due to social media, more and more people of different origins and contexts are coming into contact with one another. Amidst all of these opportunities for connection, many people have characteristics or attributes (e.g. ethnic traits) that may feel foreign and can be stigmatised by others. This has an impact on interactions between those who have a stigmatised condition and those without. We will examine these interactions from the perspectives of both groups using some of the concepts discussed earlier in this chapter.

4.4.1 INTERACTION FROM THE PERSPECTIVE OF NONSTIGMATISED PEOPLE

To start, members of the general public tend to be well aware of widespread stereotypes about those who are stigmatised (Sect. 4.1.1), and they can engage with these stereotypes regardless of whether they agree with them. Stereotypes can be activated automatically, outside of voluntary control (Sect. 3.1.6). They can also be used to scrutinise even the most minute interactions and feed into circular logics. Suppose you see a man on the street who you know has recently been treated in a psychiatric hospital for psychosis. You are familiar with the stereotype of the danger posed by people with psychoses. The man seems calm. Nevertheless, thinking of the stereotype affects your perception, and you pay close attention to signs of tension or even aggressiveness in the man's facial expression or behaviour. You yourself will likely appear less relaxed, in turn creating tension in the other person. We do not need to describe the scene in any more detail to make it clear that such a stereotype, even without agreeing with it, can become a *self-fulfilling prophecy* and have a negative result.

Related to these types of interaction is the previously mentioned fear among members of the general public when dealing with stigmatised people, and the frequent discrepancy between their attitudes and behaviours (Sect. 4.1.4). Many nonstigmatised people are concerned that others might perceive them as prejudiced and thereby try to avoid giving that impression. This concern is, so to speak, a less consequential form of a stereotype threat (Sect. 4.2.3). These people may have prejudices but do not want to show them, or they may sincerely reject prejudice. In either case, this behaviour can have a negative influence on the overall interaction: they can come across as insecure, tense and uninviting.

4.4.2 INTERACTION FROM THE PERSPECTIVE OF THE STIGMATISED

From the perspective of stigmatised individuals, interactions with members of the general public are similarly influenced by some of the factors mentioned above. Stigmatised individuals are familiar with the negative stereotypes about themselves but do not always know whether the other person in an interaction agrees with these stereotypes and/or will show prejudice or discriminatory behaviour. Nice words can be deceiving and don't always lead to positive actions (e.g. an employer can be complimentary towards an applicant with mental illness and still choose to reject them based on bias; Sect. 4.1.4). The logical thing, then, is for stigmatised individuals to be on their guard. Vague encounters can be a danger to stigmatised individuals' self-esteem, as they may have to fear devaluation or rejection. Some may choose to overcompensate and disprove the prejudice by behaving in an extremely friendly way. Others may act very reservedly to forestall rejection.

Several other factors further complicate interactions for stigmatised individuals. If the other person is unaware of their stigmatised condition, they must deal with the aforementioned difficulties of secrecy and decisions about disclosure which complicate interaction (Sect. 4.3.4). If the other person is aware of the stigma, they may suffer from stereotype threat and worry about confirming the negative stereotype through their behaviour (Sect. 4.2.3). Finally, the ambiguity of the interaction (Sect. 4.2.5) means they might be unable to identify whether a potentially negative reaction from the other person is due to them as individuals or because they belong to a stigmatised group. This also applies to positive reactions.

Alternative directions for interaction, such as when prejudices are openly expressed, can of course be harmful; making animosities explicit can rapidly escalate any situation. But opaque interactions such as those described above can also be so insecure and tense that the stigmatised condition or identity is subsequently avoided. People who are stigmatised might find it helpful to actively disconfirm stereotypes, but this is stressful in terms of the effort and overcompensation that needs to occur (Sect. 4.2.6). In an ideal world, the nonstigmatised person would not only be without prejudices but would behave calmly and positively without getting stuck in the above-mentioned pitfalls. Having shared experiences with members of stigmatised groups is the most effective solution. The topic of positive contact to reduce the stigma of mental illness (as an antistigma strategy) will be dealt with in Section 8.4.

People With Various Mental Disorders and Their Relatives

Different types of stigma and their consequences for people with mental illness are discussed in Section 5.1. Groups for which stigma differs in form and consequence are then presented in the remaining sections of this chapter.

5.1 People With Mental Illness

This section deals with the three basic forms of stigma: public stigma (Sect. 5.1.1), self-stigma (Sect. 5.1.3) and structural discrimination (Sect. 5.1.8). Biological models of illness and their influence on public and self-stigma are discussed as well (Sect. 5.1.2). Subsequent sections deal with secrecy and disclosure of one's own mental illness (Sect. 5.1.4), stigma as a stressor (Sect. 5.1.5), recovery (Sect. 5.1.6) and stigma as a barrier to seeking help and treatment participation (Sect. 5.1.7). Stigma in certain areas of society (work, housing, healthcare, media and law) is addressed in Chapter 7.

5.1.1 PUBLIC STIGMA

Public stigma manifests itself in two ways:

1. through broader attitudes of the general public, such as those expressed in representative population surveys,
2. through discrimination against people with mental illness by members of the general public.

Attitudes of the General Public

Negative stereotypes about people with mental illness contain certain key assumptions: that they are dangerous and scary lunatics, that they are rebellious spirits or that they are childishly incompetent and need supervision [155]. These concepts are often learned through media portrayals (Sect. 7.4). Many studies have examined attitudes held by the general public [156]: people with mental illness, especially those with schizophrenia or alcohol addiction, are considered unpredictable, dangerous and even less human (dehumanisation [157]). There is also a marked desire for social distance from people with alcohol and drug addiction or schizophrenia (and less so for depression and anxiety disorders). Older people and those with less education tend to hold more negative attitudes towards people with mental illness. Those who have had more contact with people with mental illness have fewer prejudices, though this principle can only be applied to a certain extent when it comes to relatives (Sect. 5.6) and professionals working in the healthcare system (Sect. 7.3.1 [158]). This is presumably because contact can (also) be stressful for these groups. Apart from them, contact under favourable conditions reduces prejudice; we will look at this more in-depth in the case of antistigma strategies (Sect. 8.4). Until a few years ago, representative data on attitudes in the general public was primarily only available from Western countries. But the above-mentioned international study on attitudes

61

towards people with schizophrenia and depression reveals a universal existence of negative attitudes across national borders, especially in the areas of childcare, marriage and violence/unpredictability (Sect. 3.3.4 [134]; on stigma in LMICs, see Ch. 13).

Recent Development of Public Attitudes

Whether from the newspaper or in discussion with audience members after a lecture, I often hear that prejudice against people with mental illness used to be a problem but isn't anymore (or, if it is, much less of one). My anecdotal experiences align with representative surveys in Germany; according to one study, the general public is of the opinion that public stigma has decreased in recent decades [159].

So, is this true? The question can be answered empirically. In numerous population surveys, members of the general public were asked repeatedly, at intervals of several years, whether they would accept people with mental disorders as colleagues or neighbours. Questions such as these gauge how individuals think and feel, rather than their perceptions of the general public. The answers are a good measure of social distance and thus of the public stigma of mental illness.

Georg Schomerus examined the development of social distance using 16 large representative population surveys that were repeated in various countries, usually about 10 years apart [160]. The results were sobering. The public's desire for social distance from those with schizophrenia actually increased significantly in the 1990s and 2000s. Public attitudes remained unchanged regarding those with depression. By the 2000s, the percentage of respondents who would accept people with mental illness as colleagues or neighbours was roughly less than half for schizophrenia and just over half for depression. These figures likely underestimate the problem; many people find it uncomfortable to admit their desire for social distance and to reveal their own prejudices in a survey. This effect is called social desirability and suggests that the actual rejection of people with mental illness is likely higher in everyday behaviour than indicated by survey responses.

A striking example of the increase in prejudice over time was provided by an American study that compared the frequency with which people with mental illness were considered dangerous during two time periods 50 years apart [161]. More than twice as many respondents in 1996 perceived people with psychosis as dangerous than in 1950. That prejudice has increased, especially against people with serious illnesses, is upsetting: this is a group especially in need of social support, not social distance.

Experience and Expectation of Stigma

For people with mental illness, attitudes of the general public are not some abstract issue. Prejudice and discrimination are everyday experiences that they have come to expect. Examining the first-hand experiences and perspectives of people with mental illness is therefore crucial. In 2009, Graham Thornicroft and his colleagues surveyed more than 700 people with schizophrenia in 27 countries worldwide and looked closely at the areas in which they had received unfair treatment because of their condition [162]. The most common areas of discrimination were personal relationships (friends, family, neighbours, partnerships), personal safety and employment (with rates of experience ranging from 20% to 50% for each area). Unfair treatment in dealing with the police, education system, housing and authorities were also reported (each between 10% and 20%). Discrimination was more often experienced by people who had been ill for a longer period of time and who had been treated against their will. The study also recorded whether people with schizophrenia had given up on achieving their life goals because of anticipated discrimination (i.e. if someone expects rejection, they can avoid its injuries by choosing to not look for new friends or work) (Sect. 3.1.5, '"Why-Try" Effect'; Sect. 5.1.3). Around two-thirds of respondents said they had given up on the idea of work or of a partnership/marriage because of expected discrimination.

The same group of researchers conducted a similar study on depression with over 1000 participants from all over the world [163]. The frequency of experiencing discrimination was comparable to that reported for people with schizophrenia in the area of personal relationships, but slightly lower in other areas. Almost half of the participants with depression reported that they had given up on their own activities in the areas of work or searching for a partner because of expected discrimination. In both studies on schizophrenia and depression, about three-quarters of the participants stated that they keep their diagnosis secret to avoid discrimination.

The true extent of discrimination was probably underestimated in both of these studies for a couple of reasons: first, only participants who were in treatment were interviewed. Those strongly affected by discrimination and who had avoided treatment for fear of stigma were thereby less likely to participate (Sect. 5.1.7). Second, it is those who suffer from self-stigma who may feel that their discrimination is fair and appropriate ('I am to blame for my illness, so I don't deserve any better'). They are the ones who may be reluctant to point out the unfair behaviour from others that outside observers would regard as discrimination (Sect. 3.3.3, 'System Justification'; Sect. 5.1.3, 'Who Suffers From Self-Stigma?')

The experience of stigma has also been investigated in qualitative studies (i.e. people with mental illness reporting on their experiences in interviews). Eighteen studies of this kind regarding people with schizophrenia from different countries have been summarised [164]. Three main areas of focus were identified:

1. stigma in the psychiatric and somatic care system (Sect. 7.3)
2. stigma and everyday social contact
3. service users' own behaviours as a result of stigma (e.g. keeping their condition hidden).

Changes in everyday, personal contact were reported: 'Yes. All my friends turned away from me. They started to avoid having contact with me. They just stopped communicating with me, broke off relations' or 'My illness was a big obstacle for me' or 'At the beginning of my illness, when my neighbours found out about it, they said: "This lunatic should be left alone".' In addition, many experienced paternalistic treatment, decisions being made for them, and their no longer being taken seriously; this occurred in their private lives, for example, with relatives who did not take their privacy into consideration or who interfered in decisions about partnership or parenthood. Negative experiences in the working environment were frequent (Sect. 7.1). Many kept their illness secret for fear of stigma: 'I don't tell anyone. I just find that telling someone ... they don't understand ... especially with schizophrenia, they think they're going to be murdered by you, so I don't like to mention anything' (quotations from [164]).

When asked about being treated positively due to the illness (positive discrimination), service users reported on people who had behaved 'nicely' towards them. A common kindness that would typically go without saying was seen by subjects with schizophrenia as something extraordinary [165]. They had likely become accustomed to not expecting, or feeling undeserving of, kindness (Sect. 5.1.3). The findings were consistent across the different countries studied. Overall, a sad picture emerges and relays a vicious cycle: the behaviour of many members of the general public is determined by prejudice and leads to discrimination; people with mental illness withdraw and keep their illness a secret. The interaction between people diminishes, and prejudice and social separation between 'them' and 'us' become entrenched.

Public Stigma as a Cause of Self-Stigma?

Are public stigma and self-stigma directly related? In theory, the answer is clear cut: self-stigma does not simply arise 'by itself' in the minds of people with mental illness. It is, as described above, a consequence of public stigma and experienced and expected discrimination. When service users agree with negative stereotypes, adopt them and turn them against themselves, self-stigma arises (Sect. 5.1.3). But is this causal link always evident, especially when comparing different countries?

Sara Evans-Lacko has addressed this question in a very instructive study, which brings together two independent data sets from 14 European countries [166]. One dataset contains information on the 14 countries' population attitudes, and the other focuses on self-stigma amongst approximately 1800 people with mental illness. In countries with more negative public attitudes and less uptake of support services, service users suffer more from self-stigma. The most influential factor is whether members of the general public feel comfortable talking to people with mental illness: the more comfortable they feel, the lower the rates of self-stigma amongst service users. The study cannot prove that public stigma is the definitive cause of self-stigma; it was done cross-sectionally, and the participants were not selected as a representative sample. But the study does point to a possible causal link. For antistigma initiatives, this demonstrates the value of promoting positive contact between people with mental illness and members of the general public (Sect. 8.4.1). It would increase the comfortability of the latter when in conversation with the former.

5.1.2 THE ROLE OF BIOLOGICAL ILLNESS MODELS

The causes of illness and who is to blame for it have been questioned for a long time. Guilt is fundamental to the stigma of an illness; those who are ill are often held responsible for their own suffering, as are their relatives (Sect. 6.2). In the Gospel of St. John (9:1 ff.), Jesus meets a man who was born blind. The disciples ask: 'Who sinned, this man or his parents, that he was born blind?' Jesus answers: 'It was not that this man sinned, or his parents, but that the works of God might be displayed in him.' He thus breaks the supposed link between guilt and illness and heals the blind man.

These days, mental disorders are often understood as genetically determined diseases of the brain. But this hasn't always been self-evident: in antiquity and the Middle Ages, mentally ill people were regarded as possessed by demons. And this belief is still held in certain parts of the world today (Sect. 5.8, Ch. 13). There were, however, early countermovements that questioned the status quo. The Hippocratic Theory of Humors (circa 400 BC), for example, was a biological model of illness that attributed melancholy to a predominance of black bile (Greek mélaina cholé, Sect. 2.1.1).

While somatic medicine, particularly infectiology, made great progress in the 19th century in deciphering and combating biological causes of illness, psychiatry was at risk of falling behind because the biological causes of mental illness remained unknown. This may be a reason why psychiatry was in fact so open to biological interventions that today are considered inhumane, brutal and nonsensical, such as lobotomy. Lobotomy involves the severance of connections between areas of the brain and often leads to severe changes in character (as presented in film, Sect. 7.4.2). The procedure was popularised across the world in the 1940s and was practised until 1970. Unsurprisingly, advocates and psychosurgeons of that era emphasised lobotomy's advantages: 'The emotional nucleus of the psychosis is removed, the "sting" of the disorder is drawn out' ([167], p. vii).

The first neuroleptics (antipsychotics) appeared in the 1950s, followed soon after by antidepressants. As a result, psychiatry increasingly saw itself as a biomedical subject, meant to treat its patients with medication just like other fields of medicine. The pharmaceutical industry contributed to this relationship with advertising campaigns, and the trend continues to grow: according to data of the Organisation for Economic Co-operation and Development (OECD), almost three times as many antidepressants were prescribed in Germany in 2015 as in 2000 [168]. This increase in prescription and use of certain medications is remarkable, as no substantial progress in psychopharmacology has actually been made during this period. The development of new psychotropic drugs is in fact in crisis worldwide [169].

This leads to a self-reinforcing cycle: psychopharmacological treatment is an ever-growing trend while one-sided results of biological research are continuously circulated by the media. A reductionist picture of mental illness, which locates the illness solely in the brain or in singular neurotransmitters, receptors or genes, is reinforced. This does not do the role and value of human subjectivity justice; the human experience can never be reduced to neurobiological processes [12].

Attribution Theory and Essentialism

Given the prevailing culture of biomedicine, a question arises as to whether and how prevailing biological explanations affect the stigma of mental illness. There are two opposing theories worth examining: attribution theory and essentialism.

According to Bernard Weiner's *attribution theory*, responses to people with a stigmatised illness depend on whether others think the illness is controllable [170]. If they do, the ill person is considered at fault for his or her illness and reactions tend to be negative, taking the form of accusations, anger or punishment. However, if the cause of illness is understood to be out of the person's control, he or she can count on an untarnished perception, compassion and support. According to attribution theory, biological and especially genetic illness models should carry less stigma because no one is responsible for their inherited genes.

In relation to attribution theory, mention should also be made here of the common attempt to destigmatise mental illness by presenting it as an *illness like any other*. For example, if people could see schizophrenia as a metabolic disorder just like diabetes, even schizophrenia would no longer be stigmatised (for an example, see Sect. 1.5.1). This message of an illness like any other has been used in many antistigma campaigns. Its effectiveness is discussed later in this section.

The second theory is *genetic essentialism* [171]: people are determined by their genes, or, as the saying goes: 'You are your genes!' Genes become the unchangeable core or *essence* of a person and his or her illness. From this viewpoint, *the mentally ill* are reduced to a category all their own, so to speak (Sect. 3.2). An essentialist perspective assumes that mental illness is unchangeable and therefore incurable, since genes are nearly impossible to change. At face value, this theory dictates that the guilt aspect of stigma (i.e. the assumption that the ill are to blame for their illness) should decrease. However, essentialism could lead to an increase in overall stigma: people with mental illness could be perceived as genetically modified, different, foreign or—to put it in exaggerated terms—a *different species*.

This distorted but widespread perception is fuelled by simplistic media reports about *the schizophrenia gene*. Genetic research findings are much more complex, and thoughtful researchers are well aware of the reality: hundreds of genes are thought to be associated with schizophrenia, but each predicts only a tiny increase in the risk of illness. Whether and how they are related and influence brain function is largely unknown. Follow-up studies often cannot confirm prior findings on so-called risk genes, and this applies to studies of depression as well as schizophrenia [172, 173]. Many risk genes are therefore false-positive, random findings. Individual genetic changes likely only have an effect when in complex interactions with other genes and various environmental factors, such as prenatal damage, traumatisation, cannabis use and discrimination. Put simply, the problem is not the genes themselves but the coincidence of genetic risks and environmental factors. And this all too often lands upon those on the margins of society. Genetic essentialism leads to a simplistic view of *the genes* as the core of the illness and the ill person, and the importance of social factors is underestimated [174].

Consequences of Biologism

We have two opposing theories regarding whether biological, and especially genetic, models of mental illness reduce or reinforce stigma. What does the data say? Matthew Lebowitz and Paul Appelbaum have summarised studies regarding the impact of biologism on the public, on professionals in psychiatry and on people with mental illness [175].

In population surveys, hardly any connection is found between the biological model of illness and blame. The stereotype that people with mental illness are responsible for their condition also seems to be less pronounced than the stereotype that they are dangerous and different [176, 177].

However, as would be expected according to the attribution theory, experimental studies present a clear link between the biological model and reduced blame [175].

The biological model of illness can reinforce essentialist ideas: mental disorders are perceived as less modifiable, their prognoses as poor and their therapies as less promising. While the direct influence of the biological model on the public's desire for social distance tends to be unclear, there is some evidence that suggests this theory increases desire for distance from those with schizophrenia [176]. Amongst the general public, the above-mentioned approach of seeing mental illness as an *illness like any other* also increases willingness to seek treatment. However, the desire for social distance remains unchanged and even increases for schizophrenia (Sect. 8.1.4, 'Normality' [178]).

Biologism also affects professionals working in psychiatry and their interactions with patients. In a series of three studies, Lebowitz and Ahn show that the empathy of practitioners towards their patients decreases if they have previously read biological explanations for various illnesses [179]. This is applicable to anxiety and obsessive-compulsive disorders as well as depression and schizophrenia and occurs even when psychosocial explanations are brought in secondarily. Accordingly, professionals who promote a biological model to explain an illness are perceived as less compassionate by their patients. Biologism is thereby likely to affect the quality of the therapeutic relationship between practitioners and patients. This approach also leads professionals to recommend drug treatment rather than psychotherapeutic treatment [175]. There is, however, much to suggest that the increased focus on biological determinism in mental illness has increased the willingness to seek professional help [160]. For those who want treatment, this is the positive side of this development.

The effects of the biological model on service users themselves have not been studied extensively. People with severe mental illness who agree with a genetic model of illness tend to express more fear of others with mental illness and report stronger feelings of guilt [180]. Because genes are considered central to one's identity [174], these service users might think of themselves as defective and thus develop an irrational sense of guilt. The biological illness model is also associated with keeping one's own illness secret [181]. Finally, experimental studies show that people with depression or eating disorders become more pessimistic about the course of their illness when told that their illness is neurobiological or genetic [175].

There has long been an expectation that the biological illness model could have strong destigmatising power in society. Recently, a biomedically oriented psychiatrist wrote to me that he had heard that biological models actually reinforce stigma, but he felt strongly that that was untrue. Everyone has a right to their own opinion (Sect. 1.5), but this question can be answered empirically. The data summarised here gives a sobering picture.

Conclusion

Promoting a biological illness model does not have positive effects, except for a slight reduction in the perceived responsibility of people with mental illness for their condition. This model in fact has many negative consequences: on public opinion, on clinical work and on people with mental illness themselves. Mental illness, of course, has biological causes and consequences. But a strict, one-sided biological view leads to what Karl Jaspers called *somatic prejudice* (Sect. 2.3.2). Instead, mental illness needs to be understood as a combined biological, psychological and social process that affects both body and soul and that requires respect for the subjectivity of the individual.

Interventions that establish good human contact with service users and embrace them—with their history, humanity and social environment—as people (and not as genetic carriers), help counter the consequences of genetic essentialism (Sect. 8.4 [175]). Practitioners should stress that genes, neurotransmitters and their consequences are adaptable rather than set in stone. In one experimental study, such an approach was found to uplift those with depression who had felt demoralised by genetic determinism [182].

5.1.3 SELF-STIGMA, SHAME, 'WHY TRY'

What Is Self-Stigma?

As mentioned previously, there are three basic types of stigma (Sect. 3.1.5): public stigma (Sect. 5.1.1), self-stigma and structural discrimination (Sect. 5.1.8). There is also a critical causal link involved: self-stigma arises as a consequence of public stigma (Sect. 5.1.1). *Self-stigma* is when people with mental illness are not only aware of negative stereotypes about their group but agree with and internalise them, thereby turning against themselves ('I am mentally ill, therefore I must be incompetent and lazy'). Self-stigma is therefore a step-by-step process, from awareness of public prejudice to agreement with it and application to oneself [183].

This process negatively impacts those with mental illness in several ways, affecting their self-concept, behaviours and emotions. In regards to self-concept, self-stigma reduces self-esteem ('I am worth nothing') and self-efficacy ('I cannot achieve my goals'). Behavioural changes are due to the above-mentioned 'why try' effect (Sect. 3.1.5 [79]): 'I am mentally ill, so I am not worthy of good treatment.' 'Why try' means that people feel a lack of worthiness or ability to pursue their life goals and thereby give them up. This is a form of demoralisation not due to depressive symptoms but as a result of self-stigma. Finally, self-stigma has an emotional impact, namely the creation of shame about one's own illness. Shame tends to be a very tormenting emotion; it can contribute to social withdrawal and secrecy. Self-stigma as an agreement with stereotypes and shame as an emotional reaction to it are—independent of depressive symptoms—associated with low self-esteem [184].

Because self-stigma can only be experienced and described by people with mental illness, two short descriptions follow. The first is by Maureen Deacon, a professor of psychiatric nursing who had experienced several bouts of major depression and was in the final stages of cancer at the time of this quote. She died in 2015. For her, depression and the stigma associated with it were worse than the cancer: 'While objectively I understand and disapprove strongly of stigma, subjectively I have internalised it.... There are two parts to this. Firstly, I tend see my mood disorder as a character flaw—evidence of my weak and neurotic nature.... Secondly, there is the guilt and worthlessness that come along for me with the depression experience: I should not feel like this, I have a blessed life, a partner who loves me, a lovely home' ([185], p. 458).

The second quote is from Kathleen M. Gallo, a woman with psychosis for whom self-stigma was agonizing and worse than any form of public stigmatisation, no matter how bad: 'I perceived myself, quite accurately, unfortunately, as having a serious mental illness and therefore as having been relegated to what I called "the social garbage heap".... Thinking of myself as garbage, I would even leave the sidewalk in what I thought of as exhibiting the proper deference to those above me in social class. The latter group, of course, included all other human beings' ([186], pp. 407 f.).

Who Suffers From Self-Stigma?

Not all people with mental illness report self-stigma. In one large European study, members of an organisation representing the interests of people with mental health problems were interviewed about self-stigma. Just under half of the approximately 1200 participants with schizophrenia and just under a quarter of the approximately 1200 participants with bipolar disorder or depression reported suffering from pronounced self-stigma [187, 188]. These numbers likely underestimate societal rates of self-stigma, which are likely to be higher amongst those who do not affiliate with interest groups such as the one studied. In other words, we should expect that self-stigma and the 'why try' mentality are less common amongst those already engaged in advocacy work, peer support and interest groups [79].

Why don't all people with mental illness suffer from self-stigma? Two models can explain this: Pat Corrigan's so-called self-stigma paradox and Joshua Correll's model of the in-group as a social resource [189, 190].

The *self-stigma paradox* explains why some people suffer from self-stigma while others remain largely indifferent to stigma or react with righteous anger. If a person does not identify with his stigmatised group, he feels unaffected and remains indifferent to stigma. But if he identifies with the in-group, his reaction depends on whether he considers stigma to be fair and legitimate [191]. If he does, he may suffer from self-stigma and decreased self-esteem (perceived legitimacy of discrimination). If he instead dismisses prejudice and discrimination as unfair, he may react with righteous anger.

The *model of the in-group as a social resource* explains how being a member of an in-group can have positive or negative effects on one's own self-concept [190]. Prerequisites for the group to be able to have any impact on a group member at all are entitativity and identification with the group. *Entitativity* refers to when a group is perceived as a 'real' and singular group, as a coherent, stable entity consisting of people who have things in common. Firefighters in a city are a group with high entitativity; people who just happen to be on the same train car are not. If a person with mental illness does not feel that others with mental illness alongside her make up a 'real' group, or if she does not identify with this group, the group membership will hardly affect her (and vice versa). Whether belonging to a group has a positive or negative effect on someone's self-image depends on whether she perceives her own group as a good and valuable part of society (group value).

For example, if a woman with schizophrenia identifies with and considers mentally ill people as a distinct group in society yet simultaneously thinks of this group as bad and dangerous, her self-esteem will suffer. However, if she considers this group to be one of value, her self-esteem will be strengthened, and she will be more motivated to engage in antistigma work or peer support. Research has confirmed the expected consequences of perceptions such as entitativity, group identification and group value for people with severe mental illness: irrespective of individuals' depressive symptoms, there appear to be both positive handlings of stigma (educating members of the public, antistigma work, helping other people with mental illness, social competence in achieving one's own goals) and negative consequences (social distance from peers, hopelessness [192]).

Empowerment and Stigma Resistance

As discussed above, not all people with mental illness suffer from self-stigma. On the contrary, some develop a sense of empowerment and stigma resistance. *Empowerment* is an important term in the recovery, peer support and mutual-help movement. Studies show five main components of empowerment in people with mental illness [193]:

1. good self-esteem and self-efficacy—in this sense, empowerment is the antithesis of self-stigma on the long continuum of whether and how people turn negative stereotypes against themselves,
2. 'power' as a departure from their own feelings of powerlessness and from leaving decisions up to others,
3. autonomy and active participation in the in-group or in their own social environments,
4. optimism and the will to shape their own futures,
5. legitimate anger about discrimination and disregard for personal rights.

Very briefly, empowerment is the attitude and process of taking control of one's own life—to determine it for oneself and not be restricted by self-stigma. This includes making choices in regards to treatment participation: if and what kinds of support to use. Studies show that more empowerment is not only associated with less self-stigma [188, 191], but also with a better quality of life, social integration and functional capacity as well as less need for support [194]. Empowerment of people with mental illness has emerged as a key goal for many societies and health systems, as well as for the World Health Organization (WHO) [195].

Stigma resistance refers to when people do not accept and apply stigma to themselves but instead resist it. Peggy Thoits developed a model of stigma resistance based on Bruce Link's modified labelling theory [196] (Sect. 3.2.4). It differentiates between two forms of resistance:
1. to block or deflect stigma from oneself and
2. to fight back against and challenge stigma.

Deflecting is a defensive approach: people can tell themselves that their illness is only a small part of who they are or that they have a problem rather than an illness. Both types of thinking reduce the effects of stigma on the person, similar to the low level of identification with one's in-group (Sect. 5.1.3, 'Who Suffers From Self-Stigma?'). People can choose the strategy of deflecting whether their illness is known to others or not. Fighting back against stigma, on the other hand, is an offensive strategy. It presupposes that others are aware of one's illness. Fighting back can consist of informing others and thus correcting prejudices, or directly contradicting stigmatising statements (Sect. 4.3.7).

Conclusion

The advantage of these active approaches is that they can also be pursued collaboratively, in a group (e.g. in associations of service users, relatives or mutual-support groups), which in turn heightens one's sense of empowerment. One summary of about 50 individual studies shows that stigma resistance is not only associated with less self-stigma but above all with improved self-efficacy, quality of life, hope and recovery [197].

Causes and Consequences of Self-Stigma

In a comprehensive review of 272 individual studies, self-stigma is associated with a number of factors that have a negative impact: reduced hope and quality of life, depressive symptoms, low participation in treatment (Sect. 5.1.7) and reduced social support [198]. It is not always clear whether self-stigma is the cause of these problems, though some longitudinal studies suggest that it is. Self-stigma is thereby a risk factor for suicidality (Sect. 5.2 [4]). Importantly, there are circumstances and experiences that promote self-stigma: shame, self-loathing and stigma stress (Sect. 5.1.5 [199]), as well as experiences of discrimination in the social environment or in the healthcare system [200]. Self-stigma seems to be more common among people with mental illness in Southeast Asia and the Middle East.

Insight and Self-Stigma

People with severe mental illness, such as acute psychosis or mania, are not always aware that their perceptions, feelings and behaviour are altered by the illness. This is also called a lack of insight. Whether insight into having a mental disorder is helpful, harmful or both varies greatly depending on the study and context [201]. Some studies have shown that people with good insight are more likely to take part in treatment, have a better course of illness and are better able to cope professionally and socially. In other studies, people with more insight tend to suffer from lower self-esteem, poorer quality of life and suicidality.

Paul Lysaker explains this apparent paradox [202]. He has studied insight and self-stigma in people with schizophrenia. Only those with high disease awareness and high self-stigma suffer from poor self-esteem and hopelessness. Conversely, those who have insight but are free from self-stigma are best at managing social relationships. Insight into illness and the associated acceptance of having an illness is therefore not simply 'good' or 'bad'; it depends on what service users associate with their illness. Similar to the above-mentioned role of group value (Sect. 5.1.3, 'Who Suffers From Self-Stigma?'), people suffer from their identity as *mentally ill* if they evaluate it negatively ('My life is ruined because I have schizophrenia.').

This has consequences when it comes to supporting service users (e.g. in healthcare settings or peer support). Hope is an important component of recovery, but self-stigma can undermine hope and recovery and, in particular, contribute to suicidal behaviour [4, 199]. It is therefore not enough for practitioners to relay a diagnosis and treat the symptoms. On the contrary, the decisive factors as to whether a person with mental illness perseveres are the conveyance of hope, reducing self-stigma and supporting the integration of the psychotic experiences into the personal biography [203].

Diagnosis and (In)acceptance

Insight is quite a controversial concept in psychiatry. It is often only understood to mean that a patient has accepted what the psychiatrist says. If a patient disagrees with or rejects his diagnosis, he is 'unreasonable'. This assessment is problematic for several reasons. First of all, psychiatric diagnoses can be incorrect; the underlying definitions of individual illnesses are not without controversy. Second, individual mental disorders are not clearly circumscribed, determinable entities (i.e. 'real things'), each with a common cause, course and treatment option. Diagnoses tend to be typologies or language rules for frequent constellations of problems or symptoms (Sect. 1.6).

This way of communicating with diagnoses can be more or less helpful depending on the situation and those involved [7]. On one hand, diagnoses can facilitate communication about psychological problems and treatment. Many service users are relieved that they can finally give their problems a name, which facilitates access to information, treatment, self-help and so forth. On the other hand, diagnoses carry the risk of stigma in any form (public stigma, self-stigma and shame, structural discrimination). People can be reduced to just their illness ('Mr Moore, the schizophrenic') and risk no longer being seen as multifaceted ('Mr Moore is a carpenter, lives with his wife and four children, is a volunteer firefighter and has had recurring schizophrenic episodes for many years').

For all these reasons, it is understandable why and when people refuse a diagnosis: from their point of view, it may bring more harm than good. The rejection of the diagnosis and its disadvantages can be seen as a form of self-assertion [204]. The process of diagnosis has therefore also been described as a negotiation [90]. It can only succeed if healthcare professionals listen and understand the personal significance of the symptoms and problems in the lives of service users. Without skilled communication and dialogue, diagnosis can be difficult: 'How can they diagnose me as bipolar if they don't even know who the hell I am, because I don't even know who the hell I am?' ([7], p. 756).

5.1.4 SECRECY AND DISCLOSURE

Keeping one's own illness secret from others is an attempt to alleviate the consequences of public stigma or structural discrimination against oneself and one's in-group (Sect. 4.3.4). If others do not know about the illness, they cannot label and stigmatise the person who has the illness. Keeping it secret can also be a result of self-stigma and shame. The tendency towards secrecy seems to be stronger when people with mental illness regard their illness as biologically caused (Sect. 5.1.2 [181]). The concern that by having treatment one's own illness will be made known is also a common reason to refuse it (Sect. 5.1.7).

What Are the Consequences of Disclosure?

The consequences of secrecy or disclosure were investigated in a longitudinal study in southern Germany over a period of six months. Three hundred people who were unemployed and had mental health problems were asked whether they would disclose their problems to an employer when looking for work or to friends and family. After six months, participants were asked how they were faring. Different links were found depending on whether it was about their work (e.g.

job searching) or quality of personal life: Participants who wanted to report their mental health problems to employers at the beginning of the study were *less* likely to have found a job after six months than those who preferred secrecy. This finding was true regardless of the extent of the participant's psychological symptoms or length of unemployment. The study shows the profound risks of disclosure when looking for work [152]. Unfortunately, the strategy of secrecy may have detrimental side effects in the long term. For starters, if employers and fellow colleagues do not know about a new employee's illness, they cannot provide support when in need.

However, participants who initially favoured disclosure amongst family and friends were significantly better off six months later in terms of higher quality of life. This finding was again independent of psychological symptoms, age, gender and so on [205]. Disclosure in one's private life thus seems to promote well-being; secrecy, on the other hand, appears to be stressful (Sect. 4.3.4). Bruce Link also investigated whether secrecy is a helpful coping mechanism for people with mental illness but found no positive effects [154].

What Does Disclosure Depend On?

What are the factors that help people with mental illness choose to disclose outside the workplace (on the work environment: Sect. 7.1.1)? According to one literature review, disclosure is more likely to occur when people perceive less public stigma and suffer less from self-stigma and stigma stress [206]. Who the person with mental illness chooses to disclose to is also critical; people are most likely to favour disclosure to their doctors and close relatives. Those with serious mental illness are less likely to favour disclosure altogether. And older people are more willing to tell others about their illness—perhaps because their lives are more stable and they have less to lose. In qualitative studies, the following factors were found to be particularly important:

- Disclosure depends heavily on the expected consequences, which can be positive (e.g. the person anticipates much-needed support) or negative (e.g. the person is scared of compulsory admission to a psychiatric hospital).
- The relationship with the other person is important (e.g. disclosure is easier if the family doctor is empathetic and trusted) (Sect. 7.3.1).
- Disclosure can become complicated for a person if he is worried about losing control over what others think about him.
- The fear of discrimination after disclosure, such as thinking that others will see the person as stupid, strange or crazy and turn their backs, is perhaps the strongest deterrent from doing so. This fear extends to catastrophic thinking: expecting one's private or professional life to collapse after disclosure (e.g. one's children being taken away).

People may opt for disclosure because they see how the positive consequences outweigh the negative ones in their own, personal lives. But some choose to do so because they believe that their personal disclosure will help to reduce public stigma [207]. Disclosure by homosexuals, for example, is considered to have been a key contributor to the reduction of stigma attached to homosexuality and the LGBTQ+ community overall. Similarly, for people with mental illness, there is a hope that a higher incidence of disclosure—especially from those well-integrated and fully functioning in society—will increasingly help the public to realise how common and 'normal' mental illness is. When it comes to disclosure, it is difficult to weigh personal consequences on one hand with social goals on the other. Taking personal risk into account, individuals should never feel pressured to talk indiscriminately about their illness. Partial disclosure in the private sphere can also contribute to social change.

Whether people are more likely to pursue personal or social goals in their disclosure seems to have an impact on their well-being. Social psychologists Julie Garcia and Jennifer Crocker have examined this choice and effect, particularly for college students with depression [208]. In the study, Garcia and Crocker asked student participants whether their decisions about disclosure were made for their own benefit, or whether they were thinking about the consequences of their choices on those around them. Participants who considered the effects for themselves as well as for their social ecosystem fared significantly better than those who made the decision to disclose solely for their own benefit.

Conclusion

In summary, disclosure has consequences but is not simply a 'good' or 'bad' choice. The decision for or against disclosure depends on the environment and the stigmatised person, and it can only be made individually. No one should be pressured into a decision one way or the other. Since (non)disclosure is a key step in coping with stigma, we will address this topic again in the field of antistigma interventions (Sect. 9.2).

5.1.5 STIGMA STRESS

The concept of stigma as a stressor for people with various stigmatised characteristics was introduced in Section 4.2.4. Stigma becomes a stressor when a person perceives stigma as a threat that exceeds his ability to cope. It is therefore important to assess the risks associated with stigma against one's own coping abilities. This does not mean that we should leave others to cope with stigma by themselves; stigma and stigma stress have social causes, and overcoming them remains primarily a social, collective task. But people with mental illness do have different ways of reacting to stigma, and this gives options in terms of its management.

How does stigma stress arise? Some studies have shown that people with severe mental illness are particularly burdened if they perceive more public stigma and if they regard their own group of people with mental illness (in-group) negatively [209]. Members of the general public who report a moderate level of mental health problems are also affected by stigma stress: the more public stigma they perceive, the more they felt part of the group of mentally ill people. And the more they consider the stigma of mental illness to be justified, the more they experience stigma stress (Sect. 5.1.3, 'Who Suffers From Self-Stigma?').

People with mental disorders are often burdened by the pressure to disconfirm prejudices and to prove particularly competent and efficient (Sect. 4.2.6). Many also suffer from the fact that their behaviours, which would otherwise be perceived as perfectly normal if shown by nonstigmatised people, are often considered symptoms of their illness. This is also called 'symptomising': 'She's reacting emotionally, so she is probably becoming ill again.'

What are the consequences of stigma stress? Stigma stress has been shown to make disclosure of mental illness difficult—due to the fear or risk of subsequent discrimination—and contributes to social withdrawal [210, 211]. Stigma stress increases self-stigma and reduces empowerment following compulsory psychiatric admission [212]. The relationship between stigma stress and reactions to this stress in people with severe mental illness has been investigated. First, stigma stress is associated with their increased shame and social anxiety. Second, their behaviour in everyday situations tends to change: the more these service users compare themselves primarily to their own group, the more they tend to physically distance themselves from 'healthy' people (when, e.g., seated in an audience), and the worse they perform in role-playing when learning to pursue their own goals [213]. Finally, in various longitudinal studies, stigma stress is shown to be a risk factor for suicidality (Sect. 5.2.2 [4]) and the transition to schizophrenia in those at risk of psychosis (Sect. 5.3 [214]), as well as an obstacle to recovery (Sect. 5.1.6 [199]).

Stigma stress decreases commensurately with the threat of public stigma or when one's own ability to cope increases. This suggests two starting points for how we might reduce stigma stress:
- programmes against public stigma (Ch. 8) and
- programmes that help people to cope with mental illness and overcome stigma.

One initiative is the peer-led group programme HOP ('Glossary'), discussed in Section 9.2. HOP helps participants with mental illness decide whether and how to tell others about their illness and reduces stigma stress [215, 216].

5.1.6 RECOVERY AND STIGMA

The concept of recovery in the field of mental illness ('Glossary') has various meanings and applications [217]. First, recovery necessitates a recognition that many people with serious mental illness do not actually have as bad a course of illness as was previously assumed. Long-term studies have proven good trajectories from being in treatment even before the introduction of psychotropic drugs. Second, a distinction must be made between the traditional, clinical concept of recovery (i.e. the disappearance of symptoms) and the life-affirming process of recovery. Many people experience clinical recovery as a remission, with or without treatment, of their mental illness. Others live with persistent or recurring symptoms, but they too can achieve recovery—not in the sense of being symptom-free but in the sense of a self-determined life full of hope. Recovery in this second sense is not an outcome but a process and an attitude towards living with one's mental illness or disability. This type of recovery involves social connectedness, hope, a positive self-image, finding meaning, self-chosen life goals and empowerment.

William Anthony described recovery 'as a deeply personal, unique process of changing one's attitudes, values, feelings, goals, skills, and/or roles. It is a way of living a satisfying, hopeful, and contributing life even with limitations caused by illness. Recovery involves the development of new meaning and purpose in one's life as one grows beyond the catastrophic effects of mental illness. Recovery from mental illness involves much more than recovery from the illness itself. People with mental illness may have to recover from the stigma they have incorporated into their very being; from the iatrogenic effects of treatment settings; from lack of recent opportunities for self-determination; from the negative side effects of unemployment; and from crushed dreams' ([218], p. 15).

The link between recovery and self-determination does not imply that people with persistent symptoms are to blame for their condition or that they simply have not made enough effort. Recovery should not be misconstrued to suggest that people with mental illness are responsible for their own happiness and need to provide for themselves; it should not be used as an excuse to cut resources. Correctly understood, recovery is not a new, fashionable term for self-optimisation (as is often touted). In fact, the recovery movement has its roots in the social and civil rights movements of the 1960s and 1970s. As the large psychiatric institutions of the era were being closed or downsized, the question arose as to what should be done with the former *inmates*. The concern was not so much a medical one, in the sense of psychiatric symptom management, as it was a social one. Leonard Stein and Mary Test, the developers of the Assertive Community Treatment in Wisconsin, formulated their basic attitude in 1980 as follows: '(1) it is better to be outside a hospital than inside; (2) it is better to work productively than to be dependent on others; (3) it is important to be effectively interdependent; and (4) it is a good thing for people to be happy' ([219], p. 396). Such beautiful language would be a rare find in today's scientific jargon. Here Stein and Test demonstrate what is truly at stake: recovery involves a life of self-determination and as much successful social participation as possible. It cannot be implemented without social justice (Sect. 7.5.1). Peer support is one way to promote self-determination and recovery (Sect. 7.3.4, 'Peer Support' [220]).

The social aspect of recovery is also critically important in the realm of disability rights [221]. Here recovery is about accessing the right to protection against discrimination (UN-CRPD, Sect. 7.5.2), as well as civil rights and certain social roles. Fully materialised citizenship for people with disabilities, including psychiatric disabilities, cannot be taken for granted: for example, until 2019, many were not allowed to vote in German elections and were thus excluded from *the* democratic right of participation (Sect. 7.5.4). Achieving civil rights and social participation for all people with mental illness requires both the initiative from them and their advocates from the *bottom up* and social, sociopolitical and legal measures from the *top down* [221].

The recovery movement espouses the idea that people with mental illness should not and must not be made to wait for the complete remission of their symptoms (i.e. 'stabilisation') in order to be active social participants of a community or claim their citizenship. This justifiably impatient attitude is also called the '*do it now*' *approach* [221]. This means giving people direct access to housing (Sect. 7.2.6) and to the general labour market (Sect. 7.1.2, 'Supported Employment') if they want it—even if they still have symptoms.

'People with mental illness don't need treatment—they need a *life*' ([222], p. 704). Recovery-oriented treatment can help lead a life of self-determination (though it is not the be-all and end-all). This approach considers people with mental illness to be *people*, first and foremost; they are not 'the others' (Sect. 3.1.4). In this respect, the recovery orientation is fundamentally destig-matising. Not all professionals working in psychiatry have internalised this attitude. Many talk about stabilisation, daily structure, increased drive or medication for hearing voices without being clear as to whether and how these 'improvements' might actually benefit the lives of their patients. Metaphorically speaking, some professionals think they have to get rid of the feedback noise on the radio, but some of their patients don't mind the noise; they want to dance to the music and go ahead with their lives, with or without the hiss in the background.

One review of recovery programmes in various countries' healthcare systems suggests that there is still room for improvement [223]. Mental health services in English-speaking countries are often redirecting towards recovery orientation and peer support. But leading German psychiatrists and coauthors of this review cite as examples of German recovery programmes the guidelines from their psychiatric professional association (DGPPN), in which recovery is in fact one topic among many [223]. Recovery could here be seen as the addition of yet another string to the bow of psychiatry—an example of what Diana Rose calls the 'mainstreaming of recovery' [224]. The recovery approach is all about achieving equality and self-determination for people with mental illness—they must be seen as agents in the process. It would be a misunderstanding to place 'recovery' on some perfunctory checklist and consider the job done.

Fortunately, genuine recovery programmes can also be found. Recovery Colleges, which promote recovery through education, have proven to be particularly valuable. In these programmes, people with and without mental illness, members of the general public and professionals alike attend courses on mental health. They learn together about dealing with illness, all kinds of treatment and support options, recovery, social integration and so on. The courses are jointly developed and led by peers and professionals (termed as co-production). From a stigma perspective, recovery colleges are a successful combination of education and contact. Contact takes place under favourable conditions; all participants are involved on equal footing, learning cooperatively, as a team and with a clear goal (Sect. 8.4.1). There are positive effects for individuals, clinical institutions and for the wider community [225]. As a manager in the UK's National Health Service once said: 'I will think, everything I do now, let's look at about how we can co-produce this ... God, my mindset has absolutely shifted' ([226], p. 483). Recovery colleges are now widespread in Britain and are encouragingly, albeit gradually, spreading across various countries. One example is an online programme called Empowerment College (https://empowerment-college.com), which started in Bremen in 2018 and has developed in part because of the peer support movement and in cooperation with several European partners. There has also been a recovery college in Berlin for a few years (https://recoverycollegeberlin.de).

Stigma in all its forms and consequences hinders recovery. Prejudice among professionals within healthcare can demoralise people with mental illness and impede their progress: 'You don't need people who say, "She'll never recover. She's for the scrapheap, she'll never work again, she's on medication for the rest of her life"' ([227], p. 801). And stigma outside the treatment system hinders recovery if, for example, employers perceive service users as unfit to work again (Sect. 7.1). Self-stigma and shame also make recovery more difficult (Sect. 5.1.3). In one longitudinal study, people with severe mental illness were interviewed after compulsory admission to a psychiatric hospital. The more burdened by stigma stress they were at the beginning, the less empowerment they felt one year later, and the less their recovery had progressed even two years later. These connections were independent of the extent of their psychological symptoms [199].

5.1.7 STIGMA AND PARTICIPATION IN TREATMENT

The Treatment Gap

When I started working in psychiatry, I worked with patients who had come to the hospital for treatment. It took some time for me to realise that most people with mental illness are *not* in treatment. This phenomenon is commonly known as the treatment gap, and the figures speak for themselves: WHO studies show that even in rich countries, only about 20% of people with depression receive some form of treatment, such as antidepressants or psychotherapy [228]. The situation is even worse in cases of drug and alcohol dependence or abuse; in rich countries, only about 10% of those affected receive even minimal treatment. These studies apply a very broad definition of treatment, including support from professionals such as doctors, psychologists, acupuncturists and self-help groups [229].

In the past, treatment was understood as a patient visiting a doctor or psychotherapist and following the prescribed treatment regime. We refer to this as compliance (with the dictated requirements or specifications). Today, views on treatment options and decisions have become more diverse. This is good for people with mental illness, as it promotes their self-determination. However, it also means that more factors must be taken into consideration; these will briefly be explained in the following section. What is treatment participation anyway? And what happens when someone refuses treatment?

What Is Treatment Participation?

Treatment is not a case of black or white, or yes or no. Seeking help and participating in treatment are processes that occur in phases. The first step is the identification of the problem (Sect. 3.1.7). Many people who have psychological problems are not aware of them. They may think their difficulties are normal or are symptomatic of a physical illness (e.g. a feeling of pressure on the chest or exhaustion due to depression). Upon feeling that one may have psychological symptoms, the next step is the subjective decision to decide on and ask for help. This is a very personal assessment: some want help after a week of poor sleep; others see no need even after years of severe symptoms. The decision to then seek and contact help (e.g. a psychotherapist) is a step of its own. This is followed, often after a long waiting period, by the start of treatment.

Those who take part in treatment do so until it is considered 'complete' or may very well end it early. Even in clinical studies in which participants are closely and well cared for, an average of 20% of those recruited terminate their psychopharmacological or psychotherapeutic treatment prematurely [230]. In online interventions for depression [231], it has been shown that about 60% of participants drop out before the programme is halfway through. To further the point, long-term treatment programmes tend to include relapse prevention (i.e. renewed contact if there are signs of deterioration). Again, all of this is based on a broad understanding of treatment, including psychotropic drugs, psychotherapy, psychosocial interventions (including help in the area of work or housing; Ch. 7), addiction counselling and self-help programmes.

Deciding Against Treatment: Self-Determination and Coercion

To clarify and avoid a frequent misunderstanding: when people with mental illness decide not to seek treatment or to end it prematurely, they haven't necessarily made the 'wrong' choice (although professionals working in psychiatry or psychotherapy may see it that way; Sect. 5.1.3, 'Diagnosis and (In)acceptance'). It may be a risky decision; in retrospect it may turn out to be a mistake. But everyone, with or without mental illness, has the right to make mistakes. Moreover, there may also be completely valid reasons for not having treatment: the treatment may not be available to a mother with young children, it may not be proven effective or the side effects may be too severe. Some people have had bad experiences with treatment or practitioners that have rightfully deterred them. The decision against having treatment is therefore often a sign of a lack of suitable and available options—it is not simply a sign of the 'noncompliance of the patient' (Sect. 7.3.1, 'Interaction'). Theories about health and decision-making behaviour, such as self-determination theory, therefore emphasise the value of *autonomy* in motivating people to adopt health behaviours. People show healthier behaviours and are more likely to participate in therapy or prevention programmes if they can choose to do so autonomously and do not feel that decisions are being made for them [232]. As mentioned previously, self-determination for or against a type of treatment is a key aspect of recovery (Sect. 5.1.6 [233]).

Self-determination is a much-discussed topic that gauges several hard truths in the realm of mental healthcare. One is that people with mental illness may be unaware of their symptoms or psychological state, especially during acute phases of psychosis or mania, and therefore would find it difficult to form an opinion about treatment options. In extreme cases, this may lead to compulsory hospitalisation if the life of the person or of other people is endangered. Such measures are often, but by no means always, judged negatively in retrospect by those admitted to hospital and can increase the burden of stigma [199]. Because these measures restrict and challenge the basic right to self-determination, they must be approved by a court in most countries.

It is worrying that the compulsory admission of people with mental illness in institutions (including residential, forensic and prison settings) increased in Europe between 1990 and 2006 [234]. During this period in Germany, the number of forensic psychiatric beds more than doubled, the number of assisted living places multiplied and the number of prison inmates increased. These figures were similar in Austria and only slightly better in Switzerland. The reasons for this trend are unclear. The widespread stereotype that people with mental illness are fundamentally dangerous (Sect. 3.2.4) could play a role; there has also been increased support among the general public for restrictive measures (Sect. 5.1.8, 'The Law and Protection Against Discrimination' [235]). That this type of admission to institutions hinders people's right to self-determination is problematic; there are well-known alternatives that are less restrictive. Knowledge about the quality standards and follow-through of these residential care facilities is also opaque: there are hardly any studies that determine whether and how they help those inside to lead an independent life, possibly leave the facility one day and avoid readmission.

In some countries, people with severe mental illness are required to attend outpatient treatment (i.e. community treatment orders). However, large randomised controlled trials (RCTs) have failed to show any advantages provided by these measures [236]. Better approaches to averting coercive measures include advance statements and crisis plans: during a nonacute and stable period, the service user, practitioners and potential third parties (e.g. relatives, friends, legal guardians, peers) discuss jointly what treatment the service user does and does not want. This is recorded in writing and serves as a guideline for any future crisis. The agreement promotes self-determination for people with mental illness and can reduce the number of compulsory admissions by almost a quarter [237]. A commentary on Article 12 of the UN Convention on the Rights of Persons with Disabilities (UN-CRPD) explicitly refers to such crisis plans as a means of supporting decisions and the ability to consent [238]. Nevertheless, they are not often used in Germany [239].

Stigma as a Barrier to Treatment Participation

Whether someone takes part in treatment is the result of a complex process, and stigma can act as a barrier to it at three different levels: at the individual level (i.e. of the person with mental illness), professional level (i.e. healthcare practitioners) and at the level of the healthcare system (i.e. its structure and financing) [240]. The first level is discussed in detail in the following section; the second and third can be found in Section 7.3. It is important to bear in mind that stigma is only one reason to explain why the above-mentioned treatment gap is so large. But unlike some other barriers, stigma is an obstacle that can be tackled through interventions.

Sarah Clement has reviewed the literature on stigma as a barrier to treatment for people with mental illness [241]. She collected both quantitative and qualitative work and found 144 relevant studies with a total of about 90,000 participants. Overall, the quantitative studies showed a small to moderate yet statistically significant negative correlation: those who suffer more from a type of stigma hold more negative attitudes towards treatment. The connection was particularly clear for self-stigma and for the stigma associated with treatment ('I feel ashamed to go to a psychotherapist'). Stigma was also found to be a greater obstacle among ethnic minorities. In some of the review's individual studies, participants were asked to rank the greatest barriers to treatment participation. On average, stigma was mentioned as the fourth greatest barrier out of ten. As obstacles to participation in treatment, just under a quarter of respondents cited stigma (mainly negative social reactions, shame, discrimination in the workplace), and around a third cited concerns about disclosure (e.g. that their illness could become known through their participation in treatment).

The answers to the questions of how and why stigma acts as a barrier (asked in the qualitative interviews) can be summarised in a simplified model (Fig.5.1). It typically begins with negative stereotypes that pervade society and which lead people with mental disorders to expect or experience various repercussions of stigma (Sect. 5.1.1): being labelled as *mentally ill*; compulsory disclosure of the illness or having the diagnosis recorded and filed (which can lead, for example, to an insurance premium increase or rejection of insurance applications); others discriminating or behaving negatively in a private or professional environment, or in the healthcare system itself

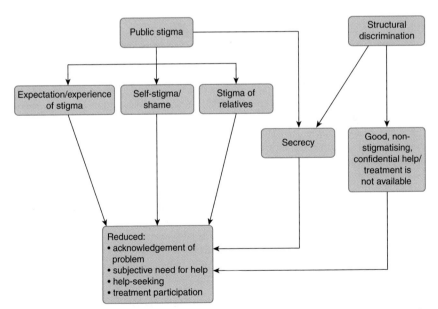

Fig. 5.1 Types of stigma as barriers to seeking help and treatment participation. (Loosely based on Clement S, et al. What is the impact of mental health-related stigma on help-seeking? A systematic review of quantitative and qualitative studies. *Psychol Med.* 2015;45:11–27. Courtesy of Heike Hübner, Berlin.)

(Sect. 7.3); self-stigma and shame (Sect. 5.1.3); or stigma faced by the family (Sect. 5.6, Sect. 6.2). An ultimate consequence of these negative stereotypes is the desire to keep one's illness a secret (Sect. 5.1.4).

All of these harsh realities can lead to avoidance of treatment. And they can be experienced very early in the process of seeking help: a person's own prejudice or shame regarding mental illness can reduce his or her awareness of the problem and perception of need [242, 243]. Even the anticipation of shame and possibility of being affected by mental health problems in the future can worsen individual attitudes towards treatment in the general public [244]. Other barriers to be discussed include various aspects of structural discrimination, such as substandard treatment or a lack of available treatments (Sect. 7.3.3).

Which forms of stigma are predictive of lower rates of seeking help? An overview of numerous individual studies with a total of over 30,000 participants has shown that personal negative attitudes towards treatment and people with mental illness are particularly influential [245]. In other words, if a person thinks that *the mentally ill* are lazy or dangerous, she likely would not want to become one of *them* by seeking treatment *herself*.

As mentioned above, participation in treatment is a process that at any point can be interrupted or stopped altogether. Do different types of stigma contribute to people stopping their treatment? Longitudinal studies, which at the baseline assess stigma and then proceed to examine participation in treatment over time, suggest that this is the case. It has been found that the more people with depression perceive public stigma, the more likely they are to stop taking antidepressants [246], and the more likely women with borderline personality disorder are to stop psychotherapy [247].

The model for stigma as a barrier (Fig. 5.1) is a simplification that leaves out four important points:

1. Symptoms can influence various trajectories of the model. In a state of psychosis, for example, one's awareness of illness can be limited. Or in a state of depression, feelings of guilt and shame (and thus self-stigma) can increase.
2. Knowledge about mental health (mental health literacy [88]), which includes prevention and treatment options, can also influence recognition of mental health problems, as well as acceptance of stereotypes and help-seeking decisions.
3. The process does not occur linearly (from experiencing stigma to avoiding treatment) but often rather in feedback loops: previous experiences of treatment or nontreatment can have a reverse influence on certain concerns, such as about disclosure or labelling, shame or expectation of discrimination.
4. Hard-to-reach and marginalised people with mental illness need particular forms of support that are sensitive to their cultural and social environments and experiences [248].

When considering the extent to which stigma acts as a barrier to treatment participation, it is important to remember that existing studies only examine particular aspects of the process. One study may deal with self-stigma and the initial search for help, while the second may examine the perception of public stigma and treatment discontinuation. However, many forms and consequences of stigma that affect people and their decisions do so in combination: a woman may seek help late because of self-stigma and shame and then stop treatment immediately afterwards for fear of public stigma. Like Proteus (Sect. 1.1), stigma takes on many forms and works in different ways at different times. Stigma's effects are cumulative, which is why individual studies tend to underestimate its overall impact.

Groups Particularly Deterred From Seeking Help by Stigma

Stigma is a particularly strong barrier to treatment participation amongst certain groups of people, namely soldiers, young people, members of ethnic minorities and healthcare professionals [241]. Soldiers are discussed here and the other groups in Sections 5.7, 5.8 and 7.3.1, respectively.

Soldiers are exposed to particular psychological stresses due to their profession: repeated military operations in crisis and war zones, the risk or experience of personal injury and the death of comrades, and frequent redeployments at home and abroad. It is estimated that hundreds of thousands of soldiers in the US, UK and German militaries face posttraumatic stress disorder after foreign missions, but that many cases go undetected or untreated [249]. For soldiers, the question as to whether and how stigma makes seeking help and treatment more difficult also arises.

A review of more than 100 individual studies has shown that psychological problems, especially posttraumatic stress disorder, depression and suicidality, are more common among soldiers than in the general public [250]. Yet only about 30% of soldiers seek help. There are three obstacles they face. First, soldiers fear that their careers will be negatively affected if they seek help, including not being promoted, not being offered permanent employment or being considered unreliable by higher-ups and comrades. Second, they may fear or experience being excluded by their unit. Finally, they suffer from self-stigma and feelings of guilt or shame about their illness. A review of qualitative studies with soldiers has confirmed these results and points to disclosure as a key issue [251]: many soldiers are concerned that their condition will become known or go on record as a result of treatment. This discourages them from seeking help. First responders who work for civilian emergency services, such as police officers, firefighters and paramedics, are similarly deterred from seeking help because of stigma [252].

In one interview-based study, soldiers of the German military reported on aspects of stigma as obstacles to seeking help (quotations from [253]). It was difficult to reconcile their own psychological problems with the image of the strong soldier: 'You're a soldier, you're strong, you must function.' Many experienced others making fun of them: 'I was laughed at, "You are not a real soldier!" and thought "Thank you, that's exactly how I feel myself."' Requests for help resulted in labelling: 'I knew there was a psychologist, but he was only ridiculed. And for God's sake, if you're seen just standing near him, they say, "Oh, look, he's nuts!"' Having mental illness and desiring help led to a feeling of weakness: 'I felt like "You're not a real man any more, not a real human, not a soldier."' 'Disclosure facilitated help-seeking and recovery; this included both mental health services and informal support by comrades: 'When you keep it secret, you cannot find help.' Yet disclosure was found to be liberating—'I feel better now, even for my self-esteem, honestly.... I don't need to hide anymore'—and could even build up new self-confidence: 'I have dealt with it [mental illness] ... and if people don't accept it or have a problem with it, I don't care.... Almost everyone has it [a mental health issue] ... and therefore I tell myself: "At least I have come out, and you haven't!"' Stigma was also understood as a problem from officers' points of view: 'It is a stain. Somehow it still carries a stigma, having a mental illness is something really bad. Nobody can deal with it.'

Various interventions have been developed to promote help-seeking amongst soldiers [251]. Most programmes focus on improving the recognition of mental health problems, speeding up referrals to mental health practitioners, psychoeducation (i.e. teaching about mental health and treatment options) or peer support. It is not yet clear, however, whether these approaches really do make it easier to seek help. A pilot study of the Honest, Open, Proud programme (Sect. 9.2) for soldiers of the German military with mental illness is currently underway. The HOP programme supports soldiers in deciding whether to disclose their illnesses and thereby in coping with stigma. But programmes that improve the attitudes of soldiers without mental illness need to be put in place alongside what is being done to support soldiers most affected. If prejudice in the public or in an institution such as the military were to diminish, these strategies to support disclosure, help-seeking and coping with stigma would be more successful.

5.1.8 STRUCTURAL DISCRIMINATION

For people with mental disorders, structural discrimination occurs, as the name suggests, in structures (Sect. 3.1.5). Unique aspects of structural discrimination in these specific areas are discussed in later sections: employment (Sect. 7.1.1) and unemployment (Sect. 7.1.2), housing (Sect. 7.2), the healthcare system (Sect. 7.3.3, Sect. 7.3.4), the media (Sect. 7.4) and the legal system (Sect. 7.5). Three additional examples are mentioned here: the consequences of a lack of legal protection against discrimination, unequal resources for treatment and offers of help, and unequal research funding.

The Law and Protection Against Discrimination

Public discourse helps to shape the vying political viewpoints that lead to legislation and regulation. For this reason, Matthias Angermeyer and his colleagues investigated changes in the attitudes of the general public regarding legal restrictions on those with mental illness [235]. In Germany, from 1993 to 2011, support for voting rights for people with mental illness fell slightly to 50% (Sect. 7.5.4). And the percentage of those who disagreed with compulsory sterilisation fell to 42%. This is a particularly sad finding given Germany's history (Sect. 2.1.2). Tolerance of disruptive behaviour in public spaces also decreased, and support for compulsory admissions increased sharply to almost two-thirds of respondents.

Discrimination in the legal system can affect physical and mental health even if it is not the intent of the law. Why? The law permeates social life in so many ways—it can pose a threat, be a source of stress and threaten a loss of status for discriminated minorities. This in turn affects the psychological state of society, leading to stress reactions and health problems over time [143]. The court ruling that granted same-sex marriage across the United States in 2015 helped improve the health of gay and bisexual men: studies show that this population suffered less from high blood pressure and depression in the year that followed that decision. Contrarily, gay and lesbian adolescents are more than twice as likely to attempt suicide in school districts without specific protections against bullying than in those that have them [254].

Unequal Resources for Services

Support and assistance for people with mental illness requires money. That being said, these illnesses create a high burden in terms of lost healthy life years (DALYs), as well as direct (treatment) and indirect (productivity losses and early retirement) costs (Sect. 2.2). When these costs are compared to the proportion of healthcare expenditure that is earmarked for mental illness, we find a considerable discrepancy (Sect. 2.2). Money may not be everything, but underfunding of care for a group of such prevalent illnesses is structural discrimination (Sect. 7.3.3).

Financial health policy decisions correspond to public attitudes. In a study by Georg Schomerus, around 1000 members of the general German public were asked where in care provision (i.e. which illnesses) could the budget be cut [255]. Most frequently mentioned were alcohol addiction, depression and schizophrenia (in that order). Almost nobody (<5%) was willing to save money on treatments for cancer or heart disease. Such findings suggest a link between public stigma and structural discrimination, because there clearly does not appear to be a plausible link between an illness' severity and the distribution of resources for it.

Unequal Research Funding

The distribution of research funding is not much better. About 1% of overall EU research funding goes to projects dealing with mental illness; within the budget for health research, it is about 5% [256]. The reality is even more gloomy, as the category of 'mental illness' includes funding for basic neuroscientific research. Therefore, only a fraction of that 1% or 5%, respectively, goes to applied clinical or health services research focused on yielding benefits in the form of prevention or future therapies. Furthermore, research funding bodies are not required to account for their priorities. Instead, they are vulnerable to lobbyists as well as the zeitgeist. We need to make more transparent the relationship between the amount of research funding available and the illness burden (e.g. DALYs) and social costs at stake for people with the disease [257]. Neglecting to take this relationship into account means that, per person suffering from the illness, about 25 times more is currently spent on cancer research than on research into mental illness. The situation is not improved by the fact that donations towards research tend to follow the public attitudes mentioned above and further distort the funding imbalance: a lot of money goes to cancer and next to nothing to mental illness [257].

5.2 People With Experience of Suicidality

5.2.1 PREVALENCE AND RISK FACTORS

Worldwide each year, some 800,000 people die as a result of suicide. In Germany in the 2010s, the figure was around 10,000 per year (with a recent slight downward trend); that is about four times the number who die in traffic accidents. In recent years, Switzerland has seen its suicide figures rise significantly due to assisted suicides. In countries such as Belgium and the Netherlands, assisted suicides are permitted for people with mental illness, which is considered a very controversial issue [258]. In most countries, more men than women die by suicide (China is an exception); in Germany, three-quarters of all suicides are among men. Women, however, are more likely to attempt suicide. According to WHO estimates, suicides are the leading cause of death among young people in rich countries (15–29 years), before traffic accidents and every type of illness [259]. In Austria, Germany and Switzerland, about 15 out of every 100,000 inhabitants take their own lives every year (in Italy about 8, in Russia about 31 [260]).

The suffering associated with suicide is enormous. Its impact can only be approximated. First of all, for every suicide, there are about 10 to 20 nonfatal suicide attempts. Second, dozens of people are affected by each individual suicide: partners, children, parents, relatives, friends, colleagues, neighbours. This means that in Germany alone, there are between 1 and 2 million people who have survived a suicide attempt in the last 10 years. A similar number have lost someone close to them to suicide during this same time period. Behind every statistic, there is a person and their community.

The reasons for suicides are as varied as people themselves. There have been many attempts to socially explain this phenomenon [261], such as the anomie and lack of social integration famously written about by French sociologist Émile Durkheim in his book *Suicide* in 1897 [60]. Psychiatrists, on the other hand, to this day see suicide primarily as a result of mental illness, especially depression. Yet regardless of diagnosis, suicides tend to occur out of desperation and in crisis, when the person sees no other way out. Many do so because they believe they are a burden on those around them or want to end their unbearable suffering. It is, however, very difficult to predict suicides and to thus assess someone's suicide risk. Risk factors found statistically in large samples are typically unhelpful for individual risk assessments. It is true that about one-third of those who die by suicide have already attempted suicide in the past. But conversely, only about 10% of people with a history of attempted suicide later die from it. So there are no ideal predictive models for suicide—this is also a problem for suicide prevention programmes that find it hard to establish a focus in the absence of good prediction models.

5.2.2 STIGMA AND SUICIDE

Suicide has not always carried a stigma in Europe. The ancient Romans did not know the neo-Latin word *suicidium*—they spoke of *mors voluntaria* (voluntary death). In Hellenistic philosophy, as practised by the Stoics and others, suicide was a widely accepted practice. Early Christianity also did not reject it in principle, partly because the boundary between martyrdom, which was revered, and suicide was blurred. The rejection of suicide by the Church Father Augustine around AD 400, whose thinking was based on the fifth commandment, was momentous but not self-evident for late antiquity [262].

My colleague Nathalie Oexle researches how the stigma associated with suicide today differs from that associated with mental illness. This distinction is not only because suicide can exist separately from mental illness. The content of its stereotypes also differs: people who attempt suicide are often considered immoral, selfish, cowardly or attention-seeking. Prejudice and behavioural reactions amongst members of the general public include fear, anger, distrust, contempt and coercion [263, 264]. Self-stigma is common among people who have experienced suicidality. The more often those affected turn public prejudice against themselves (i.e. the higher their self-stigma), the lower their confidence in recovery and empowerment [265].

Out of fear of public stigma and due to self-stigma and shame, many people find it difficult to talk about suicidality. This includes not only the decision to disclose a past suicide attempt, but also conversations about and requesting help for current suicidality. Similar to the disclosure of a mental illness, the disclosure of suicidality also carries opportunities (such as social support, help) and risks (stigma, stress or the overreactions of others) [266]. Reactions from parents and health-care professionals are often seen as particularly unhelpful [267]. Disclosure decisions are therefore complex and can only be made individually. Since stigma and self-stigma make it difficult to seek help in the private sphere, they are a central obstacle to suicide prevention and timely help.

Families who have lost relatives through suicide are also affected by stigma. Many find themselves facing the accusation—or accuse themselves—of being responsible for the suicide, or feeling that they could have prevented it. Many are regarded as tainted by suicide—a typical case of stigma by association (Sect. 5.6, Sect. 6.2). Relatives may choose to keep a suicide secret or hushed because of stigma, even within the family itself. How often do I hear in conversation with patients: 'My grandfather died suddenly. They say it was a hunting accident. But I don't know if it was really an accident.' Stigma and secrecy complicate the grief of relatives and can contribute to suicidality among those left behind [268]. Families can therefore carry the burden of silence for generations. Because reactions of people from one's personal life can often be stigmatising or accusatory, peer support is helpful—often more so than professional help [269]. In this context, peer support means support from other people who have also lost loved ones to suicide (for peer support in general, see Sect. 7.3.4).

Can the stigma associated with suicidal behaviour discourage suicide and in this way help to prevent it? Stigma is an expression of social disapproval of certain behaviours and thereby could keep people conforming to the norm, as it were ('to keep people in', Sect. 3.3.3; for addiction, Sect. 5.4.7). In Western countries, the pronounced stigma of suicidal behaviour is unlikely to play this positive role, partly because it makes help-seeking more difficult. However, it is interesting to look at East Asia, where suicide does not carry much of a stigma [270]. One approach to suicide prevention there is not the stigmatisation of suicide but rather its careful 'denormalisation' (i.e. make it seem less 'normal' as a response). That is to say, various legal and health policy measures (e.g. information campaigns) present suicide as a nonnormal, undesirable solution when in crisis. If 'denormalising' suicide is done carefully enough, such that people do not fall silent in shame and requests for help are seen as courageous, this approach could have a preventive effect [270].

Does the stigma of mental illness contribute to suicidality? The starting point for this question is the reality that many consequences of mental illness stigma (including social isolation, unemployment, avoidance of seeking help) are also risk factors for suicidal behaviour. Causal relationships are never easy to prove (Sect. 1.5). However, recent longitudinal studies have shown that various aspects of stigma do increase suicidality over time [4]. These include stigma stress (Sect. 5.1.5), self-stigma and self-contempt due to one's own mental illness [271]. There-fore, reducing the stigma and self-stigma of mental illness can help in preventing suicide (on media, stigma and suicidality, see Sect. 7.4.5).

5.2.3 SUICIDE PREVENTION AND STIGMA

How does suicide prevention specifically work, and is it affected by stigma? First off, there are two levels of prevention (Sect. 7.3.4): primary prevention for the general public and secondary or indicated prevention for persons at increased risk. An example of primary prevention is making access to dangerous tools such as deadly pesticides or firearms more difficult. Secondary preven-tion includes accessible support and counselling services for people who are in psychosocial dis-tress or have depressive symptoms. Stigma can make any of these types of prevention more dif-ficult to enact (Sect. 7.3.4). An albeit unlikely dilemma faced in suicide prevention work is that, while the stigma associated with suicide should be reduced to promote help-seeking, its reduction could help normalise suicidality and thereby lower the threshold for suicidal behaviour—an un-wanted outcome. (This is, so to speak, the Western counterpart to denormalising suicidality in East Asia mentioned in Sect. 5.2.2.)

Successful suicide prevention is possible. A combination of primary and secondary prevention strategies could prevent about a quarter of all suicides over time [272]. But we rarely see suicide prevention work implemented widely in everyday life. This is a sign of structural discrimination and neglect of one of the most vulnerable groups in society (on structural discrimination, see Sect. 5.1.8; on deficits in care, see Sect. 7.3.3). For example, the BZgA ('Glossary'), a specialist agency of the German Federal Ministry of Health, offers a wealth of information on prevention related to addiction, smoking, HIV, nutrition, vaccinations and so forth. But there is nothing available on suicide prevention. Diana Doko from the Berlin-based *Friends for Life* association for suicide prevention (www.frnd.de) once told me that she had repeatedly offered to make her organisation's materials available to the BZgA, but that she was refused. While working on this book in 2020, I called the BZgA and asked for educational materials on suicide prevention. I was told there was nothing on this subject. On the BZgA (https://bzga.de) website, I only managed to find a rather hidden link to a virtual reality project of the Robert Enke Foundation (https://robert-enke-stiftung.de; Robert Enke, goalkeeper in the German national football team, died by suicide in 2009). The project is intended to provide insight into how a person with depression might be feeling. This almost complete lack of engagement in suicide prevention from the BZgA could be explained by a lack of political will to address suicide's stigma. Nevertheless, this gap in the BZgA's range of services is not easily reconcilable with the agency's goals: 'In fulfilling our man-date, we are guided by the urgent health problems with regard to prevention that exist at the time and the developing theories and methods of health education' (https://bzga.de, accessed 24 Apr. 2020). Meanwhile, in Germany, someone dies by suicide approximately every hour.

How might the situation be improved? Nathalie Oexle has addressed this question in a review [273]: through a combination of population-wide informational campaigns on suicidal behaviour and help options (supported by the BZgA, for example); educational work in schools that reaches all age groups; improvement of the aftercare system following suicide attempts with the involve-ment of peer support; offers of easy-access help for at-risk groups (e.g. the military, police and first responders) [274]; the development of integrated help systems that link health and social services and include psychosocial interventions (Sect. 7.3.4); and the use of new technologies that can detect signs of suicide risk in social media and provide real-time information on help options [275]. Prevention of suicide and suicide attempts is definitely possible. A meta-analysis of con-trolled studies with a total of almost 30,000 participants has shown the positive effects of suicide prevention programmes in various settings, from prison to school to the general public [276]. Programmes that intervened at several levels simultaneously demonstrated an even better effect.

Three examples of suicide prevention programmes are briefly mentioned below (for Germany, see more at the National Suicide Prevention programme, https://suizidpraevention.de, a network of almost 100 German institutions and associations):

1. The European Alliance Against Depression (https://eaad.net) is active internationally, including Australia and Canada. It is well known in German-speaking countries, and active in about 90 cities or regions, as Alliance Against Depression (https://deutsche-depressionshilfe.de). The alliance combines educational programs on depression and help options for the general public with training for family doctors, direct support for those with depression and their relatives, and partnerships with community members who deal with those at risk of suicide (e.g. pastors, teachers, nurses). The approach appears to be viable, and much has certainly been achieved by the Alliance. However, a large study on the effectiveness of the Alliance in four European countries, including Germany, found that the programme did not reduce the number of suicides or suicide attempts. No difference in suicide or suicide attempt rates was found when the organization's German location of Leipzig was compared to the city of Magdeburg (where no alliance intervention took place), nor was the rate reduced on average across eight study locations, with a total of almost 1.9 million inhabitants [277]. This study shows the importance of early and thorough evaluation of such programmes. Ideally, an evaluation would come first—before energy, time and money are spent on the programme's implementation at numerous locations.

2. A second example is a primary prevention programme for schoolchildren (Youth Aware of Mental Health programme). It consists of several hours of educational material and role playing in schools on topics such as suicidality, depression, stress management and help options. Some 170 schools and 11,000 pupils took part in a major European study on this programme. The programme significantly reduced the number of suicide attempts and thoughts of suicide in the course of a year [278]. The study showed that the programme's cost for a 1% reduction in likelihood of a pupil attempting suicide was a mere 35 euros [279]. The programme is not widely used in schools in Germany (for a pilot project in Tyrol see https://projekt-yam.at). Yet recently, after the bankruptcy of a travel company, the German government decided to compensate customers for their cancelled trips with a triple-digit-million Euro amount. One wonders how taxpayer money is spent and where the priorities lie (or don't).

3. A third example of suicide prevention, which works on the basis of small donations, is the aforementioned Friends for Life (https://frnd.de). The organisation was founded by people who have lost a loved one through suicide. Friends works online and offline. They have a website, a YouTube channel, social media accounts and a podcast. In addition, Friends sets up in-person actions such as the World Day for Suicide Prevention, which takes place annually on September 10th. On that day, 10,000 candles are lit at the Berlin Memorial Church, or 600 young people lie down at the Brandenburg Gate in commemoration of the approximately 600 young people who die by suicide each year in Germany. Talk! is an art project also hosted by Friends for Life centred on suicide prevention. Does the work of this group prevent suicides? This is an empirical question, and there is no available data to answer it. The association does not receive funding for its work, let alone for concomitant research into its effectiveness. Evaluation would also be necessary here, especially since the effectiveness of social media programmes for suicide prevention is not well established [273].

It would be valuable for projects such as Friends to work with other programmes in order to achieve a combined, far-reaching approach. However, Diana Doko of Friends has relayed two difficulties which make collaboration more difficult (and are mentioned here as examples because they might also be an obstacle to others in antistigma work). Both problems have to do with the stigma and mutual prejudice of those involved. First, prominent people shy away from being mentioned by name in connection with Friends—the subject of suicide is obviously too taboo. Second, the work of Friends is criticised on various fronts: by healthcare professionals who feel it is 'only marketing' and not psychiatric or therapeutic enough, and by people with depression who feel that only those with first-hand experience should express their views on the subject. One must ask in response whether marketing is an inherently bad thing, especially if it is only one approach to suicide prevention. Is it effective to reach out to young people with poorly made films? Furthermore, why not allow people who have lost loved ones to speak out and get involved, even if they themselves have not suffered from depression or suicidality? This fragmentation and divisiveness within advocacy groups and the claims to sole representation seem harmful to me. Should we not concentrate on the task at hand instead of bickering about who is allowed to get involved? How do we achieve change without forming coalitions and strengthening each other (Sect. 14.3)?

5.3 Young People at Risk of Psychosis or With First Episode of Psychosis

Psychosis is a generic term for the state people are in when they move out of the reality they have shared with most others—this definition in itself highlights the social aspect of psychosis. In terms of symptoms, acute psychosis primarily refers to delusions, hallucinations and 'self-disorders'. Delusion means having a firm conviction that something has happened in a certain way—even if others around you have a completely different opinion. A delusion can be subjectively pleasant, for instance if someone thinks of himself as being powerful (as with Caligula, see Sect. 1.6); it can be neutral or even frightening (e.g. if someone imagines themselves being pursued). Hallucinations are perceptions not experienced by others: people can hear voices talking about them or talking to each other, or they might smell, feel or see things that others don't. As such, auditory hallucinations can also be comforting or threatening. With self-disorders, the boundary between oneself and the environment becomes porous: people have the feeling that others can read or hear their thoughts or put thoughts into their heads. Psychotic symptoms, especially mild and transient ones, can occur even without mental illness (e.g. with extreme lack of sleep or very threatening experiences). Psychosis (in the sense of a stressful, persistent and pathological condition) is understood to have many causes, such as drug abuse or the side effects of medication for Parkinson's disease. The most prevalent form of psychosis (in terms of both DALY impact and research devoted) is schizophrenia. This term was coined by the Zurich psychiatrist Eugen Bleuler, using the ancient Greek words schízein (to split) and phren (diaphragm—the seat of the soul in Homer's epic poems). By this he did not mean a split personality but rather the dissociation or decoupling of various psychological processes that are otherwise coordinated. In 1913, Bleuler spoke wisely of the *group of schizophrenias* [280]. By using the plural, he was referring to the different forms of the disorder(s) called schizophrenia. Symptoms of schizophrenia may seem very unusual, but Eugen's son, Manfred Bleuler, pointed out that psychosis is a profoundly human experience. From his perspective, a person with psychosis is someone who falls ill in the universal struggle to align one's own (conflicting) needs with often adverse social conditions. If this struggle to adapt is temporarily unsuccessful or overwhelming, a person with psychosis may exchange the reality of her life for a fantasy world ([281], p. ix).

Schizophrenia tends to evolve at a young age, with men usually diagnosed around the age of 20 and women at around 25. About 1% of the population is affected. Besides the positive symptoms mentioned above (i.e. delusions, hallucinations, self-disorders; 'positive' not in the sense of 'good' but because they are in addition to the baseline state), negative symptoms (in the sense that something is lacking from what is normally expected) include a loss of drive, energy, motivation or emotion. The course of schizophrenia varies greatly: some people have only one episode and are never affected in any way again, while others have severe symptoms and impairments from the very first episode onwards—and many forms of schizophrenia lie somewhere in between.

Even years before the first episode of psychosis, which is characterised by strong positive symptoms, early warning signs are already noticeable. These are in addition to the appearance of negative symptoms (e.g. loss of interest, social withdrawal), cognitive symptoms (e.g. reduced working memory) and typically temporary, mild forms of positive symptoms. The presence of these possible early symptoms is therefore referred to as a *risk state for psychosis*, which is often accompanied by anxiety or depression [282]. When young people who seek help for mental health problems are found to be at risk of psychosis, they have an average likelihood of around 20% of developing psychosis over the next two to three years [282].

From a stigma perspective, this suggests that early detection and intervention hold both opportunities and risks. Early intervention (e.g. providing information, cognitive behavioural therapy and social support) could prevent the risk state from developing into psychosis. This would be a form of secondary prevention (Sect. 7.3.4, 'Prevention'). It is important to note that the effectiveness of such programmes is not yet very well documented, and it is unclear whether the psychosis is prevented altogether or if only a delay is achieved [283]. Early detection and intervention also heighten the chance that many young people labelled at risk of psychosis will be 'false positives' (i.e. about 80% will not develop psychosis; for 'false positive', see Sect. 3.3.4). Early intervention can undoubtedly be very helpful, but the pitfalls of labelling must be considered and kept to a minimum.

What roles do stigma and discrimination play in early stages of psychotic disorders [284]?

1. Living in a socially disadvantaged situation (social defeat [285]) is a risk factor for psychoses. This applies to marginalised groups that may experience social discrimination and neglect on the basis of their ethnic minority status, for example, and as a result are at higher risk to develop psychoses (Sect. 5.8 [286]).

2. The fear of stigma, self-stigma and shame is a major obstacle to seeking help and support early on [287]. This is a problem, because the longer a psychosis remains untreated after presenting itself, the worse the course of the illness will likely be. Being labelled with an illness can have different effects depending on the person (on consequences of diagnoses, Sect. 1.6). It is true that young people at risk of psychosis are more willing to seek professional treatment if they consider themselves ill. However, in cases of high stigma stress (Sect. 5.1.5) due to the labelling associated with the diagnosis, this willingness decreases again [288].

3. Parents and relatives, who play an important role in help-seeking, are also burdened by stigma and feelings of shame and guilt (Sects. 5.6 and 6.2).

How do stigma and labels affect the individual's well-being and illness course? The more people at risk of psychosis can sense a public stigma, the more ashamed they tend to feel about their own potential or incipient illness; and the more they see themselves as mentally ill, the more they suffer from stigma stress—which in turn is strongly associated with a reduced sense of well-being regardless of psychological symptoms [289]. Other consequences are even more serious: it has been shown that when stigma stress increases in young people at risk of psychosis over the course of a year, their suicidality also increases regardless of symptoms [290]. In one longitudinal study, stigma stress at the baseline increased the probability that those participants deemed at risk would develop schizophrenia after one year [214]. This fits with the aforementioned models of schizophrenia development, which emphasise the role of social defeat and exclusion in the development of the illness (for migrant populations, Sect. 5.8). Finally, stigma in all its forms is a major obstacle to recovery after a first episode of psychosis because, among other reasons, it makes social support difficult [291, 292].

Conclusion

Even for young people with only the risk of serious mental illness, stigma presents serious consequences. What does this mean for early intervention? Of course, labelling and stigma are not only the result of early intervention programmes. Young people are more likely to be labelled as *sick* or *crazy* because of other diagnoses or for seeking help for anxiety or depression—not because of their participation in early intervention for psychosis. Nevertheless, early intervention programmes should carefully consider and avoid the effects of labelling. They should not paint a dreary picture of the risk of psychosis but rather, as is often the case, emphasise the possibilities of help and support for psychosis and other mental health problems.

5.4 People With Specific Mental Disorders

The topic of this book, the stigma of mental illness, is an intentional generalisation in the sense that I mostly write about *mental illness* despite there being so many specific types (for a justification of this approach, see Sect. 1.6). The following section considers the fact that there are unique aspects to the stigma associated with certain disorders (provided here in alphabetical order). The selection given is not complete. It is important to note that individuals may have several psychiatric diagnoses and thus be multiply affected by certain prejudices (Sect. 5.5).

5.4.1 AUTISM

Autism is a generic term for a variety of different conditions. New psychiatric classification systems thereby refer to it as 'autism spectrum disorder'. Common features are deficits in social interaction and communication as well as repetitive, unusual behaviours (such as movements or sounds). About 1% of the population is affected, and the diagnosis is usually made at a nursery or early primary school age [293]. While this book otherwise references 'people with ... (a disorder)', we here use the term autistic people; there is a lack of consensus in the field and many autistic people seem to prefer this term. Autistic people with normal speech development and average or high intellectual capacity have been, and often still are, referred to as having Asperger's syndrome. Other autistic people may have severe limitations in speech comprehension or expression or have reduced intellectual capacity (Sect. 5.4.6). Many autistic people prefer fixed schedules and rituals, have special interests (e.g. aircraft types, bus timetables) and are sensitive to noise and other sensory stimuli. Other disorders, such as ADHD, anxiety disorders, depression and epilepsy, often co-occur with autism [293]. The course of the illness and the need for support vary greatly: some autistic people are highly intelligent and manage their lives well without assistance. Others are unable to speak, need daily intensive support and can be severely disabled due to their autism and accompanying illnesses. The following discussion refers primarily to those with Asperger's, since for people with severe disabilities, some issues (e.g. keeping their disability hidden, employment) are not relevant to the same degree (however, see Sect. 5.4.6).

Autism cannot be 'cured' with treatment. Unlike for illnesses such as depression, treatment here is not a matter of eliminating symptoms or preventing a relapse. Instead, it provides support such that autistic people can learn to live as well as possible with their condition and achieve recovery in this regard (Sect. 5.1.6). Autistic people who are in organised self-help and interest groups often demand that autism should not be seen as an illness but as a difference, and not as something that should or must be 'treated'. This is the concept of *neurodiversity* [294], according to which autistic people are different from *neurotypically* normal people but are not ill. As is to be expected, this rejection of treatment has also been criticised: parents of severely impaired autistic people point out that they are very much in need of treatment (including for disorders associated with their autism, such as depression, anxiety or epilepsy). Taking a middle ground helps in view of autism's wide range of exhibited characteristics and functions, both recognising autism itself is not an illness that can or should be treated and acknowledging that severe autism and related conditions require medical and psychosocial support (and advocacy) [295].

There is much to be said for seeing autism not as an illness but as a disability. According to a social model of disability, the impairment is not only in the autistic person but in the environment. The focus needs to be on finding the right fit between a person and his or her space—for example, finding a suitable niche for autistic people in the employment sector. Such a disability model for people with autism helps to shift the focus from deficits to opportunities and environmental support. The use of assistive technology by autistic people to facilitate communication has become a controversial issue in this regard. Some say that while technology can indeed compensate for certain deficits, placing the onus on such tools and technical adaptation from autistic people lessens the responsibility of the environment to change. The debate about advantages and disadvantages of technology, including a neurodiversity perspective which rejects treatment, has yet to be conducted [296].

Swedish climate activist Greta Thunberg has made her Asperger's public. Politicians she has accused of climate inaction have responded by calling Thunberg 'deeply disturbed'. One has condescended: 'On the one hand the girl is admirable, but on the other hand she is ill' (Friedrich Merz, German politician, *FAZ*, 25 Sept. 2019). Such discriminatory responses, in which one's political opponent is maligned by reference to her stigmatised disability, are also diversion tactics. This behaviour is no different than avoiding a substantive discussion with a person because they are in a wheelchair or have a different skin colour. It is a strong example of how widespread the stigma of mental illness remains.

Thunberg was quick to reply on Twitter that she was indeed 'deeply disturbed'—by the hate campaigns against her and her cause. Using Thunberg as an example, psychiatrist Leonhard Schilbach has pointed out that Asperger's is often accompanied by a strong factual orientation and is therefore a strength, not a weakness, for politics and activism (*FAZ*, 20 Feb. 2019). Given the state of our planet, one might question who is truly disturbed here. We need to remind ourselves of the idea, popular in Romanticism, that so-called madness is a sign of health in a world gone mad [297]: 'And who finally decides whether we fools here in the asylum are erring more masterfully, or faculty members in their lecture halls? Whether perhaps error might even be truth, folly wisdom, death life' (Bonaventure's Nightwatches, published in German 1804, Ninth Nightwatch, Monologue of the Insane World Creator; [298], p. 74). Madeleine Ryan, an autistic person, was naturally able to express it most succinctly and soberly: 'We're in the best position to see society clearly, because we don't fit into it' (*Sydney Morning Herald*, 27 Sept. 2018).

Public attitudes towards autistic people are not well researched. Some studies indicate that autistic people often face rejection and can be regarded by others as less human (dehumanisation Sect. 3.1.4 [299]). Stigma hurts autistic people too: the more discrimination they experience or expect and the less open they are about their autism, the worse their well-being over time [300].

The approach of the media towards autism appears ambivalent. The stereotype of autistic people as people with rare extraordinary talents, a widespread view following the film *Rainman* with Dustin Hoffman, is problematic because it is an exceptional case. On the other hand, recent series such as *Atypical* on Netflix are breaking new ground: autistic people are shown not as freaks or burdens but as valuable social participants—precisely because, unlike 'normal people', they call a spade a spade. Biological models have advantages and disadvantages in the field of autism as well (Sect. 5.1.2). For example, parents whose autistic children were found to have genetic abnormalities reported less guilt but were more concerned that their child's autism was now, so to speak, set in stone [301].

Autistic people and their relatives must decide whether to disclose a diagnosis of autism. This particularly concerns autistic people with average or above-average intelligence, who can 'pass as normal' (Sect. 4.3.7). Preliminary experimental studies suggest that disclosure of an autism diagnosis improves responses from one's social environment [302, 303]. Disclosure in the workplace can also be a complex issue for autistic people, with advantages and disadvantages to doing so dependent on the work environment (Sects. 5.1.4, 7.1.1 [304]).

Autistic people have the right to the best possible supports and, if possible, training opportunities. However, very different approaches to training and education for autistic people are currently evident across Europe [305]. Autistic people with high intellectual capacity often have good educational attainment but upon graduation either cannot find work or only find work that does not match their level of education [306]. This form of social exclusion not only contradicts the UN-CRPD (Sect. 7.5.2) but is also likely to contribute to the high prevalence of depression among autistic people. There are known effective strategies for bringing autistic people into the workplace: support from social workers (job coaching, Sect. 7.1.2, 'Supported Employment') helps, as do workplace set-ups with limited distractions and scheduled tasks [307]. For employers, autistic employees should be attractive candidates not in spite of but because of their differences, as they often possess exceptional memory and concentration skills. Companies such as Auticon in Germany specifically recruit and place autistic people in the information technology sector. We can also see these skills highlighted amongst autistic doctors: 'Trainees with Asperger's have masses to offer to the medical profession; they're diligent, they're conscientious, their attention to detail is amazing, their memory tends to be brilliant. Obviously, I'm generalising, but they've so much to offer' ([308], p. 21).

As is common with mental illness, parents of autistic children are also affected by stigma (Sects. 5.6, 6.2). The vast majority witness social rejection in their children's everyday lives. And regardless of the degree of autistic behaviour, stigma contributes significantly to the social isolation of parents and families [309]. According to one systematic literature review, the more stigma parents experience due to a child's autism, the worse their own mental health [310]. These are mostly cross-sectional results that do not prove the causal effects of stigma on health. However, these findings at the very least suggest serious, negative consequences of stigma on families. Moreover, seeing a supportive figure such as a mother deal with depression could be detrimental to the autistic person as well.

Hardly any data is available on specific antistigma interventions in the field of autism. In one preliminary study, an online course for students was able to improve their knowledge about and attitudes towards autistic people [311]. In future intervention development in this area, models of autism that emphasise deficits and seek to get rid of autism through treatment, as it were, should be avoided. These types of models are associated with more stigma and are more likely to be rejected by autistic people [312]. In the 2000s, there was an American media campaign initiated by a prominent psychiatrist to raise awareness about autism. The campaign published posters styled as 'ransom notes' that said: 'We have your son. We are destroying his ability for social interaction and driving him into a life of complete isolation. It's up to you now' (pictures of the 'ransom notes' can be found online [313]). Similar to horror movies with mentally ill monsters (Sect. 7.4.2, 'Film and Online Games'), this 'ransom' tactic presented autism as a personified evil which abducts and destroys people. The campaign was withdrawn after lengthy protest from autistic people and their families. It is an example of a complete failure of a so-called educational campaign run by psychiatrists and is another reason why it is so important that antistigma work is designed and led by people with mental illness (Sect. 12.4 [312]).

5.4.2 BIPOLAR DISORDER (MANIC-DEPRESSIVE ILLNESS)

Bipolar comes from the Latin word 'bis' (twice) and 'pole'. People with bipolar disorder experience both manic and depressive phases, usually lasting from weeks to months, as extreme ends or 'poles' of mood. Bipolar disorder is also referred to as manic-depressive illness. In a manic episode, people are full of energy, need very little sleep, make big plans, are euphoric or irritable, and can cause mischief and make seemingly irrational decisions. One might do something hastily, like buy a helicopter even though they have never been in one. Such transactions cannot always be rescinded and risk financial ruin. People in a mania can also develop psychotic symptoms (e.g. in their elation think that they have superhuman powers and dangerously try to stop a tram with one hand). Mania is often followed by deep depression in which people are tormented by guilt and shame.

Bipolar disorders are challenging for those affected as well as for those around them. The German author Thomas Melle once clearly and profoundly described his experience with it:

If you are bipolar, your life has no continuity. What previously happened as a more or less continuous story, disintegrates in retrospect into unconnected spheres and fragments. The condition has shattered your past and threatens your future even more. With each manic episode, your life as you know it is made more impossible. The person you thought you knew and were, no longer has a solid foundation. You can no longer be sure of yourself [...] Who would have the strength to put together something new? ([314], p. 113)

His question at the end is, at its core, about recovery and the possibility of a new life. Melle returns to this at the end of his book and offers an almost spiritual optimism at the thought that the mania could return and 'knock him down again': 'Then I will still carry on living. Then these lines will be like a prayer' ([314], p. 348). The telling of one's own story, with all its hardship, may have the power to relieve some of the terror from the madness, avert it and give one confidence. We will return to this idea later in a discussion of narrative approaches (Sect. 9.1.3, Sect. 9.2.3).

Many people experience manic phases, especially lighter ones, as creative and enriching—and the bipolar disorder as a positive part of their identity that they would not want to get rid of even if they could [315]. Approximately 1% of all adults are affected, with roughly the same frequency for women and men. The number of healthy life years lost (DALYs) through bipolar disorder is high (about half as many as due to stroke and twice as many as Parkinson's disease or epilepsy [41]).

Public attitudes towards bipolar disorder have not been studied in depth [156]. As far as we know, they are less negative than for schizophrenia but more negative than for depression [316]. More information is available about the consequences of stigma for people with bipolar disorder [317]. According to longitudinal studies, the more public prejudice people with the disorder perceive, the worse their social functioning later on, regardless of the degree of their symptoms [318]. Much of the evidence also suggests that the stigma and fear of being devalued by others lead to social anxiety, which in turn worsens the social situation of people with bipolar disorder and the clinical course of the illness [319]. Many are understandably burdened by the decision as to whether and how they should tell others about their illness. Some recommend prudent disclosure only to those they trust (Sect. 9.2). Prejudices and the consequences of labelling make it difficult to accept one's own illness and treatment:

If my friends knew that I was taking medicine because I was bipolar, they'll say I am crazy. ([320], p. 177)

That's the way it is with mental illness. They say that there are no prejudices anymore, because people are so enlightened, but that isn't true.... They look askance at you and think, 'Hmm she's mentally ill and her behaviour is different' and at times they don't believe what you say ... and that may be the reason why I find it difficult to accept the illness. ([321], p. 126)

I am not currently aware of any antistigma interventions specifically targeted towards bipolar disorder. However, a systematic literature review has shown that psychoeducation about bipolar disorder reduces the burden of stigma for people with the disorder [322]. Self-help groups are helpful, both in educating the general public and in the fight against self-stigma and for empowerment. In Germany, the German Society for Bipolar Disorders (https://dgbs.de) is active and hosts a group for professionals with bipolar disorder working in the healthcare system.

The role of labelling in the field of early detection and early intervention for young people is controversial [323, 324]. Risk assessment, whether by genetic or clinical examination, is generally considered inappropriate for the general public. Since bipolar disorders are rare, such assessments would cause many 'false positives' or false alarms (Sect. 3.3.4). However, many researchers now advocate for early detection and early intervention in risk groups, specifically in children of parents with bipolar disorder and in young people with the first possible signs of bipolar disorder.

We face several challenges here:

- On one hand, people with bipolar disorder should be able to make autonomous decisions in regard to their risk assessments and interventions. The matter of who should be able to make these decision (i.e. a parent deciding to assess an underage child) contains several ethical considerations. What happens if, for example, a risk assessment shows that the child has a 30% chance of later developing bipolar disorder? Is the child told? What positive (i.e. family supports the child) versus negative (i.e. family is anxious or dismissive) effects could this create?

- On the other hand, the chance of early detection and treatment could result in a better course of illness and more positive educational outcomes for the person diagnosed. This opportunity must be weighed up against the risks of labelling a person 'at risk'. The latter can have a negative impact on the person's social environment, on his or her self-concept ('Am I now one of the *mentally ill*?') and even on future insurance policy options.

A social debate on opportunities and risks seems necessary—and the decisions should be left to people with bipolar disorder and their families as much as possible.

5.4.3 BORDERLINE PERSONALITY DISORDER

This disorder belongs to the group of so-called personality disorders. In contrast to episodes of depressive illness, for example, personality disorders describe a rather stable pattern of thinking, feeling and behaviour that begins in youth and leads to difficulties for those affected and the people around them. The term *borderline* comes from the fact that the symptoms were once thought to be on the *borderline* between what were considered neurosis and psychosis. A borderline personality disorder is essentially a disorder of emotion regulation and is characterised by difficulty in four areas [325]:

1. unstable interpersonal relationships,
2. skewed self-concept and self-perception, including dissociative symptoms when experiencing tension,
3. serious difficulty controlling emotions (including anger, shame, feeling of emptiness),
4. high impulsivity, leading to self-harm or suicidality. Self-harm is often used as a means to reduce agonising tension and is thus a problem-solving attempt (albeit a problematic and dangerous one).

The 12-month prevalence of borderline personality disorder in the general public is between 1% and 2%, but over the course of a lifetime reaches 5% (Sect. 2.2.1). There are more women than men with this diagnosis in psychiatric hospitals, but otherwise both sexes are affected fairly equally [325]. This may be due to the fact that men are more likely than women to end up in the criminal justice system rather than in mental health services due to their disorder-related high impulsivity and higher risk of alcohol or drug abuse [326]. For them, these behaviours can lead to multiply experienced stigma (from both the illness and a criminal record) as well as inadequate treatment or therapy. About one in five patients in psychiatric hospitals and one in seven in nonpsychiatric accident and emergency (A&E) care has a borderline personality disorder [325]. Traumatisation in childhood is the most prevalent and important risk factor. The disorder was long considered untreatable, which in turn contributed to its stigma. But this attitude is now outdated. First, the effectiveness of psychotherapy is well-documented (psychotropic drugs, on the other hand, rarely seem to help). Second, large follow-up studies over the past several decades have shown that many people with borderline personality disorder only present a few symptoms in the few years following the initial diagnosis (hence the lower prevalence mentioned above, if one considers only the period of a single year). In addition to a reduction in symptoms, many people achieve a comprehensive improvement in their sense of recovery (i.e. they face fewer problems socially and professionally [327]).

Shame and self-stigma are common among women with borderline personality disorder [328] as well as among parents of adolescents who self-harm [329]. The fact that self-stigma and shame are strongly pronounced in people with borderline personality disorder has two causes. First, people with borderline personality disorder experience more labelling due to frequent visits to A&E and hospitals, interpersonal conflicts or visible scars. Second, shame as a result of traumatic childhood experiences may increase susceptibility to self-stigma when people with borderline personality disorder encounter renewed devaluation [184]. A woman from Munich, Dominique de Marné, has lived experience with borderline personality disorder. She has chosen to disclose her illness, not least to break down shame, self-stigma and public stigma. This can be read about in her impressive book [330] and online (https://mentalhealthcrowd.de). In Munich, she has opened the Berg & Mental 'mental health café' (https://bergundmental.de).

Stigma towards this diagnosis is also present within the healthcare system. Many professionals in the somatic or psychiatric-psychotherapeutic fields consider people with borderline personality disorder to be 'difficult'. This may lead to outpatient psychotherapists refusing to treat or inpatient facilities declaring themselves neither responsible nor capable. This correlates with survey findings in which many professionals feel they are not qualified to treat people with borderline personality disorder [331]. Experimental studies also suggest that professionals hold a more negative view of a patient and his prognosis if he is labelled 'borderline'. In one study, about 250 practitioners watched a video of a patient with panic disorder who had been motivated to undergo therapy [332]. One-third only saw the video; one-third additionally received (false) written information that this patient also suffered from borderline-typical symptoms (without mentioning borderline personality disorder); the last third, in addition to the video and description of symptoms, received the (also false) information that the patient had a borderline personality disorder diagnosis. In comparison to the first two groups, practitioners in the last group presented significantly more negative assessments of the patient, particularly in regards to motivation, treatability and prognosis.

Professionals may be reluctant to inform their patients about a diagnosis of borderline personality disorder in order to protect them from stigma and self-stigma [331]. However, this is usually perceived by patients as paternalistic and limits their options for orientation regarding self-help and treatment. People with borderline personality disorder are likely to be reluctant to seek help again after encountering such behaviour from professionals. Practitioners often describe people with borderline personality disorder as 'manipulative' or 'splitting'. This is comparable to substance use disorders, where there is a tendency to morally evaluate behaviours as character flaws rather than as signs of illness. But alleged 'splitting' can also be constructive: one can appreciate the fact that these patients are often able to point out contradictions and issues in their treatment, such as communication failures between team members. In worst-case scenarios, patients are blamed for their symptoms or lack of success in treatment by their therapists (which increases shame and self-stigma). Patients in good psychotherapy, however, cannot 'fail'—the only possibility is that this psychotherapy programme is not the right one for this person at this time.

A vicious cycle is thus at stake: professionals react negatively because they expect 'difficult' patients and tend to feel overwhelmed by the diagnosis; patients feel rejected and react just as negatively—and in the end, both sides feel vindicated. There is also a structural problem at hand: for example, there is a very effective form of psychotherapy called Marsha Linehan's dialectical behavioural therapy. Yet it has not been made sufficiently available across Germany or anywhere else, especially in the outpatient sector. This makes it considerably more difficult to find qualified psychotherapists outside of the university towns where they are trained.

Since the behaviour of professionals towards people with borderline personality disorder can contribute to stigma and self-stigma, professionals are an obvious target group for antistigma interventions. Researcher Stephanie Knaak conducted a three-hour workshop for professionals that, based on Linehan's therapy, contained information and first-person accounts from people with borderline personality disorder about their recovery, as well as a combination of education and contact strategies (Sects. 8.1 and 8.4 [333]). The study showed that the attitudes of the professionals towards people with borderline personality disorder were initially more negative than towards people with other mental disorders and that the workshop seemed to improve attitudes.

5.4.4 DEMENTIA

Dementia is a generic term for a number of illnesses that lead to disorders of memory, orientation, thinking, speech and coping with everyday life. The most common types of dementia are Alzheimer's disease (approx. 60%) and the so-called vascular forms of dementia that are based on circulatory disorders and numerous mostly small brain infarctions ($\sim$20%), as well as mixed forms of both types ($\sim$10%). Prevalence of dementia increases from around 3.5% amongst those 70 to 74 years to around 25% amongst those between 85 and 89 years, further increasing with higher age. Whether the number of new cases will rise sharply in future decades due to the ageing population in rich countries is unclear [334]. Although dementia usually occurs at an advanced age, it is responsible for the second greatest number of healthy life years lost (DALYs) among neurological and psychiatric illnesses, behind depression [41]. The WHO has thus made dementia a public health priority [335].

There are currently around 1.7 million people living with dementia in Germany, around three-quarters of whom live at home. According to figures from the Federal Statistical Office, the cost of this population's medical and nursing care was around 15 billion euros in 2015. (Due to higher life expectancy, 11 billion was spent on the care of women with dementia and 4 billion on that of men.) However, many estimate the true cost to be three times higher because most nursing work is performed unpaid at home by relatives (often spouses and daughters) [336]. Even this may very well be an underestimation—more than half of all dementia disorders go undiagnosed, and the costs incurred are therefore not correctly assigned. The costs arising from dementia needs and services are expected to roughly double by 2050.

Historically, there have always been very different views regarding dementia specifically and ageing in general. The two cannot be completely separated—dementia used to be considered a normal symptom of old age rather than an illness (and often still is today due to the high prevalence of dementia among the very elderly). In his essay, *Cato the Elder—On Old Age* from 44 BC, Cicero has Cato disprove various prejudices against ageing. For example, Cato calmly responds to the common lament about weakness in old age: he says that even as a young man he had not wanted the strength of an elephant, and that one should instead make use of what is available and act according to one's strengths ('agere pro viribus', ch. ix). When it came to ageing, Cicero relied on acceptance and serenity, on quiet commitment, further learning and exchange of knowledge. This Roman approach is not far off current recommendations.

Dementia has come to be understood as a brain disease—for example by Alois Alzheimer, who in 1906 described the form of dementia named after him. In the 20th century, there was a countermovement that saw dementia as a psychosocial problem and argued that older people live in a society that does not sufficiently support them [337]. This perspective has helped to build and improve care and social welfare systems for older people outside of institutions (and corresponds to modern concepts of disability, see Sect. 7.5.2). Other cultures' views of dementia add further dimensions to the picture [338]. In India, for example, the classification of 'turning 60' describes a state of forgetfulness, stubbornness, resentment and mistrust that is socially tolerated. And yet severe forms of dementia, particularly with aggression and psychotic symptoms, are strongly stigmatised as insanity.

Social media and literature can reinforce or reduce stigma (Sect. 7.4). One evaluation of around 30,000 Twitter messages regarding dementia showed that, besides many helpful and informative messages, about half of the tweets were stigmatising (in particular by making fun of the illness) [339]. A wide net of threatening metaphors for dementia are used in media and political discussions: the disease is a tidal wave, an epidemic, a monster, an enemy or the plague of the 21st century, against which a war or crusade must be waged [340]. Such images shape what we associate with dementia: fear, danger, terror, contagion. The worst of these metaphors is the depiction of people with dementia as the undead (zombies). Susan Behuniak has shown that this depiction is common and leads to strong reactions of fear and disgust [341]. It is particularly harmful because it denies the humanity of those who are ill. One can and must counter such images with the perspective that people with dementia are above all *people* who have feelings and dignity.

The media can also help to raise awareness and reduce stigma. Besides motion pictures like *Iris* (Sect. 7.4.2), documentaries like *Every Three Seconds*, which was produced by the organisation Alzheimer's Disease International (https://alz.co.uk/everythreeseconds), shares the perspective of people with dementia and their families. The title of the film refers to the fact that a new person falls ill with dementia every three seconds worldwide. The film itself combines information on ongoing research and social support with a focus on the strengths and dignity of people with dementia.

Population surveys show contradictory reactions to dementia: compassion and willingness to help are common, but so is fear [342]. Rejection is likely to be reinforced by a fear of infection, by the incurability of dementia and by the fact that dementia reminds us of our mortality (terror management theory, see Sect. 3.3.1). A worldwide survey of almost 70,000 people found that many people with dementia experience discrimination in everyday life: their opinions are ignored, others make fun of them or they are socially excluded [343].

Negative attitudes towards people with dementia increase scepticism towards screening and early detection of the illness. Both people with dementia and professionals alike are ambivalent about such tests [344]. Early diagnosis of the illness allows for its earlier treatment and preparation (with the limitation that current treatments neither stop nor cure cognitive decline). But early detection can also lead to (self-)labelling and anxieties about the future, culminating in suicidality [345]. Dehumanisation due to disturbing (e.g. zombie) metaphors, fear of loss of control and social pressure can accumulate as drivers towards suicide assistance. A Dutch health minister is quoted as follows: 'It would be wise for people in the early stages of dementia to draft an advance directive requesting euthanasia' ([346], p. 379). Our society attaches a great deal of importance to independence. But this overgeneralised value can be problematic and unhelpful: we in turn view the need for help too negatively and define it narrow-mindedly. But humans have always been intrinsically dependent on the help of others at the beginnings and ends of our lives.

How do people with dementia face its stigma? 'It's a strange life when you "come out"—people get embarrassed, lower their voices and are lost for words' author Terry Pratchett, who suffers from dementia, writes of the reaction of those around him [347]. The decision to disclose one's own dementia diagnosis is complicated—it can lead to support and understanding as well as discrimination. Similar to people with other illnesses, the decision depends on the context and addressee (Sect. 5.1.4, Sect. 9.2). Some people see in disclosure an act of self-determination and a way to reduce stigma: 'You take control, so you're basically taking control of your diagnosis, and in freely talking about it, plus the fact that you get to educate people because part of the stigma is the sort of unknown' ([348], p. 49). Jem Bhatt is currently working in London on a programme to help people with dementia on their disclosure decisions (Sect. 9.2).

People with dementia often feel ashamed and devalued, withdraw socially and do not want to be seen [349]. Added to this self-stigma is the fear of a worsening condition and unknown future [350]. Reports of friends and neighbours withdrawing from their relationships are also common. Fortunately, many people with dementia try to make their voices heard in society to reduce stigma and structural barriers [351]. That they supposedly do not have anything else to contribute postdiagnosis is in itself a prejudice. By finding a voice and talking about themselves, they defy social prejudice and self-stigma. Similar to disclosure, telling one's own story can be an act of resistance and self-determination. In Martina Zimmermann's beautiful monograph, which contains stories of people with dementia, there is a quote from Arno Geiger about his diagnosed father: 'It is said that every narrative is a dress rehearsal for death, because every narrative has to reach an end. At the same time, narrative brings back what has disappeared, because it is dedicated to disappearance' ([352], p. 118).

Narratives about having dementia are obviously diverse in style and messaging. Some conjure gloomy images like the black hole, the labyrinth, or the journey without return. But there are also more encouraging approaches: 'Alzheimer's is a tough thing—but since it is so tough, I feel I don't have to be afraid of anything anymore. And this opens up opportunities and chances' ([352], p. 96). Christine Bryden, who has dementia, suggests possibilities for growth to 'find the pearl hidden within us. Like the pearl that is formed through the irritation of a grain of sand within an oyster, our pearl has formed through the challenge of living with dementia' ([352], p. 104). She thus draws a counter-image to empty shells and zombies. These are not isolated examples: an overview of almost 30 qualitative studies showed that many people with dementia are fully capable of living a good life despite and with the illness [353]. People report acceptance ('I've accepted it, you know, just do the best you can and that's all you can do') and gratitude ('I've had a lovely life and I feel satisfied'; [353], pp. 688 f.).

The families of people with dementia are also affected by stigma. Like those diagnosed, many report that their friends and families withdraw. In addition to the practical severities and challenges of dementia, shame is a major contributor to the burden on family members [354]. They feel shame about their relative's illness and keep it hidden—from their communities as well as from the healthcare system [355]. Because of concerns about labelling their patients, and their knowledge of public stigma and self-stigma, healthcare professionals even hesitate to give people the diagnosis of dementia [356]. Though it is well intentioned, some people with dementia see this behaviour as paternalistic and restrictive of a patient's right to self-determination.

In the legal system, the consequences of a dementia diagnosis vary widely. The diagnosis can facilitate access to treatment, care and support, including legal guardianship. However, people with dementia often report that once they are diagnosed, they may not be heard at all: judges or caregivers go over their heads and decide for them. This disregard does not do justice to the abilities of those affected by dementia, which may be limited but not completely absent [357]. In the legal sphere, a human rights perspective which considers dementia a disability is increasingly important [358]. People with dementia are entitled to the protections provided by the UN-CRPD ('Glossary'). This includes the right to be informed about the diagnosis and treatment options, and to have a say in treatment decisions.

What can be done to counter all of these challenges, beyond personal narratives? No cure for dementia is expected in the foreseeable future. And so as stigma significantly increases the burden placed on people with dementia and their families, interventions in this area are all the more important. Billions of funds have been spent on (largely unsuccessful) biological research into dementia in recent decades. Yet little is known about psychosocial interventions for this category of illnesses due to a lack of studies [359]. Promising approaches involve bringing people with dementia out of their isolation through participation in art, poetry or storytelling. These projects have a positive impact on people with dementia and their families—as well as on medical students, if they participate [360]. One such project brings together poetry by people with dementia (https://alzpoetry.com), such as the poem 'Celebratory Confetti' by Stuart Hall.

'CELEBRATORY CONFETTI'

My mind's not at all a blank slate,
Though I cannot keep track of the date
Or the day of the week,
And facts play hide-and-seek,
For my mind to be blank would be great.
Instead it is wired like spaghetti;
It conflates the important and petty;
The connections of things
Are like tangles of strings
Or like celebratory confetti.

Correlating with the title of this poem, a campaign in Germany called 'Konfetti im Kopf' (confetti in the head) campaigns for education and against the stigma associated with dementia using photo competitions and parades (https://konfetti-im-kopf.de). Other initiatives take place in museums, where people with dementia are accompanied by trained cultural mediators, encounter works of art and take part in workshops in which they themselves become artistically active. Rotraut Krall has established such programmes at the Vienna Kunsthistorisches Museum: participants meet in the public space, they take on an active role and their old memories are reawakened and exchanged [361]. There are also programmes where people with dementia meet each other, telling and sharing stories based on artistic images. Milan is home to the Alzheimer Fest association, which organises parties and meetings in Italy for people with and without dementia through music, art, etc. ('like the Oktoberfest: perhaps with less beer, but with more hugs'; https://alzheimerfest.it). In Austria 'people with forgetfulness' and their supporters meet at the organisation Promenz (www.promenz.at). These are examples of successful social inclusion of people with disabilities. One such programme participant with dementia summarised the effect it had on her nicely: 'The revelation that I can't remember but I CAN imagine blessed my mind, heart, and soul' ([360], p. 710).

Such activities, local and at a grassroots level, are likely the best way to reduce the stigma and social isolation of people with dementia and their families. The advocacy work of organisations for people with dementia and their relatives fits in with this [362]. Internationally, there are various national dementia strategies [363]. Amongst those in German-speaking countries, one in Switzerland does not focus on stigma. In Germany, a national dementia strategy published in 2020 mentions awareness-raising as a way to reduce stigma [364].

A wide range of activities will be needed to alleviate the stigma of dementia and its consequences. Alongside initiatives by and for people with dementia and their relatives, this includes work with the media and healthcare professionals, the development of dementia strategies at a national and European level that prioritise stigma, the development of integrated care models that link different professional groups and forms of treatment (hospital, family doctor, nursing, etc. [365]), a heightened and critical consideration of poverty and loneliness in old age, and increased research on psychosocial care and antistigma interventions in this area.

5.4.5 EATING DISORDERS AND OBESITY

Eating disorders include bulimia and anorexia. Being severely overweight (obesity), while not considered a mental illness, is more common in people with mental illnesses. Weight gain can also be a side effect of many psychiatric medications. Whether being overweight should be con-sidered a physical illness is itself controversial. Some people support this view by pointing to the serious consequences and disabilities associated with obesity [366]. Opponents argue that being overweight is only a risk factor for a very diverse and indeterminate list of illnesses (including cardiovascular disease and depression) but is not an illness itself. From this perspective, the clas-sification of obesity as an illness would not reduce its stigma, but rather lead overweight people to feel labelled as ill instead of as 'normal people in big bodies' ([367], p. 1266). Because obesity is not only stigmatised but can also be a cause and consequence of mental illness, it is briefly discussed in this section following an overview of eating disorders.

Eating Disorders

In newer psychiatric classification systems, three common eating disorders are differentiated: anorexia, bulimia and binge eating. People with anorexia consume as few calories as possible, which can lead to becoming severely underweight; a person with anorexia may be afraid of be-coming fat and/or feel fat despite being extremely thin. Bulimia refers to recurrent eating fits in which a person will lose control over the type and amount of food he or she eats and then induce vomiting or take laxatives to avoid weight gain. A person with bulimia can be of normal weight and the condition, unlike anorexia, is often not bodily visible. Binge eating is similar to bulimia, except that it is not followed by vomiting; those affected are often overweight. Eating disorders usually begin in adolescence. On average about 1% of the total population is affected, but eating disorders are much more common among young women. These are life-threatening illnesses: about 5% of all people with anorexia die within 10 years of the disorder's development [368].

There is a common view and discourse amongst the general public that people with eating disorders are responsible for their condition and should thereby pull themselves together. Men seem to be more prejudiced than women in this regard [369–371]. There also exist contradictory attitudes: empathy and helpfulness as well as the desire for social distance. Occasionally, those affected by anorexia are admired by people around them because of their slimness [372]. These reactions indicate that the stigma of anorexia is different from the stigma of other mental disor-ders. In light of the socially widespread ideal of thinness, young women with anorexia tend to overfulfil social norms, so to speak. Positive reactions to anorexia make clear why it can be so difficult to distance oneself from the disorder. This 'achievement' fits with the perfectionism and high-performance expectations that are common among people with this disorder. Some people with anorexia consequently see their thinness as a sign of strength: 'It [anorexia] shows that you have a strength that others don't, because, let's face it, not many people have the ability to starve themselves to death' ([371], p. 10).

Many people with eating disorders feel guilty and ashamed of their illness [371]. In some longitudinal studies, stronger shame at the beginning of the study led to increased eating disorder symptoms later on [373]. People with eating disorders may feel inferior and marginalised by oth-ers, become socially withdrawn and develop more severe symptoms [374]. Fear of stigma or discrimination and shame are the biggest barriers to seeking help and treatment. Many fear that they will be seen as weak by seeking help, so they avoid it. Being stigmatised by friends, family or caregivers is also often cited as an obstacle [375].

'The Outdated Stigma of the Anorexic' was a recent headline of a renowned German daily newspaper. The article reported on a study on the genetic make-up of people with anorexia [376]. Unsurprisingly, the authors of the study concluded that anorexia is a *metabo-psychiatric disorder*. However, the term only describes the well-known fact that anorexia affects metabolism as well as the psyche. It is unclear why the newspaper concluded from this one study that the stigma of this illness is outdated. This optimistic interpretation ignores the fact that biological models of men-tal illness reinforce stigma (Sect. 5.1.2). Amongst the general public, the belief that eating disor-ders are due to biological causes increases the desire for social distance from people who have them [377]. In addition, many people with eating disorders fear that biological disorder models will label them as terminally ill because of their defective genes, so to speak. 'It makes it sound like ... that's who I am. And I don't like that. Because I don't see my eating disorder as who I am. I see it as something that's, like, invaded my life and that I want to get rid of' ([378], p. 1413; Sect. 5.1.2, 'Essentialism').

The newspaper report draws a conclusion (regarding outdated stigma) that neither fits the research nor has been made by the authors of the original study. Such media reports are based on a Cartesian (17th-century) dualism according to which the body and soul/psyche are completely separate from each other, leaving little room for nuance. However, it is not the soul or brain alone that suffers, but the whole person in both body and soul [12]. This applies to all mental disorders and is particularly obvious in the case of anorexia. This type of media coverage is also an example of the frequent overestimation of individual studies. Many genetic findings cannot be confirmed in later studies; they are (false positive) chance findings that are exaggerated for sensationalism [172, 173]. Causes of eating disorders are complex and thereby lend themselves less to headlines: in addition to biological factors, personality traits and prevalent societal standards of slimness contribute to the development of eating disorders [379].

Traditional media outlets (i.e. television and magazines) are often accused of being partly responsible for the development of eating disorders by depicting extreme slimness as a beauty ideal. The argument in response has been that the media only follows cultural trends and public preferences. Self-control is highly valued in rich, Western societies where food is abundant; slimness is thus considered a visible and prestigious sign of self-control. This could help explain why the ideal of being slim promotes the development of anorexia [380]. There is a double bind at play here. On the one hand, weight control is considered a medical problem of the individual. On the other hand, we live in a society in which the food industry provides affordable, fast, fatty, sweet or salty food on a large scale. When consumers make use of these services, they behave in a system-compliant manner but are simultaneously stigmatised for being overweight. Increasingly, demands are being made for eating disorders and obesity to be seen more as sociopolitical problems rather than (just) individual ones [381]. Experimental studies suggest that images of slim people aggravate eating disorder symptoms, especially in people at risk [382]. It has been shown that the more the media ideal of slimness is internalised by young girls, the less satisfied they become with their bodies over time and the more they compare themselves to others [383].

Almost all young people use social media, which has many features that can promote the development of eating disorders [384]: they are highly visual outlets, and images (of the body) are often more important than words. Advertisements for diet programmes, for example, can be embedded and aimed precisely at susceptible users. Online social interactions and evaluations are more intense (e.g. mocking obesity or praising slimness). Groups and forums that represent extreme positions are formed online (e.g. glorifying anorexia as a lifestyle). There is a lack of moderation or quality control (e.g. apps that encourage behaviours that can be harmful to health, like calorie counting, can be advertised to young girls). Significantly, social media app sales and commercial advertising are largely controlled by corporate interests. For all of these reasons, it is unsurprising that activity online is associated with the development of eating disorder symptoms. However, the effect and cause are not entirely clear; only a few longitudinal studies have begun recording the consumption of social media and correlating it with subsequent symptoms [384]. Two mechanisms for harmful effects on eating behaviour are important to consider in future research: social comparison—whereby users compare their figure or eating behaviours with those of others online—and feedback from others (e.g. comments on one's own figure).

Besides the usual forms of social media, there are, as mentioned, websites that explicitly advocate eating disorders as a lifestyle (rather than treating them as an illness). This position paradoxically corresponds to the attitude, not uncommon in the general public, that people with anorexia are not ill (Sect. 1.6). In the case of anorexia, these websites are called *Pro Ana* sites and show countless images of very skinny young women. They give encouragement to continue starving oneself and tips on how to lose weight or hide your anorexia from the offline environment. Like other websites, Pro Ana sites offer mutual support and exchange within the in-group. But the goals are fundamentally geared towards maintaining anorexia rather than overcoming illness. Disclosure in the online environment also proceeds differently on Pro Ana pages. In these spaces, a sad or anxious disclosure of one's own eating disorder can often be followed by very negative reactions from forum members. These reactions interpret ill behaviour as positive ('Avoid them [your worried family members] like the plague and fight your urges. You should starve just like Ana'; [385], p. 223). Peer support (Sect. 7.3.4) is important for recovery and overcoming (self-) stigma (Ch. 9). In this respect, Pro Ana sites are a perverted form of peer support that can lead further into social isolation and illness.

A meta-analysis has shown a clear connection between visits to these websites and stronger eating disorder symptoms [386]. Due to the above-mentioned life-threatening nature of eating disorders, there have been repeated attempts to block such websites. But any success in doing so is temporary, as another site will quickly pop up. A more promising approach could be the widespread production of online groups for mutual support on the pathway to recovery. The internet can also be used for healing purposes, and data suggests that this can be a successful way to combat eating disorders [387]. A study about YouTube found videos in favour of anorexia as well as against it. The latter were commented on more positively and viewed more frequently [388]. It seems that along with all of the drawbacks of social media, there is also self-regulation.

Many people with mental illness find it helpful to hear stories of recovery from others that can serve as a model or inspiration and provide hope [389]. Unfortunately, stories of people with eating disorders seem to be the exception. When people with eating disorders hear recovery stories, they seem to trigger harmful social comparisons and/or imitations of the narrator's past unhealthy behaviours [390].

Similar to addictions, the stigma of eating disorders also serves as an obstacle for programmes on prevention and increased public awareness. These campaigns seek to create negative attitudes towards eating disorder *behaviour* in order to promote healthy eating. However, they thereby run the risk of reinforcing negative attitudes towards *people* with eating disorders. An experimental study with healthy students has shown this side effect: an educational video about anorexia with stigmatising content as intended deterred students from disordered eating behaviour, but the study participants also wanted to have less to do with those who were affected [391].

In one meta-analysis, various interventions were examined with regard to their effectiveness in reducing public stigmatisation of eating disorders [392]. There were three approaches: education, contact and communicating illness models (for antistigma strategies, see Ch. 8 ff.). A combination of education and contact, whereby people with experience of an eating disorder talked about themselves and informed members of the general public, proved to be effective. Communication of different causal illness models was also effective in reducing stigma. It should be noted that the communication of biological models likely worked because stigma was narrowly framed and measured as an issue of guilt attribution (i.e. blaming people with eating disorders) [392]. Specific interventions for self-stigma among people with eating disorders do not seem to exist. However, programmes that strengthen understanding and compassion for oneself (self-compassion) have, in pilot studies, reduced shame around personal eating behaviours [393]. Overcoming often-tormenting shame can be a major turning point on the way to healing.

Overweight (Obesity)

Obesity is one of the world's most pressing health problems, and it has a lot to do with the food industry. Obesity, malnutrition (in poorer countries) and climate change are linked globally by a wide range of common causes and consequences, which is why the complex is also known as a *global syndemic* (Sect. 1.7 [17]). Obesity is thus not just an individual problem.

Even though obesity is not a mental illness, stigma in regard to being overweight abounds and is discussed here. The controversial approach to food addiction as an illness and cause of obesity does not seem to reduce stigma [394]. Belittling or even shaming overweight people is not a new phenomenon, though this impression may arise when viewing Rubens' paintings of sensually beautiful and fuller figures from the Baroque era. As early as the 18th century, 'fat shaming' emerged and continues to this day [395]. This stigma is pronounced because obesity is seen as a moral failure, a character defect or a lack of self-control [396]. Negative attitudes towards people who are overweight are even more pronounced in the United States than in Germany, even though obesity is more common in the United States [397]. Such prejudice is taking on shocking proportions: in one international online study, participants classified people who are overweight as less human. On a scale depicting the evolutionary development from apes to humans as a continuous process, overweight people were placed closer to apes than normal-weight people. This assessment correlated with participants' support for structural discrimination (i.e. to make access to healthcare more expensive and less accessible for overweight people) [398]. It has also been shown that parents seem to be prejudiced towards their own overweight children [399]. All of this means that those affected know rejection only too well: 'So, you know, people think you're lazy, people think you're stupid, people think you're dirty. When they see that you're fat they think all those things' ([400], p. 8). Consequently, self-stigma and shame are common. The stigma of being overweight is rarely an isolated problem (Sect. 3.1.8): if people also have a low social status, they meet with even more rejection [401]. Discrimination on the grounds of obesity seriously affects people at school, in education and at work [402].

Public stigma and self-stigma are harmful to health and often inextricably linked. Social stress factors such as poverty and discrimination based on other characteristics and statuses initially promote the development of obesity [403, 404]. And once obesity is present, the experience and expectation of discrimination can further increase food intake [405]. Discrimination harms the health of overweight people in many ways (including further weight gain, stress hormones, diabetes, depression and anxiety). Self-stigma further impairs psychological well-being, particularly in the form of anxiety and depression [406]. And stigma is also toxic in the long term: out of approximately 1000 young women in a study, those who suffered most from drug addiction were those who had been teased as teenagers for being overweight 10 years prior [407].

The stigma of being overweight also has negative effects within healthcare provision [408]. Healthcare professionals are not free from prejudice influencing their behaviour when dealing with overweight patients. This may emerge explicitly, in the form of derogatory statements, or implicitly, by having lower expectations or spending less time with these patients. These reactions can make overweight people feel stressed by and avoid contact with therapists.

Representations of obesity in the media cover a wide spectrum: from denigration and sensationalism ('housewife Helga [40] weighed an incredible 374 pounds'; [409], p. 657) to positive reports about acceptance and self-confidence amongst people who are overweight. Those affected can also find support online (e.g. through blogs in the *Fatosphere*) [410].

Obesity prevention programmes face a dilemma: they can improve eating habits but at the same time risk reinforcing prejudice against people who are overweight [411]. This makes prevention difficult, and careful evaluation of such programmes and their unintended side effects are all the more important [412]. Finally, it should be noted that programmes to reduce obesity are vehemently rejected by some *fat activists* [413]. They oppose the medical view of obesity as well as prevention and treatment programmes, which in their view are basically attempts of 'fat hatred' to eliminate overweight people from society.

5.4.6 INTELLECTUAL DISABILITY

Idiocy or *imbecility*—these and other terms used in the past are deeply tied to stigma. The World Health Organization's (WHO) International Classification of Diseases 10th Revision (ICD-10) uses the term mental retardation; intellectual disability is also commonly used. Unlike the ICD-10, the more recent ICD-11 refers to disorders of intellectual development. It is doubtful, though, whether this name change will reduce stigma as intended (Sect. 8.2 [414]). Intellectual disability is defined by an intelligence quotient below 70; incidence in the population is estimated at about 1% [41]. The causes are diverse, from genetic changes (trisomy 21/Down syndrome and many others) to complications at birth. Mental illnesses, including depression, autism and psychosis, can exist comorbidly with intellectual disability (but do not have to).

Negative stereotypes about people with intellectual disability are common. This means they are often trusted with less than what they can actually handle, and are seen as childishly cheerful or as aggressive fools. This can lead to an ambivalent mixture of discomfort, pity, condescension, paternalism, fear and disgust from those around them (Sect. 3.2.4, 'Content Dimensions of Stereotypes' [414]). Experiences of discrimination by people with intellectual disabilities are unfortunately common in many areas. Only a few examples are given here:

- In standard schools, they can be bullied and harassed by nondisabled classmates (Sect. 5.7).
- In the healthcare system, they regularly encounter professionals in somatic or psychiatric care who are not sufficiently trained to treat people with intellectual disabilities and do not promote their independence [415].
- In the labour market, they are often regarded as unemployable and therefore work in sheltered settings for disabled people.
- Finally, many are denied independent living with support, even if they want it (end of Sect. 7.5.2).

These different aspects of social exclusion mutually reinforce one another: a young person with intellectual disability who attends a distant, special school instead of the nearby, mainstream school will find it very challenging to build up a local social network—and this could have an impact far into his adult life [414].

Many people with intellectual disabilities suffer shaming and humiliation at the hands of others [416]. This triggers their own feelings of shame, self-reproach and low self-esteem, which in turn leads to depression and reduced quality of life and further limits their self-confidence in social contacts. Families are also affected by self-stigma and shame [417], often leading to secrecy and social withdrawal, and from there further into the vicious cycle of silence and isolation.

Attitudes of the general public are closely linked to structural discrimination. A US study of 325,000 members of the general public examined the extent of implicit prejudice against people with intellectual disabilities as well as the number of people with intellectual disabilities living in institutions in each of the 50 states (e.g. in separate residential homes [418]). The stronger the prejudices were in a state, the higher the number of people with intellectual disabilities living in its institutions. What is cause and effect, however, remains unexplained: prejudice can lead to people with intellectual disabilities living less independently, while accommodation in separate, possibly remote buildings reduces opportunities for everyday contact with the general public and thus prevents the dismantling of prejudices. One qualitative study that examines the views of people with intellectual disabilities on life in a large rehabilitation institution included one man's rejection of his categorisation: 'In this hospital you're classed as patients ... I thought how was you to get treated just the same as anyone else outside. It should all be stopped—classed as patients ... we're no dogs or animals or that. We're just the same as anyone else. They should stop all this' ([419], p. 722).

What antistigma interventions are known for this area? Only a few studies have been conducted [420]. First and foremost, the involvement of families is helpful—also for prejudice or shame among families themselves (Sect. 6.2). Some programmes rely on education (Sect. 8.1) to reduce the stigma of intellectual disability through information. They address students, teachers or healthcare professionals specifically, and usually with moderate and short-term success. Contact between the target group and people with an intellectual disability seems to be more effective.

The contact can be direct (face to face) or indirect (e.g. via videos); either way, those with the intellectual disability are meant to talk about themselves and expose the target group to their experiences. Online campaigns working to fight stigma, such as the British initiative End the Awkward (https://scope.org.uk/campaigns/end-the-awkward), show cheerful yet serious films on the subject well worth seeing. The cultural magazine *Ohrenkuss* (German for 'ear kiss'), with pieces submitted by people with Down syndrome, has been published in German-speaking countries since 1998. Their writing is dedicated to various topics, be it fashion, experienced miracles or the origin of the world. 'It has to be said: one must read Ohrenkuss. All of them' (https://ohrenkuss.de).

As far as self-stigma and shame are concerned, programmes to build up positive self-compassion (not self-pity; Sect. 8.1.4) could be helpful for people with intellectual disabilities, but robust data is missing [416]. At the structural level, initiatives usually refer to and rely on the UN-CRPD (Sect. 7.5.2), which guarantees protection against discrimination for people with all types of disability, including intellectual disability. Such programmes are helpful at reducing discrimination in the areas of housing, education, employment and healthcare.

5.4.7 ADDICTION AND SUBSTANCE USE DISORDERS

People can take substances, with or without a doctor's prescription, that alter awareness. Some of these substances are legal, including alcohol, nicotine and prescribed sedatives and opioid painkillers. Others, including cocaine and heroin, are illegal. A distinction should be made between abuse and dependence. Abuse is a type of use that damages body and/or soul. Dependence or addiction refers to the consumption of ever-larger quantities over a long period of time, whereby the craving for the addictive substance can hardly be controlled and consumption becomes increasingly important. About 5% of adults in Europe are addicted to alcohol, cannabis or opioids; men are more often affected than women. Of all mental disorders, alcohol dependence is responsible for the greatest number of healthy life years lost (DALYs) among men [41].

Attitudes of the general public towards people with alcohol or drug addiction are more negative than towards people with other mental disorders [421, 422]: they are more often blamed for their illness and encounter anger and social rejection more frequently. More than other mental disorders, addictions are seen as character defects and are morally condemned [178]. Members of the general public also believe that spending on treatment for alcohol addiction should be reduced (compared to other conditions) [255]. Public attitudes are less negative towards people with addictions if they are successfully treated [423]. Many people with drug addiction often report discrimination within and outside the healthcare system and therefore try to keep their dependency hidden [424]. Treatment centres are also affected by public rejection: protests in neighbourhoods or from local media against the opening of such facilities evoke the NIMBY phenomenon ('Not in my backyard!'; Sect. 7.3.3, 'Architecture'). The shared mentality of 'it's fine everywhere else but not near me' is a very prevalent aspect of structural discrimination.

People with addictions can suffer from self-stigma and shame, an emotion that has long held the reputation of only leading to negative behaviours such as social withdrawal and secrecy. Shame usually goes hand in hand with a generalised devaluation of oneself ('I'm a complete failure'), unlike guilt, which refers to a specific instance ('I have made a mistake in this situation'). However, a meta-analysis has shown that shame can also have a constructive effect [425]: it is an emotion that signals to oneself when misconduct threatens social contacts. The social network has always been essential for human survival, and shame of this type leads to a desire for personal improvement such that one no longer has to feel it. However, the prerequisite for this functional, constructive type of shame is that the person is confident enough to improve and change his or her behaviour. The results of a further meta-analysis of the connection between shame and addictive drug use are consistent with this view [426]: shame becomes associated with increased substance use if people think they cannot make amends for the consequences of their addictive behaviour. Whether shame is the consequence or cause of substance use is not entirely clear. Only one longitudinal study points to shame as a sustaining factor: people with alcohol addiction who had recently become sober were asked to describe the last drink that had made them feel bad. The more they showed physical signs of shame in the first few seconds of their story, such as bending forward and lowering their gaze, the more likely and sooner they were to later relapse [427]. As is often the case, empirical research lags behind the wisdom of literature: in *The Little Prince*, Antoine de Saint-Exupéry tells the story of a man who drinks to forget the shame about his drinking, and who is ashamed because he drinks [428].

Like people with other mental disorders (Sect. 5.1.7), people with substance use disorders could be deterred from seeking help because of their fear of public or self-stigma. However, a systematic overview of more than 60 individual studies did not reveal the expected correlations [429]. Longitudinal studies that assessed stigma variables at the baseline and help-seeking behaviours later on were also contradictory. Only in certain subgroups was stigma a clear barrier to treatment, for example among people in Russia or China who wanted to avoid being registered as drug addicts, or among women who feared losing custody of their children. The fact that stigma did not have an effect on treatment participation in these studies might have methodological underpinnings. Georg Schomerus pointed out to me that people with addictions can spurn being *mentally ill* because of their own prejudices: 'I am not addicted after all! I can manage by myself.' Refusal of help or treatment because of this attitude is an indirect consequence of stigma, yet is difficult to demonstrate in a study. A related concern is whether the public stigma or self-stigma associated with addictions lead to worse treatment outcomes. Qualitative studies suggest that stigmatising attitudes of the staff and/or certain procedures in treatment centres deter those in need of help. Quantitative studies suggest that stigma has an indirectly harmful effect by contributing to negative emotions and reducing the hope for recovery amongst people with substance use disorders [430].

The stigma of addiction could serve the function of helping people adhere to or 'keep in' the socially expected norms and thereby give up their addiction (Sect. 3.3.3). Conversely, stigma can lead to stress and even more substance use as a strategy to alleviate it. Studies show that experiences of discrimination make it difficult to regulate one's emotions, which in turn increases susceptibility to depression and alcohol use [431]. These two consequences of stigma—being deterred and complying with standards on the one hand and increasing consumption on the other—lead to a paradoxical effect. A well-researched example is alcohol use amongst black people in the United States, who statistically drink less than white people on average yet have a higher rate of 'alcohol problems' [432]. This is in part due to the different social and religious norms in African American communities that sanction alcohol consumption. In addition to this, black people with what would be considered 'a drinking problem' are more strongly sanctioned by the dominant white culture than white people with the same addiction. This cumulated stigmatisation of drinking behaviour makes their consumption (and perceptions of it) worse, especially among poor or older black men. This explains why lower average consumption rates and more frequent individual alcohol abuse rates within black communities can occur simultaneously.

Are healthcare practitioners prejudiced against people with substance use disorders? An overview of 28 (mostly quantitative) studies unfortunately supports this [433]: professionals were shown to have predominantly negative attitudes, especially if they were not specialists trained in substance use services. Many feared violence and manipulation and found empathy difficult. Addictions were often seen as controllable and people with substance use disorders as responsible for their own condition. These more negative attitudes from professionals can contribute to treatment being discontinued and patients losing self-esteem and a sense of empowerment.

Alongside the NIMBY phenomenon previously mentioned, structural discrimination of those dealing with addictions is evident in the healthcare system. For example, caring for people with addictions separately, in addiction centres, can complicate the quality of care of anyone with co-morbid psychiatric or somatic disorders. From experience, it is evident that people with addiction, including those with a dual diagnosis (e.g. depression and alcohol addiction, or schizophrenia and opioid abuse), have particular difficulties in finding outpatient psychotherapy.

Which interventions reduce the stigma of substance use disorders and its consequences? The available data on effective interventions is encouraging but scant [434], and the small number of studies is distributed among very different target groups and approaches: some have tried to reduce public stigma, while others are directed at people with substance use disorders or have focused on healthcare professionals [435]. Similar to antistigma programmes in the field of mental illness (Ch. 8 ff.), there are educational and contact-based approaches for fighting public stigma, self-stigma programmes with a cognitive approach, programs that deal with disclosure decisions and peer support groups. One group programme with an aim to convey acceptance and mindfulness was shown to reduce shame and self-stigma [436]. These initiatives also differ according to their overall objectives: increasing participation in treatment, reducing discrimination or boosting empowerment and self-esteem (Sect. 1.3 [437]).

So, what can be done? Emma McGinty has recommended that people with lived experience of substance use disorders should be given the space to talk about themselves and their recovery, including the problems of structural barriers and treatment underfunding [438]. Georg Schomerus and colleagues in Germany have proposed a comprehensive approach [439], which consists of awareness raising, media guidelines (Sect. 7.4.7), development and evaluation of programmes for people with addictions and their families, and structural improvements in prevention and care (Sect. 7.3.4). In comparison to other mental disorders, substance use disorders bring with them a number of unique challenges that need to be considered: local communities and leaders have legitimate interests in changing the behaviour of those affected; the public dangers of addiction, such as violence or traffic accidents, must not be downplayed (Sect. 1.4); prevention in this area can be a slippery slope, as sending negative messages to deter substance use can in turn encourage prejudice. There is a lot to be done and a long way to go to counteract the stigma of addiction.

5.5 People With Multiple Stigmatised Identities

People can hold more than one socially stigmatised identity. The interconnection between, for example, mental illness, poverty and membership of an ethnic minority is also known as intersectionality (Sect. 3.1.8). The result is often persistent and pronounced discrimination. What is known about intersectionality in people with mental illness? First and foremost, it is incredibly common: mental illness is closely associated with poverty, unemployment (Sect. 7.1.2), homelessness (Sect. 7.2) and membership in socially disadvantaged or marginalised groups (including migrants, see Sect. 5.8). The concurrence of several stigmatised characteristics thus tends to be the rule rather than the exception. Especially for those who are disadvantaged in multiple ways, there is a risk of falling through the cracks in the health and social systems [6, 49].

Good data on these intersections is surprisingly rare. For example, there are hardly any studies on intersectionality and structural discrimination in (and across) the fields of mental illness, HIV and physical disability [440]. A qualitative study of homeless people who were of an ethnic minority and had a mental illness revealed pervasive experiences of discrimination based on both of these attributes. Some completely withdrew socially because they could no longer cope with the stigma: 'I don't get myself involved in any situation I can't come out of, I stay by myself' ([441], p. 5). Because of the violent stereotypes they are affiliated with, people convicted of criminal offences in the context of their mental illness are also particularly affected by stigma. A study in New York examined the self-esteem of people with severe mental illness who had been treated in forensic psychiatry after criminal offences and who belonged to an ethnic minority [442]. Self-esteem was found to be multiply affected by three forms of self-stigma: in relation to the mental illness, the offence and one's own ethnic group.

Members of stigmatised groups can suffer physical or verbal attacks because of those group memberships. Depending on the context and severity, these are also known as hate crimes or identity-based victimisation/bullying. The consequences of such attacks are often devastating over time, including the onset of posttraumatic stress and other mental disorders [55]. In a study of nearly 1000 teenagers and young adults in the United States, those who were members of either (or both) a sexual and ethnic minority were most often affected by violence and discrimination [443]. In turn, experiencing violence was associated with higher levels of depression and poorer school performance.

A study in southern Germany examined the consequences of the concurrence of mental illness and long-term unemployment. Among some 300 unemployed people, most of whom were depressed, those who reported discrimination due to their illness *and* due to unemployment were particularly affected. It was found that they had less confidence in finding work and avoided seeking help for their illness due to stigma [444].

Peer support is an important way to help those who, in addition to physical and mental illnesses, are affected by substance abuse and homelessness (Sect. 7.3.4, 'Peer Support' [445]). Peers in this sense are people who have their own personal experiences of homelessness and substance abuse. However, peer workers' own prejudices towards clients can stand in their way and affect relationships: 'When people stopped coming I thought they might be out partying when in fact some were getting jobs, going to rehab, or in the hospital getting better. At times we stigmatise our own community and ourselves' ([445], p. 11).

These are only a few examples of studies that have specifically addressed the topic of intersectionality. But more or less explicitly, the concurrence of illness and other aspects of life on the margins of society plays an important role in many of the discussions in this chapter and Chapter 7.

Conclusion

Sociological stigma researchers have pointed out that, because of all of these intersections, the consequences of stigma are underestimated [446]. Most studies examine only one aspect or consequence of stigma despite the reality that there are often several stigmatised characteristics at play, with multiple consequences.

5.6 Families and Relatives

Stephen Hinshaw, a psychologist and stigma researcher from Berkeley, California, has written of his own experiences with his father, a professor of philosophy with severe bipolar disorder who was in and out of psychiatric hospitals throughout Hinshaw's childhood [447]. In his book, Hinshaw describes how no one in the family talked about it—a psychiatrist had forbidden Stephen's mother to discuss her husband's illness, and Hinshaw only found out where his father had been once he became an adult. In this way a deafening silence descended on the family and, more than his father's illness itself, almost shattered the author. The book is a moving testimony to the burden brought on by stigma, shame and silence. It is also a reminder to professionals of how harmful it can be to recklessly prescribe secrecy (Sect. 7.1.1).

Family members are affected by the stigma of a relative's mental illness (see also Sect. 6.2 by Janine Berg-Peer). This constitutes a significant portion of the general population, as every person with mental illness has, on average, several relatives. The stigma of an illness affects relatives because it rubs off on them, so to speak. Often, they are also stigmatised—a phenomenon referred to as stigma by association, family stigma or courtesy stigma (Goffman's expression for the stigma suffered by relatives as a 'courtesy' or consequence of the association) [8]. Vicarious stigma is a slightly different concept, whereby family members suffer because they feel for their relative with mental illness who is stigmatised.

It is wholly possible for parents or partners of those with mental illness to hold prejudices against their ill relatives. This is comparable to professionals in the healthcare system possibly being prejudiced against those with mental illness whom they are trained to care for (Sect. 7.3.1). Both relatives and professionals are often present in stress-inducing crisis situations, which may explain why they sometimes have negative attitudes [158].

Various details regarding the issue of stigma and relatives have to be broken down:

1. the different types of relatives—parents, partners, children, siblings or more distant relatives
2. the type of stigma:
   a. public stigma ('My classmates don't invite me home since my mother went into psychiatric care.')
   b. self-stigma ('Because my son is mentally ill, I must be a bad mother.')
   c. structural discrimination (e.g. lack of support for families in the healthcare system)
3. the source of discrimination, particularly from one's private life or healthcare professionals.

Many families share that their close friends and communities tend to withdraw from them: 'It's not like he had cancer ... If he had cancer, everyone would have rallied around, but not with mental illness. It's a choice to keep it a secret anyway because of social stigma, because ... people have an idea from television and movies about who gets mental illness. There is always horrible child abuse in the family, so they are looking at you differently. Only bad people or people from bad families get [mental illness]' ([448], p. 12). As a result, relatives, especially those of people with severe mental illness, suffer from loneliness and social isolation. They often face accusations that they have caused the illness through their behaviour (onset responsibility) or are to blame for the fact that the illness has not gone away (offset responsibility). Negative public attitudes seem to be particularly marked towards relatives of people with addictions (Sect. 5.4.7 [449]).

Biogenetic illness models (Sect. 5.1.2) do not help to reduce the stigma here either: in the Belgian region of Flanders, it was found that parents with concerns that their child's psychosis would be hereditary were more likely to suffer from stigma [450]. Children too hold concerns about a hereditary burden: 'I was wondering if it was hereditary then, because if I felt down or something ... then I was worrying, well, am I going to be like that too' ([451], p. 2711). In the public sphere, children may also be avoided by others when considered genetically or socially 'contaminated' [452].

Children of mentally ill parents find themselves in a uniquely difficult situation. They may suffer and even mourn the fact that a once healthy parent has been lost to them, as it were: 'When she got ill we just wanted to get away. We didn't want to know. She wasn't our mum then.... I used to cry every night, you know. I used to pray to God at night and say, "Give us back my old mum. I don't want this person. This isn't my mum.... She's not acting right."' Stereotypes spread by the media make anxieties worse: 'I've heard many times lately about people with mental problems who have killed family members. My mom isn't that bad now, but you never know' ([451], p. 2711). Many children can be overwhelmed, especially if there is no healthy parent in the household. Some may have to assume the roles and responsibilities of the ill parent (*parentification*). For all of these reasons, it is critically important to support children of parents with mental illness in overcoming stigma—both in dealing with public stigma and with regard to self-stigma and shame they may face [453].

Families of those with mental illness often feel abandoned by the healthcare system and can be confronted with judgement and accusations from practitioners (if approached at all) (Sect. 6.2). It is an unfortunate reality that support for these families is far too rare (Sect. 7.3.3). Family therapy can be incredibly helpful: it not only relieves the burden on the family as a whole but also reduces relapse rates, for example in young people having their first incidence of psychosis [454]. Family therapy also significantly increases an individual's likelihood to recover from anorexia [455]. That family therapy is not offered in many countries is a prime example of structural discrimination in the healthcare and benefit systems (Sect. 7.3.3). A review article has shown that the active involvement of relatives in the treatment of children with mental illness is possible and considerably improves treatment outcomes and the situations of the families [456].

Fear of stigma and shame about a relative's illness is an obstacle to seeking help at an early stage. That concern particularly affects parents, who decide whether their children participate in the treatment. Indirectly, stigma can affect children as early as their birth: expectant or young mothers with mental illness are deterred from seeking help because of stigma [457]. This is unfortunate; mothers with mental illness typically respond very well to treatment after giving birth. Stigma here, however, leads to worse outcomes and thus burdens mother and child (Sect. 2.2.4, 'Mothers').

All of this has an impact on families. A long-term study in the United States, which followed parents of children with developmental disorders or autism, found that the more these parents suffered from discrimination and shame (due to the child's condition), the worse their own health outcomes were 20 years later [458]. When dealing with the burden of stigma, families must develop coping strategies. Many, like Stephen Hinshaw's parents, choose to keep the illness secret. But while secrecy can offer protection against discrimination, it is often burdensome in the long term (Sect. 5.1.4). Some families succeed in rejecting stigma: 'They don't hurt me anymore. If you say like, "I think addicts should die", I just think, I will pray for you and your family that you will never have to experience this, because you would have such a shift in what you think ... you'd be singing a different tune if you walked in my shoes' ([459], p. 472).

One possible approach to reducing the burden of stigma on family members within the care system is the trialogue, an exchange as equals between people with mental illness, family members and healthcare professionals (Sect. 7.3.4 [460]). Antistigma interventions for families and relatives exist and include a version of the peer-led group programme Honest, Open, Proud (HOP; Sect. 9.2) for parents of children with mental illness, which is intended to support parents in making a decision for or against disclosure of their child's illness and thus in overcoming stigma.

5.7 Children and Adolescents

About one in six children and adolescents in Germany has a mental illness [461]. The Robert Koch Institute examined the prevalence of mental disorders in over 13,000 children and adolescents (aged 3–17) in 2005 and again in 2015. Within this period of ten years, the average prevalence of mental illness decreased from 20% to 17% [462]. As in 2005, boys were affected slightly more often (19%) than girls (15%) in 2015. It is not entirely clear why the prevalence decreased in both sexes: possible explanations range from an improvement in the healthcare system to a decrease in unemployment and thus better living conditions for many families during this period. The importance of social conditions is shown by the pronounced link the study found between mental illness and socio-economic status: children from poorer families were almost three times more likely to suffer from mental illness (26%) than those from wealthier families (9.7%).

Children and adolescents are in a unique position with regard to the stigma of mental illness in several respects [104]:

1. The majority of all mental disorders begin at this age (Sect. 2.3). Many are therefore either newly affected themselves or have siblings, friends or classmates in their immediate environment who have recently been diagnosed.
2. Stigma takes place within an imbalance of power, whereby the less powerful or disadvantaged are the ones stigmatised (Sect. 3.1.4). Minors have less power and a lower social status than adults, making them more vulnerable to discrimination.

3. Adolescents naturally distance themselves from their parents and orient themselves more towards people their own age. This has two consequences relevant to stigma: in case of mental health problems, parents are less available or welcome as a possible resource. Additionally, adolescent concerns about being rejected by friends or a social group due to being *different* makes dealing with mental health problems all the more challenging.
4. Personal beliefs and attitudes (e.g. on the subject of mental illness) are significantly formed in childhood and adolescence.
5. Identity and self-concept develop in childhood and adolescence, thus heightening the risk and impact of self-stigma in the case of one's own illness. If a child experiences poverty, violence or neglect and subsequently (mistakenly) considers himself inferior, he may be less able to counter the prejudice of others regarding his own mental illness.

For all of these reasons, the concepts and findings about mental illness stigma among adults cannot simply be transferred onto children and adolescents.

What do members of the general public think about children and adolescents with mental illness? The general attitude towards children with depression seems to be even more negative than towards adults with depression. In one American study, depressed children were considered to be potentially violent more often (40%) than depressed adults (30%) [463]. Young people often encounter incomprehension in their personal relationships as well; a girl with an eating disorder recalls an exchange with her grandmother, who had survived the period of hunger following the Second World War: 'Once I was really not hungry, but my grandmother would always say: "We were always hungry!... Nowadays there is so much food and you don't eat it?" And I said to her: "Grandma, you don't understand"' ([464], p. 299). Studies show that children and adolescents with mental illness encounter social rejection more often than not only healthy peers, but peers with physical and intellectual disabilities as well [465]. In the general public, there is widespread prejudice that children and adolescents with mental illness are responsible for their condition (e.g. because they do not *pull themselves together*), which in turn strengthens the desire for social distance. Young boys in particular are often considered dangerous. As far as confrontation with negative public attitudes is concerned, the fear of stigma after discharge from a child and adolescent psychiatric hospital is, understandably, particularly strong [466].

How early do prejudices develop, and what do children and adolescents without mental illness think? This question is important because stigma could also be tackled preventively if these issues were better understood (Sect. 7.3.4, 'Prevention' [467]). Today's antistigma programmes tend to focus on adults, but their prejudices are likely harder to change than the malleable attitudes of young people. Children learn to categorise faces as early as the first year of life; at primary school age, facial categorisation becomes linked to perceptions of status difference between social groups and personal preferences for one's in-group [95]. Studies show prejudice against other children with mental illness as early as primary school age [104]. Children adopt pejorative expressions (e.g. freak, lunatic, schizo, retard, spastic) early. And the media contributes: in many children's films as well as on social media, mentally ill characters are portrayed as dangerous, evil or repulsive (Sect. 7.4 [107]). Knowledge about mental illness (Sect. 3.1.7) is often poor, and many adolescents cannot recognise case descriptions of mental illness (e.g. depression). About half of adolescents cannot distinguish between mental illness and intellectual disability [104]. All of this shows how beneficial it would be to make mental health/illness a taught subject (Sect. 8.4.5). Bavaria took a step in this direction in 2019 with a so-called 10-point plan: teacher training and programmes for pupils would focus on mental health, stress prevention, depression, anxiety and ways to help pupils with mental health problems.

Ignorance and negative attitudes have consequences: the more negative their own attitudes, the less willing adolescents are to seek help for their own problems or help peers with their mental health problems [104]. The desire for social distance is great: when children were asked to draw the distance between themselves and members of various stigmatised groups, the greatest distance drawn was between the child and a convict, followed second by the *'madman'*. With adolescents, the distance drawn to the *'madman'* was the greatest. These examples alone show that the summary presented here on the entire group of children and adolescents is itself a gross simplification [104]: a 5-year-old will perceive their diagnosis, stigma and coping options very differently from a 15-year-old.

How do adolescents with mental illness react to stigma? First of all, their individual handlings of diagnostic labels varies greatly (just as it does for adults: Sect. 5.1.3, 'Diagnosis'). Some adolescents are relieved because diagnoses provide an explanation for confusing and frightening symptoms and may facilitate treatment and help-seeking. Others reject a diagnosis and being labelled; they may prefer nondiagnostic terms such as 'tantrums'. Whether they have been labelled diagnostically or not, many children and adolescents feel self-stigma and shame about their often painfully felt otherness [468].

Overcoming stigma is difficult for children and adolescents. Apart from their weaker social standing mentioned above, they are particularly dependent on the acceptance of others in their same age group. The decision for or against disclosure is therefore all the more difficult (Sect. 4.3.4). Among the many risks of telling others about one's illness is social rejection at school. Yet disclosure allows for social support and exchange, and frees one from the burden of secrecy. Secrecy can lead to social isolation: 'I would be happy if someone had said to me: "You should tell your close friends about it." Because now I have lost all my friends' ([464], p. 300). Stigma is ultimately the strongest obstacle to help-seeking for young people with mental health problems [104, 243]. The fear of public stigma, self-stigma and shame as well as the fear of being considered inferior or weak by asking for help all act as deterrents [468]. Stigma therefore contributes to the fact that mental disorders among young people often go untreated for years. This not only worsens the course of the illness but often has bitter, long-term consequences for school, professional training and social networks.

How can the stigma of mental illness in young people and its consequences be reduced? Some programmes have been designed to improve teachers' knowledge of the subject. They show positive results for reducing stigma, but there are few robust evaluations [469]. Offering low-threshold psychological counselling and help in schools could make help-seeking easier for adolescents with mental health problems. In these situations, however, stigma remains an obstacle—many young people fear that taking advantage of such offers means they will be labelled and subsequently discriminated against [470]. Another approach is Mental Health First Aid, a programme that provides information about symptoms, recognition of mental illness and ways to help. It is discussed in more detail in Sections 8.1.5 and 8.1.6. In one large Australian study, a Mental Health First Aid programme targeted towards teenagers showed that participants subsequently became more aware of peers' suicidal crises and were more willing to help them [471]. The positive effect was still ongoing, albeit slightly weaker, a year later. A version of the peer-led group programme HOP designed for young people with mental illness has proven to reduce stigma stress and self-stigma (Sect. 9.2 [472]).

Any and all programmes that aim to effectively reduce prejudice among adolescents who are not ill should contain the following three elements [473]:

1. The programme should be implemented by peers (i.e. young people with lived experience of mental illness) (Sect. 8.4).
2. The content should convey hope and a recovery orientation (i.e. it should not focus on symptoms, deficits and diagnoses).
3. Exchanges, including through social media and the use of online resources, should be part of the programme.

Last but not least, it is important when working with youth to make people with mental illness recognisable as *human beings*. This is the best remedy against the dehumanisation caused by stigma (Sect. 1.4). The school projects Irrsinnig Menschlich and Irre Menschlich are successful examples of this approach (Sects. 8.4.5 and 8.4.6).

To this discussion belongs the hot topic of school and the inclusion of children and adolescents with psychiatric or intellectual disabilities (e.g. autism with or without intellectual disability). Article 24 of the UN-CRPD (Sect. 7.5.2) establishes the right of people with disabilities to access an inclusive education system with individual support (i.e. children with disabilities have the right to attend the same classes as children without disabilities). Some German federal states have abolished 'special needs' schools as a result, but in many places there are now dual structures in place and parents can decide what kind of school to send their child to. The implementation of these choices is not always easy, not least because qualified personnel for the support of disabled children is lacking in mainstream schools. From a stigma perspective, certain dilemmas arise:

- By attending a special school for students with intellectual disabilities, children are automatically labelled. But being labelled as needing support is also necessary to receive support in a mainstream school and its effects are thus unavoidable.
- In addition, behavioural problems or learning disabilities in mainstream schools can lead to labelling and social exclusion by classmates—possibly more than in special schools.
- In mainstream schools, pupils with disabilities are more directly socially compared to other children without disabilities (in their self-evaluations and in their evaluations by others), which can impair their self-esteem.

The danger seems to be real: many parents refrain from getting support for their children in mainstream schools to avoid the label—even when the child would be entitled to it due to his disability needs. But successful inclusion can lead to children with and without disabilities living and learning together. And social contact can reduce prejudice or prevent it from arising in the first place (Sect. 8.4). To achieve this, the contact must be positive and this in turn depends on resources (including staff). Given the complexity of this situation, the question of attending a mainstream or special needs school should remain an individual decision. I am not aware of data on the consequences of the dual structure system's implementation within German schools.

5.8 Migrants and Refugees

We live in an age of global migration. While the term *migrant* is not well defined, it is primarily used to describe a person who has left their home country for one or several reasons (e.g. to find work or education in a new country, to look for a better life, or to escape hunger or violence). According to the International Organization for Migration (https://iom.int [474]), there were approximately 270 million migrants worldwide in 2019 (3.5% of the world's population). About three-quarters of all migrants were of working age, with an equal ratio of men and women.

The term *refugee* is defined by the UN Refugee Convention of 1951 [475] as a person who has left his or her home country for fear of persecution based on ethnicity, religion, political opinion and other characterisations. According to the UN High Commissioner for Refugees (https://unhcr.org), there were around 71 million refugees at the end of 2018; 26 million were refugees outside their home country, and around 41 million were internally displaced people (e.g. Syrians who had fled from their hometown to other parts of Syria). About half were under 18 years of age. The countries of origin of most refugees in 2018 were (in descending order) Syria, Afghanistan and South Sudan.

For the sake of simplicity, only migrants (whether or not they are also refugees) will be discussed here. However, the distinction between the two is critical, not least in regards to complicated issues of asylum and rights to stay. For example: depending on the German federal state, the health services to which people are entitled arise from a combination of factors including their length of stay, the status of the asylum procedure and the respective framework agreements between that federal state and health insurance companies. This is a maze that even experts find hard to negotiate. Fortunately, access to the labour market in Germany—a key pathway to integration for refugees (Sect. 7.1.2)—has recently been made much easier.

What role does stigma play for migrants? In the following section, a few selected issues are discussed. First and foremost, migration and migrant status in the country of arrival can contribute to the development of a mental illness. Second, there is a dual stigma attached to migrants with mental illness: that of their illness and that of their migrant status. Third, there may be discrimination against migrants in the healthcare system. Finally, interventions for migrants can include the issue of stigma and structural disadvantage of this group.

Mental illness is more common amongst migrants in a country of arrival than amongst its general public. Particularly common are depression, anxiety and, depending on the reason and course of the migration, posttraumatic stress disorder. This is because migration, especially due to fleeing or displacement, is associated with danger, uprooting and numerous material and social losses. However, the prevalence of mental illness continues to rise in the years after arrival in the new country, which indicates a continuing stress due to lack of social integration and unemployment [476].

Psychosis, which psychiatry regards as a predominantly biological illness, is also more frequent among migrants (another argument for the greater inclusion of social factors into our understanding of mental illness [477], Sect. 2.3.2). This fact has been known since studies were conducted on Norwegian immigrants in the United States at the beginning of the 20th century. A review of individual studies with a total of about 10,000 first- and second-generation immigrants with psychosis showed that psychosis was twice as prevalent among immigrants and their offspring as among the population of the host country [478]. Therefore, it is not the process of migration but rather the immigrant status with which both the first and second generation (who were born in the host country) identify, that seems to increase the risk of psychosis. This points to discrimination and low social status as risk factors for psychosis. This conclusion is in fact strengthened by its exception: Jewish immigrants to Israel. Unlike in their countries of origin, Jewish immigrants are no longer members of a discriminated minority. In Israel, their risk of psychosis has not been found to increase [478].

Migrants with mental illness have to struggle with the stigma of their illness as well as that of their migrant status. This has several consequences, listed here:

- Multiplied and intersecting discrimination has a stronger impact on mental and physical health, particularly through stress reactions and harmful coping reactions (Sect. 1.8) that hinder recovery.
- Some migrants come from cultures where mental illness and mental health service use are highly stigmatised [479]. Therefore, many suffer from self-stigma or shame and do not seek help [480, 481]. Different illness concepts can also make communication more difficult (Sect. 3.1.7). A man from Somalia said the following about professionals in his arrival country's Western healthcare system: 'They don't understand what this problem is. This is Djinn [spirit]. You need another prescription. Something like the Quran' ([482], p. 11). A German population survey compared attitudes on depression amongst Germans to those of first- and second-generation Turkish immigrants. First-generation immigrants born in Turkey held the most negative attitudes, both in terms of keeping their distance from people with depression and in terms of self-stigma and guilt regarding their own depression [483]. Recent interventions have therefore specifically targeted self-stigma as a barrier to help-seeking amongst immigrants. One such online programme, which was designed for male refugees mainly from the Arab world with posttraumatic stress disorder, was shown to reduce self-stigma [484].
- There may be discrimination against migrants with mental health problems in the healthcare systems of countries of arrival. Four issues are important for equal access to healthcare for migrants: accessibility and availability of help and treatment; financing of their treatment/health insurance; addressing linguistic and cultural needs; a health policy focus on migrants' health, including in-depth research on the group's general health and evaluation

of the effectiveness of improvement measures [485]. An overview of 38 countries, including all EU countries and Switzerland, showed a very mixed picture in regards to immigrant healthcare. The vast majority of those working in the psychiatric-psychotherapeutic care system appeared to have no significant intercultural knowledge to help conduct work with migrants. Particularly pronounced deficits were found in countries that joined the EU after 2000. The situation was better in countries that addressed the health of migrants across different policy areas (for an overview of 'health in all policies', see [486]).

A straightforward example of a structural barrier to good care of migrants with mental illness regards interpreting services in Germany that are not reimbursed by health insurance companies. I recall seeing a migrant who had been admitted to the psychiatric hospital during a night-time emergency. He held out his cell phone to me the next morning and though we did not speak a common language, he showed me the phone's German translation of what he had just said; in turn, it could translate my spoken words into his language. In such a situation, many questions arise: from the befuddling reliability of translation algorithms to the confidentiality of the data.

What interventions are available for migrants with mental illness? First, cognitive behavioural therapy can improve symptoms of anxiety, depression and posttraumatic stress disorder [487]. These therapies should be made available, but because our healthcare system is overstretched in this respect, a staged approach is often recommended: in the case of moderate symptoms, self-help (including via smartphones) should be promoted, and counselling by other trained refugees (so-called peer-to-peer counselling) should be offered. Professional psychological help should only be pursued in the event of more severe symptoms. From a stigma perspective, current problems are clear: refugees are fobbed off with second-class care, whereas the German public receive better, more direct treatment [488]. Outreach work, whereby practitioners visit the homes of migrants, especially refugees, is also often recommended. Unfortunately, outreach work in the German mental healthcare system is elusive (Sect. 7.3.4), especially for this target group.

There are, however, rays of hope: the Lower Saxony project, refuKey, integrates low-threshold outpatient counselling into a psychosocial centre designed for refugees. It is a 'cooperative competence centre' that advises and accompanies patients and professionals across the different care sectors and offers psychiatric hospital care. Initial results indicate that offering such comprehensive care more effectively addresses mental health problems in refugees than the usual undersupply (Evaluation report, 3 Aug. 2019; https://refukey.org). School-based programmes are a special form of staged care that can be aimed at students who are refugees. These include various forms of assistance with varying degrees of complexity: for the families of schoolchildren and for schools as well as for different types of need [489]. The approach is plausibly effective, particularly because all refugees of school age (and indirectly, their parents) can be reached through schools. More research is still needed on the effectiveness of this approach.

Adequate care for refugees requires integrated care first and foremost. Housing, education, employment, individual needs and legal issues need to be covered along with psychosocial support [476]. This is because both mental health and successful integration depend to a large extent on these social factors—not least the experience and feeling of acceptance rather than discrimination in one's country of arrival [490]. The language barrier and unfamiliarity of a care system mean that migrants in general and refugees in particular are often dependent on coordinated assistance. Unfortunately, their needs are likely (un)met by a fragmented, rigid care system divided into sectors that even locals find difficult to navigate (Sect. 7.3.3). Vulnerable migrants with mental disorders facing this type of structural discrimination are at a particular disadvantage.

CHAPTER 6

Personal Perspectives

6.1 Stigma in the Lives of Service Users

MARTINA HELAND-GRAEF

Hello, I am Martina Heland-Graef, a service user and professional—I worked in psychiatry for many years as a nurse and then became ill myself. What a blow it was to suddenly stand on the other side and watch everything around you change. Family, friends and work colleagues were suddenly a little different. The family was confused and didn't understand anything at first. Friends and work colleagues became a little distant, unsure, concluding with: 'Yes, you do belong on the other side now.' Life was a balancing act that lasted for four years before I decided to live with my illness, to live with the voices. From then on, many things became easier, including with family, former work colleagues and friends.

Service users can decide how they want to live, just like everyone else. But they do have to make a decision—that's the most important thing. Decisions are not set in stone and can evolve, and you can adapt them to your way of life. Service users must carry on with being the makers of our own lives—not our relatives, society, hospital, therapist or, even worse, legal guardian. Stigma and discrimination are parts of our lives. But if we do not let ourselves be affected by them, we make it harder for others to behave in a stigmatising or discriminatory manner. It is not an easy journey, but one for all and all for one: service users join together and organise amongst themselves, and do so successfully. The awareness of a service user to be different, to be valuable and to defend oneself, is a tremendous life experience that others will never have. Many service users organise themselves in the area of self-help and thereby gain new hope, a new self-image and a sense of personal responsibility. This means that I am able to learn through self-determination how to better deal with stigma. Through experiencing that I can make it and cope with problems, stigma loses its power. This is uniquely helpful.

Stigma in Different Areas of Life

In different areas of my life, be it my private life, at work, in public, in politics or amongst others with mental illness, it is important for me to assert my position—including against stigma and discrimination. For this I lean on friends and a stable environment: a support group can be a constant source of strength. Family or life partners can also be important mainstays. When my husband says: 'I think you need to be alone', I know that he doesn't want to get rid of me but rather realises sooner than I do that I am in need of a break. I used to think that he didn't want me to have a part in his life because I would react differently than before the illness. In my personal life, I know I am not the only one who experiences stigma as something terrible. In self-help group discussions, I have heard stories of others' children turning their backs on their parents and trying to protect the grandchildren from these 'dangerous' service users. Sometimes nothing can be done: you can't force your children's partners to try and understand service users or let us be part of their family life. But I have learned that we service users are able to grow from these heartbreaking experiences.

Thoughts on Getting Started

Stigmatisation occurs when a group with otherness is marginalised. Nowadays, even the poor or people living on a basic income are stigmatised (i.e. labelled and pushed away). Stigmatisation is

113

particularly terrible for service users because we are immediately classified as a threat that others should be afraid of. Human rights are supposed to ensure that no one stigmatises someone else (though I think they imagined this to be easier). Human rights laws and legal protections against discrimination (Sect. 5.1.8) need to be better explained to people. Why must stigma hold me back? I already feel restricted by my voices. If others, who really have no idea what I go through, want to marginalise me, I am prevented from living a fully self-determined life. Stigma prevents me from fighting for my rights.

Fear, Fury, Fight

The fight against stigma often feels like Don Quixote battling windmills. Regardless of the challenge or outcome, you have to do something about it: awareness raising, speaking positively about mental illness and recovery, media dissemination of more positive stories. Every single person should know that it is wrong to label, and thereby paralyse, the weak. It frustrates me that stigma is tolerated and that often nobody stands up in support. Helping others to help themselves does not have to be a difficult task. I always have the feeling, which has been confirmed by many other service users, that we must do more than others to prove ourselves … but what do I have to prove? That I can work? That I can live my life?

I've been told that when I'm loud and defend myself, I'm radical. But we service users need a loud voice so that we can be heard in regards to our rights to self-determination, to reasonable accommodations, to have a say, to nonviolent treatment. We do have a right to treatment and to protection from public assault. But people need to know we're not dangerous. It helped that I came out with my illness—it was like a weight had been lifted and life became a lot easier. However this kind of initiative took courage, strength and time. Let's continue with our fight.

Stigma Within One's Own Ranks, Among People With Mental Illness

Stigma is unfortunately also evident within our own ranks, amongst people with mental illness. At first I really didn't think there would be, but I had it wrong. This type of stigma was a terrible blow. When I became affected by mental illness, I was excluded by my new peers because I had worked as a nurse in a psychiatric hospital and had therefore been part of 'the system'. This exclusion was more humiliating and worse than anything I had experienced before. If I had experienced this from others (i.e. from professionals or society), I certainly would have defended myself. But how does one do so against one's peers? I cannot answer that question—it still hits too close to home. But I find it important to honestly address this issue here, just as I have in other areas of my life.

My Private Life Is Not Only About Stigma

The biggest issues regarding stigma that service users encounter are at work and in their private lives. I tend to prioritise my private life because that is where most problems arise and where the impact can feel most devastating. Unfortunately, the people who are closest or nearest to you are particularly difficult to face: family members withdraw, in-laws find it difficult, children side with their partners … all for legitimate reasons. But for people with mental illness, it is difficult to cut those connections. Family is the smallest, most intimate unit of all, and of all people they show you how stigma works.

Many service users decide not to disclose for fear of losing friends. Unfortunately, it tends to happen anyway. How are people with mental illness supposed to deal with this? Most receive psychotropic drugs that involve visible side effects (e.g. weight gain, repetitive movements), and so they stand out (which affects them as well as others). I know many service users who do not want to come out about their condition. They are concerned about their status and perception from others, or don't want to put up with others' reactions. It's especially upsetting when their best friends abandon them and only one or two are left in the end. Of course, new friendships can be made amongst peers with mental illness. But this is unfortunately an already special and distinct kind of world, as we are not accepted elsewhere. Through our otherness we experience stigma even if it is not openly stated. Case in point: I once booked seven single rooms at a hotel and then requested an invoice for our Bavarian alliance of service users. All of a sudden, according to the hotel, the rooms had become occupied.

Stigma and Work—'How to Get Rid of Me?'

I believe that service users are different, but we are assets if you allow us to be. Psychiatry is with us throughout our lives, each and every one of us. We've all been at a crisis point in our lives, some more, some less. I figure that whoever is hell-bent on ruining me must have a much bigger problem with life than just me. They say that barking dogs never bite—well, someone who stigmatises does both.

I asked a colleague if I could relay her story here. She agreed but does not want to be recognised, which I gratefully respect. A few years back, she held a really good job in which she was proficient and gave 100%, and sometimes more. She was respected by her colleagues and appreciated by her supervisors. Unfortunately, at some point, the synapses in her brain became muddled (as she still refers to it) like a storm in a teacup. She heard phones ringing and people talking that had not previously been there—it was monstrous. She no longer sat with the others at their breakfast break and refused to comply with her supervisors. She was admitted to a hospital, and the stigma took its course, all by itself and without mercy.

She joined our self-help group, but she and her mind hovered listlessly. She always looked like she was about to give up for good. It was unspeakably sad. At one point I was able to persuade her to take a weekend trip with me, to a place that is quiet and uneventful. On that very same day we began to sort out the muddled synapses in her mind; we differentiated between her favourite and least favourite parts of the muddle, and we later gave the parts she liked the names of people she could imagine talking to about the confusion in her head. Through conversation, she would be able to convince her colleagues that she could work as well as before, as long as her workplace environment could be adjusted and demands could be moved to different times of the day. While planning for this conversation, she repeatedly reminded herself that things can go wrong, that they don't always work out. She set her priorities, and I was pleased to see that she could again do various tasks almost the same as before, with little to no impairment. I watched with great contentment, happiness and excitement as she realised her capabilities as well. It was as if I was witnessing a rebirth—which is what it was in the end.

We were pleased, and she had made a plan. Her direct supervisor had to be the first one told; he agreed with nearly all of the suggestions she came up with, and was impressed by and curious about her openness. She did immediately come to grief with two colleagues and had to put up with them not wanting to have anything more to do with her. It was her first run-in with stigma. What a tumble it was—but we celebrated the successes she did have. She resumed her work and kept in touch on the phone when necessary. She only called three times, and after a few weeks she stopped phoning all together. At the next self-help group sessions, she sat up straight and proud, satisfied and happy, with her head held high. She thanked everyone who had believed in her.

For me, this woman's story shows that everyone has the right to take a chance (or several) at having a job. Two years on, she now has an advisory role at her workplace for people in crisis. She is taking very few psychotropic drugs. Being given a chance, help and some courage brought her back to live her life despite the stigma. She still won't disclose her illness, but this is to be respected. For her, stigma was both a challenge and an opportunity, which perhaps she understood only much later.

Society and Politics in the Life of a Service User

Upon becoming a service user, I was asked by a peer if I would want to join a regional alliance of service users. My voices said no; there was first a battle to be won against them. After, I discussed it my husband. He was sceptical, but he didn't fight back. And so I became a board member of a national association that looks after the interests of service users. I learned through this work that the general public is certainly odd—socially as well as politically.

I worked politically and became more widely known as a service user. I quickly found my way around my responsibilities and began to develop strategies for myself, to know what I absolutely had to listen to and what was more flexible. I didn't hide my challenges with concentration in meetings: I couldn't bear it when everyone talked at the same time, so I chose to be upfront about it and most people understood. Nevertheless, whenever I'd speak up, I always had the feeling that several of those sitting in on the meeting would not listen, instead looking at their mobile phones. And there they were again, the voices that said: 'They don't take you seriously, you're nothing to them, they don't care what your opinion is about what service users need.' After I'd paused to put a stop to the voices, which was just long enough for someone else to chime in, I finally spoke up: 'It's rude to look at a mobile phone when I have something to say. I feel like I'm not being taken seriously here.' I then got up and said: 'A break after two hours of sitting is important too', and walked outside. That moment was a breakthrough; from then on everyone knew what stigma is and what effect it can have on me.

I have learned that it doesn't really help to whine and rant about the existence of stigma—it will always exist as long as people are different from one another. It is up to us, those with mental illness, to inform others about what stigma does to us. We service users need to work with strong allies to figure out how to stop this ogre. We cannot and must not give up, be it politically or amongst our families or at the hospital. I never cared that much about stigma before, but I know that it can hurt and even kill in the long run. We can't let that happen, and neither can society. I work every day to minimise stigma through my work, and I am confident we can affect change. All peers and professionals should be able to stand up and say: 'Hey, we're all human beings, nobody should lay negative words (stigma) on another person.' Let's call upon society to find more positive terms and messages about mental disorders. Help people with mental illness to rise up! We need to find various ways to appeal to people in all areas of life and make them aware in order to reduce stigma.

Stigma in the Life of Service Users—How Do We Deal With It?

It is important that we get to know ourselves well. This is an individual's greatest defense against stigma. If I myself know who I am and what I can do, then nobody in the world can doubt me. An example: a village, a festival, a woman, a discussion about mentally ill people. I heard someone say the following: 'I wouldn't let people like that save my children in a dangerous situation.' The man she was talking about used to be a fireman but had to leave the job because of his mental illness. It was cruel. It nearly took my breath away. I was quick to tell her that a few days earlier, her nursery-school-age children had wandered far outside the village with the dog and that I was one of *those* (mentally ill) people who had noticed and informed her as a concerned mother. Many people, I think, don't even realise what they are doing to us with their ignorance, thoughtlessness or disrespect. I know what I am capable of and what is appropriate—even if I am a service user.

I think that a lot depends on a person's own resilience or psychological resistance, which is what is needed now! What is also needed is discovery of one's own abilities to mitigate harmful behaviour or reactions prevalent in society, so that he or she will find it possible to be part of society again. Unfortunately, psychiatry does not teach us to figure out on what our own resiliencies may be. It's just interested to see who reacts in what way to which medication. Research trials are continually being made to prove this scientifically. Yet humans get a raw deal; we're often forgotten and unfortunately not taken into account as whole beings in our treatment.

Service users can find this kind of care in self-help groups or, if they are lucky, in a doctor's outpatient practice. In a group with peers who all have similar problems and shared goals but who hold different approaches to solving them, individuals can decide for themselves how to find an

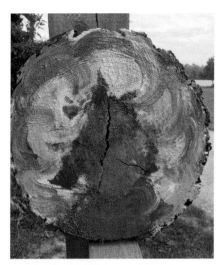

Fig. 6.1 I painted this myself: a picture and puzzle. I am in it, as well as an image of a horse. I painted it on a good day. I would like to see mutual respect, conversations with each other, listening to each other. I would like to see positive debate in all areas of life. (Courtesy of Martina Heland-Graef.)

appropriate solution (Fig. 6.1). Good solutions are found through conversation, and then self-healing can begin. I have set up a self-help group and still attend it regularly because time and again it helps me to start a project with renewed vigour and knowledge of what I have to do. Many colleagues and peers feel the same way. Resilience means being resistant to life crises. This is best learnt from like-minded people in a self-help group. In my own group, I fed off the courage of others, was able to come out about my illness and realised that I can be strong for others.

Stigma is bad. But through dealing with it, I have grown. I realised that I can defend myself. In this sense, learning to cope with stigma has actually changed my life in a positive way. I know things about myself today that I never would have experienced otherwise. I finally felt free when everyone knew about my illness; I no longer had to play hide and seek. I now had all the strength and attention I needed for work and for my peers. I would never have known that I could speak in front of large groups of people and also share personal information. I have experienced and learned first-hand that I can help 'normal' people better understand those of us with mental illness. I have been given a great deal of support in my work to bring a certain amount of open-mindedness and freedom to this world and to convey to service users and others in peer support settings that a mental illness does not have to mean failure even when it feels like one. I have enough energy for all of these self-help projects because I no longer have to concentrate on my secrecy.

Family and Stigma

I was allowed to witness an affected family's story that, at first, seems terrible and sad. The mother had a mental illness and had tried for a long time in hospital to get used to her voices and overcome the psychosis. When she arrived back home, her youngest son (about six years old) started bringing other children home from school for lunch. The mother would ask each morning how many would be coming over so that she could adjust the amount of food. She began to notice that the children would initially eye and observe her very carefully but later would be very friendly, thank her for the food and leave. One day, however, she observed that the children were giving gifts or money to her son at the front door. She told me it seemed very strange and that she didn't really know what to make of it. I encouraged her to ask him. The son explained that at school they had to talk about what their parents did for a living and how things were at home. Her son, fascinated by her illness, just told his class that his mother 'is nuts'. That was his matter-of-fact tone about it. Because he could not explain everything properly and the children were asking questions, he decided to show-case his mother. The son said: 'Well, if we go somewhere else, we have to pay too, in a museum or something.' He informed his mother that he had done nothing other than what those places did.

It took me a long time to consider that this son had actually acted in a destigmatising way. So did the mother, by the way. Strictly speaking, his experiences with his mother (who was not quite the same as before but still impressive and sweet, and not dangerous or mean or terrible) were something he could share with his classmates. By charging the so-called entry fee, he could pro-mote the fact that his mother, albeit different, could also cook food and be kind. His mother and I talked about it at length, and we came to the conclusion that the son had acted very self-confi-dently and in a way that destigmatised himself and his environment. The fact that he made some pocket money—well, no one was hurt. By the way: during the summer, most of the children would come around every day and were not afraid of contact with the mother—unlike their parents. In an uncomplicated way, they enjoyed cooking, playing or simply being with her.

That this son later wanted nothing more to do with his mother is another story. Another one of her sons wants his mother to leave the family; he claims that if he could, he'd have her locked up. What is a mother to do in this case? All she can do is activate powers of self-healing and strengthen her resilience in order to make life without children worth living. It's sad, but who really knows what experiences like these are meant to teach us at the end of the day? Who knows what life will bring, even for a service user?

Self-Acceptance and Authenticity

One doesn't need to receive self-acceptance and authenticity from others. I am convinced that all of us already have self-acceptance within ourselves—otherwise we would question ourselves every day on every decision we make. Yet only those of us who have supposedly lost it, because of illness or difference, actively think about it. The capacity for self-acceptance, self-respect and authenticity were given to all of us at varying degrees from birth. It is important to apply them and surround yourself with people who recognise the struggle and thereby offer support. Many people have relayed back to me that it is good to hear that everything in life has meaning, that I have to be just as I am in order to connect with others. Acknowledging and talking about it helps—if you're authentic, you're believable. People want to be accepted for who they are. There is a power difference and distance between a government department and service users. But there is no such gap between us service users and peers.

Politics and Public Relations

My courage and work encourage others and give them the energy to fight against exclusion and stigma. I found strength in this way, and unfortunately many people find this frightening. I've been able to make a difference in many ways. For example, I have actively collaborated with the Bavarian Mental Health Care Act (Sect. 7.5.5). I have worked in public relations for the German National Alliance of Service Users and even longer for the Bavarian Alliance of Service Users. I have talked to politicians and other decision-makers and explained our problems. I have fought against power structures, violence and coercion, for open psychiatry and for non-violent work in psychiatry. In this work, I make it clear that you have to listen and talk to us, that we also want to listen and that together we can bring about change. I remember the people who died due to psychiatry, the victims of euthanasia (Sect. 2.1.2). For a long time, I remained unaware of this history, but this year at the Aktion T4 event in Berlin, I was taken back to a time when I prob-ably would have died as well. I now work with others to make sure these events are not forgotten. I also write reports for our service user group newsletter, to let our members know what we do all year round: that we are vigilant, also regarding political parties and their agendas; that the UN Convention on the Rights of Persons with Disabilities is implemented; that we want to respect human rights; and that no security forces should be allowed to enter psychiatric institutions. By participating, we are heard and give a voice to those who cannot or do not want to disclose but are suffering. We want to be allowed to live independently—even if we do so in unusual ways.

Recently, I was at an event in which the Bavarian Mental Health Care Act was once again under discussion. To be honest, I was under the impression that I didn't need to go at all—I already felt I knew everything I need to know. But someone at the event said that ever since the new law had been enforced in Bavaria, it had become harder to place people in hospitals against their will. Hooray, I thought, the problem has been acknowledged. However, what came next was a kick in the teeth. The man said that those who are no longer accommodated by institutions live a neglected and shabby life. Hello, I said, psychiatry would have to accommodate a third of Bavaria's population if you admitted all people who appear 'neglected' or 'shabby' for all kinds of reasons (although it is not even true that they are neglected). And just because after this new law they cannot be forced into the psychiatric system, they are not admitted—can you believe it? This man's views and our exchange is exactly why we service users and advocates have to continue to participate in such events. I argued that people's mindsets have to change; we have to find other solutions, such as supporting the Salvation Army with more money or donations. People are freer under this law, and freedom in every sense is the highest good. Well, I hope I didn't talk my head off.

My Life as a Professional and Person With Experience

I trained as a nurse in psychiatry from 1980 to 1983. Before that, I caught up on my school-leaving certificates, boarding at a preparatory nursing school to bridge the time until I was allowed to start my training. In total, I trained for five years—not because I was too stupid, but because I was too young. At barely 15 years old, I got started at the preparatory nursing school of the Bayreuth district psychiatric hospital. Away from home for the first time, I entered a world I would come to see as normal; I never felt pity and focused on what my help could look like. People would walk through the hospital parks laughing and seeming to have a great time. I once gathered up my courage and dared to ask a gentleman why he was laughing and what he found so amusing. He immediately froze and stopped laughing; his face, which had been cheerful just a moment before, was marked by fear. He began to run away, but I tried to stay next to him. Panting, I asked him why he was running and told him I meant no harm, I just wanted to have a conversation. But I didn't stand a chance. Continuing on my own way, I realised that he must have been experiencing something special to make him look so happy, joyful and satisfied.

Eventually, my training came to an end, and I still had not learned what the man who was happily laughing to himself had been thinking about. Time and again I would remember him without being able to figure out his secret. After three years as a registered nurse, I trained as a specialist nurse in psychiatry. We had to learn the theory in our free time, which meant many extra hours of study. But the additional weekends didn't matter; I wanted to do the training because I thought it would help me to solve the mystery of the gentleman in the park. I was always asking doctors and other colleagues about it, but none of their answers was satisfactory. One answer I was given was about the heard voices and other phenomena that some people experience that we cannot. The doctor said we have to take away the suffering of those types of patients: 'You can see that they live in their own world.' I wanted to know how she knew that these people would be willing to have their worlds taken away from them. I told her about the encounter with the smiling and laughing gentleman. The doctor assumed that he was hearing voices and was receiving medication to counteract them. I was a nurse and, yes, I was in the field of psychiatry, and, yes, I understood what I had learned, but that was a line of thinking that frustrated me to no end. Why are people not asked? I didn't think that the gentleman was suffering—he was afraid of me and my question.

I decided to try and gain the confidence of the gentleman. It took a long time and required many 'bribery attempts'. At some points I thought it was all for nothing, but then one day he asked me if I liked it there, at the hospital. I did not fully understand but said, 'Yes, I think so. I like my work.' He looked at me and then at his hands for a long time, placing one on top of the other. He then asked me: if I had to live there like him, would I also like living in one room with four people whom I couldn't stand? I backed down and told him that I probably wouldn't like that. Then I said: 'But I always see you smiling when you go for a walk, you seem relaxed and somehow happy.' He smiled: 'You are the first person to ask me why I smile when I go for a walk. I listen to the voices, they talk, they're funny and are always ready with a joke, and they laugh at the people I meet.' I wanted to know that he wasn't afraid, but he immediately went rigid and said to me that he was very afraid of the doctors who wanted to take his voices away. He needed them—they were the only ones who talked to him.

Why take away the happiness of this person? Why not instead make a contract with him (e.g. if his voices want something bad from him, he could still take medication)? Since that encounter, I have always, truly always, asked the people I am responsible for what they believe could help them. And their wishes are not always unreliable. In this work, I have become closer to many more patients than the doctors have (even if the doctors refuse to believe it).

When I fell ill and was able to admit to myself that I heard voices—and mine were not friendly, as much as I wanted them to be—I thought a lot about that gentleman. I thought that I perhaps just have to be nice to the voices, without wanting to get rid of them. That's how I eventually accepted my arrangement with the voices. I once tried to explain this to a doctor, and he increased my medication without being asked. When I protested … well, that's another story. All I'm saying is that stigma is everywhere, but you don't always have to take it seriously.

Conclusion

I sometimes find it easier to put up with stigma and then bring it up at a later time as a topic of discussion to try to get 'normal' people to understand it. Tackling this issue is not so much about immediately responding to something threatening everywhere as it is about delving into conversations to make others aware of stigma and its consequences. If society has no opinion on the inclusion or stigma of service users, it is up to us to change it. We always have the opportunity to talk to one another. Amidst the service landscape for service users, much could still be changed to combat stigma more effectively. Community mental health services (i.e. services that are close to our living environments) enable us to find better help; we need shorter distances to multifaceted services that strengthen resistance and courage. Dorothea Buck once said that as long as we talk to each other, we do not kill each other (Sect. 7.3.4, 'Peer Support').

6.2 Stigma and Relatives
JANINE BERG-PEER
'You Have a Symbiotic Relationship With Your Daughter!'

It was 60 years ago that I first experienced mentally ill people and their relatives being stigmatised. My mother, who suffered from a manic-depressive illness, attempted suicide. As a consequence, she and our family were not exactly shunned, but people whispered. At school, there were knowing looks between teachers and students. On social occasions, the conversation would suddenly fall silent when my mother turned up. Still today I come across people from my youth who, when I greet them, suddenly exchange looks and cautiously ask me if it wasn't my mother who…?

From my estimation, little has changed in my lifetime. Coverage of almost every criminal act resulting in death shows the extent to which people with a mental illness are still stigmatised. The media's knee-jerk reaction is to raise the question of the perpetrator's psychological stability. A headline such as 'Perpetrator in Psychotherapeutic Treatment?' immediately establishes an unspoken agreement between journalist and reader. Psychotherapy? All right, then. We know what people with a mental illness are like: dangerous and unpredictable. This is quickly followed by questioning why such people are not locked away earlier. The implicit demand is clear: protect society from crazy violent criminals. Not only must the stigmatised group be rejected, but stigma itself should lead directly to concrete discrimination.

What Is the Function of Stigma?

People turn their backs on other groups because it strengthens their own group affiliation. This behaviour, also known as *othering*, highlights the positive characteristics of one's own group over the negative characteristics of another. The *other* group is devalued to demarcate one's own group from it. People distance themselves from the mentally ill and their relatives in order to be protected from becoming like *them*.

What Does Stigma Do?

People with mental illness have a wide range of stigmatising characteristics attributed to them: they are seen as dangerous, unpredictable, crazy or even stupid—a group of people one should stay away from. Those diagnosed with schizophrenia allegedly have a split personality—Dr Jekyll and Mr Hyde—which at certain stages will cause them to do scary and cruel things. They hear voices that supposedly force them to kill other people. Although these attributions apply especially to people with psychoses, all mentally ill people tend to be subject to similar prejudices.

Negative perceptions of mentally ill people carry consequences: they are shunned by colleagues, friends and often also by family members. The illness is kept secret, and the ill person is not invited or is kept 'hidden' when a family celebration takes place. Those with mental illness can also be treated brutally by police officers during compulsory hospitalisations if and when the police officers are convinced they pose a danger.

These negative perceptions of mentally ill people can lead to difficulties in finding housing and work. They often experience scant understanding in social situations—with authorities, in shops, on buses and trains. Their confusion, slowness or awkwardness are perceived as harbingers of dangerous behaviours or outbursts, and they correspondingly face unfriendly, hostile or harsh reactions.

A Mental Illness Takes Away One's Self-Confidence!

The effects of stigma on the self-confidence of people with mental illness are particularly serious. Social exclusion or harsh reactions make people with mental illness feel insecure and create a sense of inadequacy. 'A mental illness takes away all self-confidence', my daughter aptly put it a few years ago. My mother suffered so much from the stigma of mental illness that she was actually 'pleased' to later get the diagnosis of breast cancer. She could tell people about this somatic illness; suddenly she was given advice and friendly support. Stigma of mental illness has particularly grave consequences for the long term: it requires great emotional and cognitive effort to work one's way out of the crises and accompanying social slumps that mentally ill people are susceptible to time and again. After a crisis, people with mental illness must try to reconcile with friends, lovers, neighbours or colleagues. They often have to look for a new place to stay, find a new job or recommit to their interrupted education. All of this requires great strength and, above all, the confidence that it will work out. But those who repeatedly experience stigma can easily become discouraged in the long term.

Families and Relatives Are Also Stigmatised

Although there is widespread agreement that people with mental illness are stigmatised, the stigmatisation of families is less frequently addressed. As family members, we are also stigmatised when we are blamed and attributed with characteristics and behaviours that have purportedly driven our children into mental illness. Perhaps we family members would have been better off when evil spirits, the devil or excessive masturbation were considered the causes of mental illness. But ever since the discovery of the schizophrenogenic mother by the psychoanalyst Frieda Fromm-Reichmann in the 1940s, families have been seen as the perpetrators of schizophrenia in particular and have been condemned. Mothers are perceived as having an ambivalent attitude towards their children, which in turn leads children directly to schizophrenia. Autism can also allegedly be caused by mothers: cold-hearted 'refrigerator mothers' are to blame for the autism of their children. Although experts today repeatedly stress that these concepts are outdated, in my experience the schizophrenogenic and cold-hearted mother is still very much alive in the minds of many psychiatrists, psychotherapists, service users and even lay people. The schizophrenogenic mother is further developed within double-bind theory and high-expressed emotions theory, as well as in systemic theory. The focus is always on the fact that dysfunctional behavioural strategies, especially those of the mother, force the child to take refuge in a mental illness.

'But You Are a Very Dominant Woman!'

Twenty-two years ago, I was unaware that we mothers had the power to drive our children into schizophrenia—but I learned this quickly. When I first encountered psychiatry, a quite friendly psychiatrist tried to assure me: 'Your daughter has schizophrenia, but you don't have to feel guilty'. What an introduction to the minds of these practitioners. Of course, nobody told me explicitly that I had caused my daughter's illness. Implicitly, however, this conviction appeared in many comments made by experts and lay people. 'But you have a very symbiotic relationship with your daughter', a young psychiatrist told me 10 days after the diagnosis of her schizophrenia. 'That's not at all good for a psychotic. Every time you come to visit, you hug and kiss each other. It's not normal in a mother-daughter relationship.' When I told a colleague who had noticed my red and tear-stained eyes that my daughter was in a psychiatric hospital, his response was: 'You certainly are a very dominant woman!'

When my daughter insisted on wanting to do her secondary school leaving certificate, we were not only warned about taking such a 'dangerous' step, but I was also accused of wanting to transfer my career ambitions onto my poor, seriously ill daughter. After reading my book *Schizophrenia Sucks, Mum* (in German: *Schizophrenie ist scheiße, Mama*), a friend of mine said that it was perfectly clear to him why my daughter had developed a mental illness: 'She wanted to take revenge on you for sending her to a boarding school!' In the psychosis seminar, a social worker sighed: 'Terrible, these overprotective and controlling mothers. My poor client.'

I once had an unforgettably remarkable experience at a conference. Before my turn to speak, a friendly and young psychotherapist concluded her own talk with the words: 'No child with a mental illness could ever build a positive relationship with their mother in childhood. And now we are delighted to welcome Mrs Berg-Peer, who will tell us about her life with her mentally ill daughter.' We families are seen as overprotective, unstable, domineering, hostile or clingy. This is what many professionals think of us—even those who invite us to give lectures.

The schizophrenogenic mother is also immortalised in the media (Sect. 7.4). Few people have gotten to the heart of it the way movie director Alfred Hitchcock did. In his 1960 film *Psycho*, Norman Bates (played by Anthony Perkins) suffers from a mother complex: he kills women to whom he feels attracted, undeniably signifying a strong identification with his dead mother. The film is one of the most-watched thrillers of all time. Think of the number of people, including psychiatrists, who have since seen this film, in which the psychiatrist in the final scene explains the madness of Norman Bates to the court with a sentence about Bates' mother: 'She was a very clinging and challenging woman.'

How do professionals know that our behaviour is the cause? I have often wondered why, for many professionals, the schizophrenogenic mother still seems to play a role. Many tell me about conversations with service users who talk about their 'terrible' mothers and fathers. The professionals believe them. But I have heard just as many stories about 'terrible' psychiatrists and psychotherapists from service users. If I were to believe everything my daughter told me about professionals in times of crisis, I would never have let her go to one of them again. Personal encounters influence how we, the relatives, are seen by professionals: 'They really exist, those terrible mothers', I hear, and then I'm given examples of parental behaviours observed by psychiatrists. But are the few meetings with an agitated mother who has just brought her child to hospital in the middle of a serious crisis enough to warrant these 'diagnoses'? Is she crying? Unstable mother! Does she insist on talking? Domineering mother! Is she worried? Overprotective mother! Does she kiss her child when she greets them? Symbiotic relationship! But couldn't it be that we are simply feeling overwhelmed and helpless amidst our children's psychological crises? Psychiatrists judge us on the basis of an exceptional situation without having any idea of the coping strategies we exhibit in our normal, everyday lives. As families, we should be aware that patients are not the only ones diagnosed by psychiatrists—we mothers are, as well.

One could argue that psychiatrists' assumptions about us as families are irrelevant. However, stigma is most effective when there is an asymmetrical relationship (i.e. a power gap) between the person who is stigmatising and the person who is stigmatised (Sect. 3.1.4). This also has a negative effect on the dynamic between psychiatrists and relatives: psychiatrists have the power to allow us time to speak with them about our children. They also have the power to reinforce negative attitudes—often caused by the illness—of children towards their families. This power is certainly not exploited by all psychiatrists, but it does play a role in our communication. We are helplessly subjected to assumptions of psychiatrists in situations of fear and weakness.

But it is not only experts who stigmatise families. How often do we hear in our circles of acquaintances that someone has always known that certain past behaviours of other parents were not good. Divorce, early schooling, working mother, strictness or permissiveness—everything is used to explain why the mental illness occurred. 'How old was your daughter when you divorced her father?' 'So you've always worked?' 'Yes.' 'I see!' Everything is immediately clear. Now everyone knows why the poor child got sick. Cautious responses that such parental behaviours also produce many perfectly healthy children are only perceived as transparent defence strategies dictated by our feelings of guilt.

Even families with healthy children turn their backs and make us into *others* because they see the cause of the illness in the fact that our families are *different* and thereby not as good. This attribution has an important function for families with healthy children: if children only become mentally ill in bad families, then they are immune to it. Since they belong to the good families and behave properly, it cannot happen to them. I hear time and again that psychiatrists and relatives alike assume that many families feel guilty for their relative's mental illness. These feelings of guilt can be explained: if research has proven that people with mental illness are stigmatised in society, then all families in society, whether or not they have a relative with mental illness, are not free from it either. Those who have long assumed that only children from 'bad' families become mentally ill will suddenly find themselves confronted with their own prejudices when their own children are diagnosed (despite thinking they have done everything correctly).

People With Mental Illness Also Stigmatise Us

I was introduced to the conflict between service users and their relatives at my first conference, when I was asked to speak on the situation of families. Before I could say my first word, service users in the audience shouted loudly at me: 'If you have relatives, you don't need enemies!' Since then I have heard and read time and again that many service users exclusively blame their bad parents for their illnesses. They were too solicitous; they did not let go; they did not care (or cared too much); they failed as parents. To my knowledge, the exact causes of schizophrenia, for instance, remain unclear. But these service users seem to know for sure. From a psycho-hygienic point of view, I can understand why it might be a relief to be able to blame someone else for such a dreadful illness. But blaming families can also have a negative impact on people with mental illness.

What Effect Does Stigma Have on Families and Relatives?

No matter what you see as the cause of mental illness, nobody who works towards the recovery of the mentally ill can remain indifferent to the consequences of families being stigmatised. Publications, guidelines and lectures point out how important the involvement of families can be for the recovery of people with mental illness. But we as families must be enabled to offer meaningful support to our sick children. Does anyone truly believe that people who have been blamed for causing such a serious illness in their child can now be empathetically concerned about the care of their child? It is a heavy blow to families when confronted with this kind of accusation. We feel horrible and become increasingly insecure in our interactions with our children. These accusations are so distressing that we have to defend ourselves against them. And they are particularly hurtful because most families are already constantly, secretly asking themselves what they have done wrong.

It is almost unbearable if this accusation of blame comes from outside the family. Parents begin to defend themselves by pointing out that they have always been good parents, that their other children have not developed any illness, that they know other families in which the children were badly treated and yet no mental illness had occurred. We are so busy defending ourselves against these allegations that it can prevent us from thinking about whether there may in fact be some behavioural patterns of our own that were and are dysfunctional for a vulnerable child. We often fend off well-intentioned hints about changing our behaviour when dealing with our ill children because we fear that this will lead to accusations that we are responsible for the illness.

Some peer advocacy groups also want to defend themselves against being stigmatised by reinterpreting their otherness in a positive way; in turn, they try to stigmatise people without mental illness. With a book with an unhelpful title, *We Treat the Wrong People: Our Problem Is Normal People*, German psychiatrist Manfred Lütz has initiated a trend in which those who are marginalised retaliate against their exclusion and portray their own group as better. The slogan 'rather crazy than normalised' or T-shirts with the inscription 'Dangerous are those without diagnosis' follow this trend of devaluing those without mental illness. This approach is understandable from a human perspective, but I am sceptical that this way of dealing with stigma will actually help mentally ill people.

Consequences of Stigma for Relatives of People With Mental Illness

Stigmatisation of us as relatives is not only painful but can also have serious consequences for service users:

- Parents feel guilty and may wait too long before seeking professional help for their child.
- Psychiatrists and psychotherapists, as well as some social workers, do not want to have any contact with the parents, because they choose to always take the side of the service users.
- Families do not seek help for themselves because they don't feel they deserve it.
- Families do not want to accompany their children on a visit to a therapist because they are afraid of accusations and condemnations.
- Families hide the illness from colleagues and their friends because they are afraid of stigma. However, this does not offer them the possibility of receiving support and relief from stress.
- The feeling of guilt can affect them so badly that they permanently distance themselves from their children.

What Can One Do Against Stigma?

It is a good development that service users as well as psychiatrists and families want to do something against stigma, but the stabilising functions of stigma (Sect. 3.3) make me sceptical about large-scale antistigma programmes. It is not only a deficit in information that makes people need or want to distance themselves from mentally ill people. At big events like the Mut-Tour (courage tour) or at sporting events like 'Der Lauf und Markt für seelische Gesundheit' (The Run and the Market for Mental Health), I rarely see people who were previously sceptical about mentally ill people suddenly dissuaded from their stigmatising attitudes by these wonderful events. Having said that, I am in no way opposed to such efforts. On the contrary, they have a positive and supportive effect on service users. This is exactly what I think is important: instead of prioritising the reduction of public stigma, which at best can only be successful on a very long-term basis, we should help people with mental illness deal with being devalued. They should be able to develop counterstrategies in order to learn not to let every devaluation take a toll.

Similarly, I wonder whether it is useful to talk about stigma all the time and to refer to it as more and more widespread. Even if research has shown this to be true, people with mental illness must live in this world and find their way around their illness despite social rejection. We should support them not by sensing stigma in every rejection or stupid phrase but by emboldening them to depend less on the opinions of others. If they avoid all contact or arguments with 'normal' people, they cannot experience anything new and find out for themselves that not all people have negative attitudes towards mental illness. The American stigma researcher Patrick W. Corrigan has developed the peer-led group programme Honest, Open, Proud (Sect. 9.2), in which participants can learn to overcome their fears and deal with their illnesses in their own environments, with more confidence. Peer support can also help (Sect. 7.3.4). As peer counsellors or peer support workers, people with mental illness demonstrate a competence that gives them a unique selling point: only they have access to this sector of the labour market and can offer valuable skills to many institutions that complement the work of nurses, social workers and doctors.

Do Not Leave It to Others to Present the Image of the Mentally Ill

Above all, I believe that we should encourage people with mental illness—as well as their families, by the way—to speak publicly about their experiences as often as possible. In this way, much can be done to reduce stigma. If service users and relatives do not want others to talk about them and attribute certain characteristics to them, then they must step up and determine the narrative about people with mental illness themselves with their own personal stories.

CHAPTER 7

Stigma in Different Sectors of Society

Stigma operates in social contexts by way of specific norms, rules, and power structures. The various consequences of stigma for people with mental illness are therefore examined in this chapter by sectors: work (Sect. 7.1), housing (Sect. 7.2), healthcare (Sect. 7.3), media (Sect. 7.4) and law (Sect. 7.5). Different aspects of structural discrimination are highlighted for each of these five areas; for other areas, see Section 5.1.8. This chapter not only illustrates how widespread stigma is but also discusses opportunities in each area to reduce stigma, build positive attitudes and promote inclusion.

7.1 Work

'There is nothing more inclusive than work. Only work makes it possible to realise the membership to society—that is, participation in the narrower sense,' said the English social psychiatrist Douglas Bennett ([491], p. 4). Work can give a lot: a meaning and task for the body and mind, opportunities to learn, success and self-confidence, social contacts and income and thereby better conditions in the social sphere. Work can simply be a reason to get up in the morning. It is therefore unsurprising that most people with mental illness want to work in some way. Article 27 of the United Nations Convention on the Rights of Persons with Disabilities (UN-CRPD; Sect. 7.5.2) ensures people with psychiatric disabilities the right to work. Stigma, however, leads to social exclusion and is an obstacle in the field of employment. This section deals with the different ways in which stigma makes it difficult for people with mental illness to work. The first part is about the role of stigma for those who are employed (Sect. 7.1.1); the second part is focused on those without work (Sect. 7.1.2).

An individual's course of work and unemployment is determined by both economic and social factors. The pressure on the labour market during the global recession after 2008 has been an example of this. Researcher Sara Evans-Lacko has examined the impact of this recession on people with mental health problems across the EU, comparing average unemployment rates from 2006 to those in 2010 [492]. In 2006, unemployment was higher amongst people with mental health problems (12.7%) than those without (7.1%). But perhaps more importantly:

1. From 2006 to 2010, unemployment rose much more sharply amongst those with a mental health burden (to 18.2%) than those without (to 9.8%).
2. In 2010, unemployment amongst people with mental health problems was higher in countries where the general public tended to consider people with mental health problems as dangerous.

Conclusion

Public attitudes have concrete and harmful consequences for employees with mental health problems. Unemployment aggravates their situation and further increases the risk of social exclusion.

126

7.1.1 PEOPLE IN EMPLOYMENT

Addressing mental health problems in the workplace is critically important. In addition to the suffering experienced by people with mental illness and their relatives, their productivity is also affected. In highly industrialised countries with low unemployment, this either leads to desperately needed workers being absent due to illness *(absenteeism)* or to low productivity even when they are present in the workplace *(presenteeism)*. In Germany, mental disorders result in more lost workdays due to inability to work than any other type of illness, including musculoskeletal and respiratory illnesses [493]. When people become mentally ill, they are unable to work for longer periods of time than when faced with any other illness (at around one and a half months on average). The productivity losses due to presenteeism are many times higher [494]. Therefore the self-interest of employers on economic grounds alone should suffice for increased investment in screening and treatment of employees' mental disorders. A model calculation based on German data showed that timely spending on screening for depression in all employees of a company plus spending on treatment (e.g. antidepressants or psychotherapy) for depressive employees would be a good investment: the total costs would be less than the productivity losses due to sick employees [495]. International organisations such as the Organisation for Economic Co-operation and Development have long recognised the importance of the issue, but much remains to be done.

What Does the Public Think?

Attitudes in the workplace towards people with mental illness seem to have deteriorated over the last few decades. In repeated German population surveys, around half of the employees surveyed in 2011 (even more than the number originally surveyed in 2001) were not prepared to recommend a person with depression for a job [496]. A summary of numerous population surveys from different Western countries since 1990 shows that willingness to accept people with depression as colleagues has stagnated at a low level. For people with schizophrenia, it has even declined considerably [160].

The reasons for this prejudicial trend are not entirely clear. Presumably, the increased prevalence of biological models of mental illness (Sect. 5.1.2) in combination with the increased pressure on productivity in the workplace contribute to this.

What Do Employers Think?

How individual employers respond to employees with mental illness can vary widely. Most of us likely know from personal experience cases of obvious discrimination by employers as well as cases with evidence of great support and flexibility. There are, however, a few studies that indicate what the average attitudes of employers are.

EXPERIMENT

In one experimental study, managers and human resources staff in German companies received a case description of an employee who did not sleep well. Each quarter of participants received additional information that the employee suffered from either depression, a burnout, a private crisis or a thyroid disease. The study participants expected that the employee with thyroid disease would have a higher performance capability than that of the other three groups [497].

In a Swiss study, employers were faced with the choice between one unreliable healthy applicant and several reliable applicants with various chronic physical or mental disorders who had been symptom-free for years. The applicants with mental illness were the last to be chosen to hire [498].

Both studies show the reservations that exist amongst employers and also more subtly demonstrate that even *burnout* can be a harmful label.

But attitudes can improve: it was found that in England, during the *Time to Change* antistigma campaign (Sect. 12.1), employer awareness regarding employees with mental health problems increased. Willingness to then hire and support these employees in the workplace increased as well [499].

Experiences of Discrimination by People With Mental Health Problems

In England, around 6000 employees with various mental health problems were interviewed about discrimination in the workplace. One-quarter had experienced discrimination first-hand, half had expected discrimination to occur and three-quarters had decided to keep their illness a secret in their workplace [500]. People with depression were more affected than people with, for example, schizophrenia, which contradicts the common opinion that depression is less stigmatised in the working environment. A worldwide study on discrimination against people with depression from 35 countries came to a similar conclusion: almost two-thirds of all participants with depression experienced and/or expected discrimination in the workplace [501]. Here, too, the expectation of discrimination was particularly high—this fits with models of stigma as a stressor, according to which stigma has an effect even when discrimination is not explicitly apparent in individual cases (Sects. 4.2.4, 5.1.5). Since discrimination can happen at any time, it is understandably anticipated. This can have a crippling effect: almost a third of those interviewed had stopped applying for jobs because they expected discrimination. Experience and expectation of discrimination was thus also associated with higher unemployment rates. Discrimination was found to be a particularly big problem in Western countries.

Disclosure of Illness in the Work Environment

A prominent German psychiatrist once explicitly advised lying in an interview in a weekly magazine: employees should not tell their employers about their mental illness and instead fake bronchitis. This advice is certainly well intentioned and refers to the risks of disclosure. However, the recommendation is problematic for three reasons:

1. Everybody is different: Some supervisors want to know about and support their employees. And for some employees, keeping something hidden or lying is not helpful.
2. It hinders service users' self-determination and empowerment (Sect. 5.1.3) when healthcare professionals or experts dictate whether or not to disclose.
3. A blanket strategy of secrecy in the workplace reinforces workplace awareness of those mental disorders that cannot be concealed because of their severity. However, the vast majority of mental illnesses that follow a manageable course and that people can work well with tend to go unnoticed.

Taboos and silence reinforce the prejudice that the *mentally ill* do not work well, and thereby aggravate a vicious cycle of stigma and secrecy.

Making disclosure decisions is more complex in reality. From the perspective of employees with mental health problems, the advantages and disadvantages of disclosure must be weighed [502]:

- Disclosure of one's own mental illness carries the risk of long-term discrimination: lack of promotion, exclusion from collaborations, gossip or social distancing from colleagues, even loss of employment.
- But disclosure also brings opportunities: social support and exchange, reasonable accommodations and adaptations of work processes (e.g. adjustment of work shifts), and the opportunity to stand up for oneself and no longer have to hide anything (i.e. greater authenticity).

Weighing up the pros and cons will always be an individual process and will have to take into account one's own vulnerability. Not everyone will be able to fend off nasty comments from colleagues or superiors without any consequences. Caution is advisable, as disclosure is usually irreversible.

What Can Healthcare Professionals Do?

Doctors should always keep the issue of employment in mind. This does not mean that they should push service users to work; some patients decide not to work temporarily or to stop work altogether. But most do want to be employed. It is therefore advisable to make decisions at the start of treatment about the circumstances under which to work and when, what type of work will be possible, what kind of support is appropriate and how an existing employment contract can be maintained. Some practitioners hold an unhelpful prejudice that service users cannot or should not work anymore. But it is better to concentrate on strengths and resources. Almost anyone can work if they want to—not necessarily full-time and not necessarily in any kind of job, but something suitable can be found. For young adults, additional attention is needed to make the transition from education to working life smoother.

Structural Barriers in the Treatment System

Working with mental illness or keeping a job after a period of illness-related debilitation is made difficult by structural problems. First, there are the waiting times of the outpatient system: depending on the type of disorder and where they live, service users can wait from weeks to months for an appointment with a registered psychiatrist and from several months to half a year to start outpatient psychotherapy. Some people with serious mental disorders, so-called dual diagnoses (e.g. addiction and psychosis), or a borderline personality disorder considered 'difficult' (Sect. 5.4.3) often do not find outpatient psychotherapy at all. This is detrimental to the workplace and the service user's ability to maintain work; the later the start of the treatment, the more difficult this becomes. This barrier to accessing treatment is unacceptable (Sect. 7.3). A further issue is the restricted access to rehabilitation services, which is discussed in Section 7.1.2.

Finally, it should be mentioned that there is not an allowance in Germany for part-time leave. During my time in Zurich, Switzerland, I was able to give a patient with depression a part-time sick note, which could be very helpful if the person could and wanted to work part-time instead of full-time. In Germany, I have to give a patient in the same situation full-time sick leave. This often means the patient loses contacts, tasks and daily structure—and the depression does not get any better by brooding at home from morning until night. It is not clear to me why a regulation for part-time leave from work is not possible in Germany, even with the consent of the employee. Especially for people with mental illness, this could be an important instrument to reduce the risk of job loss and, indirectly, the risk of social exclusion.

What Can Companies Do?

For employees with mental illness, stigma is a threat to their professional identity [503]. Coping responses, such as secrecy or disclosure, take a lot of effort and can affect their work. Prejudice in the workplace becomes a self-fulfilling prophecy when employees with mental illness are overloaded and fall ill or are absent. Since discrimination is not only due to the behaviour of individuals but is also affected by the atmosphere of the workplace and the interactions between mentally stressed employees and their environment, interventions that only address discriminating 'perpetrators' or the 'victims' are likely insufficient [504]. Instead, there needs to be a change in the culture of the workplace, whereby disclosure of an illness is seen as 'normal'. In light of the prevalence of mental illness, this kind of culture should be self-evident—but it is not, because stigma and taboos persist. Companies must therefore actively demand and promote an attitude of this kind.

This shift includes clear policies such that employees with mental illness are supported by *reasonable accommodations* in the workplace [505]. Employers are obliged to make these adjustments, but only if they know about the psychiatric disability (a disability is present when a mental illness is long-lasting and causes impairment at work [506]). This should be borne in mind when considering the aforementioned disclosure decisions.

Since 2004, the German Social Security Code (§ 84 para. 2 SGB IX) has provided the possibility of *workplace integration management* for all employees. The aim is to support employees who have been absent from work for a long period of time due to illness and are planning to return. As mental illness can lead to lengthy periods of absence from work, this is an important aid. In consultation with the employee and employer, as well as with the company physician, staff council and representative body for disabled people if necessary, a steady return with a gradual increase in the number of work hours is planned. The employee continues to be on sick leave during this period, and there are no wage costs for the employer. The success rates are considered to be high. But the success of this model depends on the company culture. The best legal framework is useless if there is prejudice in the workplace and if the problems of employees with mental illness go unaddressed. Stigma should therefore be seen as a critical barrier for such integration management [507].

What Antistigma Interventions Are There in the Workplace?

An overview of 10 individual studies showed that training courses can improve the attitudes of superiors when dealing with mentally ill employees. It is not clear whether these training courses also have positive effects on employees [508]. Antistigma interventions for healthy employees generally seem to be helpful: they improve knowledge, attitudes and willingness to support colleagues who have fallen ill. The Australian *Mental Health First Aid* (MHFA) programme has been one of the most frequently examined (Sects. 8.1.5, 8.1.6). The MHFA programme trains course participants on how to help others with mental health problems. It has been shown that MHFA leads to better knowledge and stronger intentions to help amongst trainees; known effects on stigma are limited. But it is unclear whether those in distress who receive help from MHFA-trained first aiders (i.e. from course participants) actually benefit [509]. *Working Mind* is widespread in Canada and is based on the *Road to Mental Readiness Programme*, which was developed for soldiers and civilian first responders. Both have an educational approach and aim to improve knowledge and attitudes. However, the first controlled trial on these programmes is still pending, so the effectiveness remains unclear and is considered weak at best [510]. In principle, contact-based antistigma interventions are also a promising approach for employers and employees (Sect. 8.4). There is, however, hardly any research on this topic [511]. Another promising approach, the effectiveness of which has also not yet been well investigated, is the employment of peers who help to reduce stigma as actual examples of recovery and contact opportunity (Sect. 7.3.4).

7.1.2 PEOPLE WITHOUT WORK

Unemployment and mental illness often go hand in hand. According to estimates for Germany, only about 10% of people with severe, chronic mental disorders are active in the primary labour market. About 40% have a sheltered job (i.e. work in a supportive setting with, depending on the country and institution, therapeutic elements) or are in an adult day care centre, while approximately 50% lack employment or any work at all [512]. Employment rates of people with mental illness are lower than those of people with physical disabilities [513]. Almost half of all early retirement on health-related grounds is due to mental illness and occurs on average at only 48 years [512]. The problem is widespread: in 2018 alone, over 70,000 disability pensions due to mental illness were newly approved in Germany, and almost half of them were due to depression.

People who are unemployed have a fivefold increased risk of also having a mental illness. Unemployment can be both the cause and consequence of mental illness—individuals often find themselves in a vicious cycle: unemployment and mental illness become a dual burden. The fact that they are both stigmatised contributes to the challenge. People who are unemployed and mentally ill often face multiple discrimination (Sect. 3.1.8). A study from southern Germany has shown that the search for work and treatment is particularly difficult for those who experience dual discrimination due to their mental health problems and their unemployment [444].

Disclosure in the Job Search

The stigma of mental illness is one of the biggest obstacles to finding work again [514]. Unemployed people who are mentally ill therefore face the difficult decision of whether to disclose their illness when they apply for a job. If they do, they risk not getting the job. If they do not, they cannot expect support in the workplace; keeping the mental illness hidden can become increasingly stressful.

One longitudinal study has shown that caution is required when deciding whether to disclose one's illness in the job hunt. Around 300 unemployed people with mental health problems from Bavaria and Baden-Württemberg were asked whether they would disclose their illness when applying for jobs. Six months later, they were asked whether they had found work in the general labour market. Those who did not want to disclose at the beginning were more likely to have found a job within half a year, regardless of the severity of their psychological symptoms or the length of their unemployment [152]. One could conclude from this that disclosure when looking for a job is 'bad', but it is not that simple. The study did not examine how the respondents fared after the study's end: perhaps those who disclosed their illness and found a job were better able to cope later on because they did not carry a secret and were able to get support in the workplace more easily if needed.

Claire Henderson, Graham Thornicroft and colleagues in London have developed a guide to provide targeted support to mentally ill unemployed people when making these tricky disclosure decisions in the job search. It helps to weigh up the opportunities and risks of disclosure in the working environment. A social worker is meant to work through the guide with the participant. Simple assistance of this kind seems to make the job search easier; participants feel less burdened by the conflict and stress of the disclosure decision [515]. Because making the decision about disclosure is important in dealing with stigma, we will return to the topic of support in this area later (HOP, Sect. 9.2).

What Interventions Are There?

When talking about interventions for people who are unemployed and have a mental illness, two distinctions are necessary. First, a distinction must be made between specific antistigma interventions on the one hand and programmes that get participants back to work and thus contribute to social inclusion on the other. Second, not all mentally ill unemployed people find themselves in the same situations. Some people with serious illnesses cannot leave their house because of anxiety or other symptoms. For them, the first priority should be to find effective help or treatment. For others, the symptoms may persist but do not prevent them from visiting a job centre or looking for work. Because of these differences in experience, one intervention does not fit all. Due to often complex and overlapping problems (also called multiple placement obstacles), programmes are needed that bring together different sectors (in particular, the systems of treatment, employment agencies and job centres, employers, rehabilitation services, benefits and integrated care). Unfortunately, these integrated cross-sectoral programmes are rare finds. To give just one example: unemployed people with mental illness in Germany today are usually seen by job centre staff. This staff, however, has neither the time nor the qualifications to take care of their clients' psychological problems. The medical–psychological service of the German Federal Employment Agency has the necessary qualifications but is mainly concerned with giving written expert opinions, typically on the basis of the client's file status. Here, as at many other interfaces, there is a lack of integrated care from one primary provider that can address work, social support, healthcare and mental illness. There is also a lack of job coaching within the healthcare system. The fact that this integration is necessary, highly effective and cost-efficient is undisputed in research [66, 516]. But there is a lack of political will to implement it.

Antistigma interventions can be directed to three addressees (according to the three basic forms of stigma): employers or employees of a company to improve the environment for applicants or colleagues with mental illness (public stigma), people with mental illness themselves to help them make disclosure decisions or to help them cope with public stigma and self-stigma [517], and company rules or pension/care schemes that make integration difficult (structural discrimination).

Supported Employment

There are basically two approaches to getting people with mental illness back into work if they so wish: the traditional and, in Germany, predominant way of *first train, then place*, and the newer approach of *first place, then train*, also called *Supported Employment*.

Traditional work rehabilitation consists of participants first practising skills (e.g. a software program on a PC) and then completing a supported internship in a company. This rehabilitation can take months or a year but has an eventual time limit. It often takes place in so-called rehabilitation facilities for mentally ill people as inpatients and can be far from the participants' places of residence. At the end of the programme, the participants are on their own.

Supported Employment takes the opposite approach. Participants wanting to work are placed directly in the primary labour market by job coaches. These coaches support them during the job search and subsequently advise on a long-term basis once in the workplace. The employer can also be advised. No participant who wants to work is turned down, and the participant's wishes with regard to the type of work and degree of disclosure are taken into account. Vocational support through job coaches and treatment (e.g. with community mental health teams) takes place locally and in an integrated fashion. A clearly defined version of Supported Employment is *Individual Placement and Support* (IPS, see 'Glossary').

Which approach works better? The new version of Germany's guidelines on psychosocial interventions summarises the available evidence [66]. Randomized controlled trials (RCTs) from around the world clearly show that Supported Employment brings about twice as many participants into the primary labour market as do traditional work-based rehabilitations. This success rate has been similarly observed in routine evaluations [518]. Depending on the study and context, the success rates of Supported Employment are around 50%. Participants not only find jobs but find them faster and hang on to them longer. Jobseekers' characteristics, such as their psychiatric diagnoses, are not seen as decisive factors. Supported Employment also has a positive effect on non-work–related factors, particularly on quality of life and psychological symptoms. This approach refutes the widespread prejudice among professionals that work is too hard or too stressful for people with serious mental illness.

On the other hand, evidence of the effectiveness of traditional work-based rehabilitation ('first train, then place') is rare. Two uncontrolled studies from Germany show that participants in such programmes are more likely to find sheltered work than employment in the general labour market [66]. Overall, traditional work-based rehabilitation shows hardly any advantages over standard hospital treatment with regard to the primary labour market [491]. In fact, there are considerable disadvantages:

- Traditional work rehabilitation is expensive.
- Participants are preselected, and people with serious mental disorders who are in particular need of support are often excluded.
- The rehabilitation is lacking in everyday experience and is only for a limited period.

Besides the lack of evidence for its effectiveness, the reasons as to why 'first train, then place' is less effective are intuitively understandable: participants train for a long time, at great expense and without much targeting their own skills for a hypothetical future placement that is yet unknown. They are on their own after the rehabilitative intervention—and likewise when they find work. In contrast, one of the great advantages of IPS is the support given to participants at the time when questions arise and when it is needed at the new workplace.

Supported Education

Mental disorders usually begin in adolescence and young adulthood (Sect. 5.7). They can therefore lead to the interruption or discontinuation of school, training or university. Due to the long-term importance and value of professional qualifications, the idea of *Supported Education* was born. The approach is similar to that of Supported Employment (see previous page), except that here it is a question of direct access to teaching and training rather than a question of access to the general labour market. Supported Employment is more clearly defined, as in the form of IPS ('Glossary'), than this more recent concept of Supported Education. In most cases of Supported Education, attempts are made to adapt IPS to the field of education and to younger participants. As with IPS, the decisive factors are the integration of coaches into the clinical team, an orientation towards the wishes of the participants, the goal of rapid placement in school or training, and continued support once placed.

Is Supported Education effective? The few available RCTs indicate that about twice as many participants enter into education with the programme than without it [519]. This approach is particularly useful as an early intervention for people in their first psychotic episode (Sect. 5.3) to prevent the discontinuation of their training and career paths [520]. Supported education could also be important at universities as a support for students with mental illness or any kind of life crisis before they drop out of their studies. Psychotherapeutic counselling centres cannot do this alone. Peer support (i.e. support from other students with their own experiences of such crises) is helpful here as well (Sect. 7.3.4, 'Peer Support, Trialogue' [521]).

Is Supported Education used in German-speaking countries? This is not easy to answer—as mentioned, the approach is not clearly defined. Supported Education and the broad field of inclusion of people with mental and intellectual disabilities are two closely linked topics (Sect. 5.4.6). The German Federal Institute for Vocational Education and Training (https://bibb.de/en) offers a regularly updated bibliography with literature on structural conditions and programmes for inclusion and promotion in the field of education.

Structural Discrimination and Exclusion From Working Life

There are two issues that put people with mental illness at a disadvantage in working life and make them encounter structural discrimination: a lack of supported employment in the form of IPS and a lack of implementation of the 'rehabilitation over disability pension' principle.

Despite the overwhelming evidence of its effectiveness and its clear recommendation in the guidelines [66], IPS has a niche presence in Germany. Since 2009 (§ 38a SGB IX), there has been so-called Supported Employment that is based on 'first place, then train'. However, it does not meet the IPS criteria, is not tailored to people with mental illness and is not widely adopted [491]. This means that the most effective measure to get people with mental illness back into the primary labour market has not been implemented outside model projects: for example, a Swiss working group led by Holger Hoffmann has established the Berne Job Coach Project with great success and demonstrated its long-term effectiveness and cost-efficiency [453, 522].

Why IPS is not implemented on a large scale in Germany can only be explained by the inertia of policymakers and by the efforts of lobbyists for traditional work rehabilitation who may feel threatened by new approaches. Cynical arguments are sometimes used: IPS is ineffective, or IPS has already been offered as part of traditional approaches. Such arguments are misleading and are often used in debates on health policy. This denies not only the clear data in favour of IPS but also the fact that Supported Employment works best when it is offered in line with the IPS model.

Conclusion

The lack of political will to implement IPS puts up a permanent structural barrier for people with mental illness who want to work, thus contributing to their social exclusion.

As mentioned, another mechanism of exclusion from working life is that people with mental illness, unlike people with physical disabilities, are not cared for according to the principle of 'rehabilitation over disability pension'. Data from the German Pension Insurance show two trends from 2000 to 2018:

- The share of new disability pensions granted on the basis of mental disorders almost doubled in that time period (from 24% to 43%). Conversely, the share of disability pensions due to musculoskeletal disorders decreased sharply (from 28% to 13%).
- The share of medical rehabilitation for mental disorders, however, increased only slightly during this period (from 15% to 19.5%). In comparison, the share for musculoskeletal disorders remained stable at just over 40% despite declining cases of disability pensions for these disorders.

This means that people with mental illness are much more likely to be withdrawn from the labour market in the long term through early retirement, without any attempt at rehabilitation. Hans Joachim Salize once dryly stated that 'the path to chronification is favoured by the structural conditions of the realities in our healthcare and rehabilitation system' ([488], pp. 9 f.). For people with mental illness, rehabilitation should be offered much earlier and more frequently. Conditions for eligibility and access should be simplified [491]. That this is not happening is a bizarre systemic failure not only for individuals and their families but—in a time of very low unemployment and a lack of available skilled workers—for the national economy as well.

7.2 Housing and Homelessness

7.2.1 EXTENT OF THE PROBLEM

Homelessness is more common than is assumed by the general public. There is no consistent definition as to which people are affected. The European Federation of National Organisations Working with the Homeless (https://feantsa.org) includes amongst the homeless all those who have no roof over their heads, people in homeless shelters or refugee resettlements, people who are acutely threatened by the loss of accommodation and people in unacceptable housing conditions. In Europe, however, homelessness is not consistently defined. There are no reliable figures available for Germany; nationwide reporting of homeless people only began in 2021. The federal working group, Homelessness Assistance (https://bagw.de), calculated that there were approximately 300,000 homeless people or people threatened by acute homelessness in Germany in 2017. This figure does not include the more than 300,000 recognised refugees who do not have permanent housing. A study commissioned by the Federal Ministry of Labour and Social Affairs estimated somewhat lower figures for 2018 [523]. There is, however, an underreporting of the number of people who have temporary accommodation with acquaintances but whose housing situations remain precarious. The number of homeless people in Europe has increased in the 2010s with the exception of Finland, which consistently follows the *Housing First* approach (Sect. 7.2.6 [524]).

7.2.2 HOMELESSNESS AND HEALTH

Living as a homeless person or under precarious housing conditions is, unsurprisingly, associated with poorer health. Mental disorders are more frequent among homeless people than in the general public: the values vary by study but fall between 20% and 50% for individual disorders; namely, depression, psychoses, substance use disorders, posttraumatic stress disorders and dual diagnoses (e.g. psychosis and substance use [525]). The vast majority of homeless people are affected by some form of mental illness. However, the figures from individual studies are often controversial, not least because homeless people who are already in the health and social care systems are typically the ones surveyed (and mental disorders are overrepresented among them).

It cannot be concluded from the high incidence of illness in these reports that all homeless people have a mental illness. However, the figures indicate a high need for support that is largely unmet and point to a particularly vulnerable subgroup that is affected by illness and homelessness at the same time.

Many homeless people have suffered physical or sexual abuse during childhood [526] and therefore have a higher risk of mental illness. More than a quarter have survived suicide attempts [527]. Poverty, and resulting rent debts and unemployment, are among the risk factors for the loss of one's home [528]. The period after release from an institution (e.g. prison, hospital, youth welfare) is associated with an increased risk of homelessness. In individual cases, mental illness can be the cause or consequence of poor housing conditions. Just as with unemployment, there is often a vicious cycle of illness and homelessness. A review of 12 longitudinal studies from around the world has shown that precarious housing conditions can cause later development of anxiety and depression [529].

7.2.3 MEDIA AND PUBLIC OPINION

Media coverage of homelessness fluctuates between a fixation on negative stereotypes combined with winter-induced pity on one hand and reasonable reporting and interviews on the other. The Austrian daily newspaper *Der Standard*, for example, printed an interview (13 Mar. 2018) with the Vienna Neunerhaus Project for homeless people (https://neunerhaus.at). The article explicitly addressed the shame and stigma associated with homelessness, which has further marginalised those affected and made it more difficult to seek help for illnesses.

Public attitudes towards homelessness were examined in a study from eight European countries involving over 5000 participants [530]. Negative attitudes were evident in about one-third of the respondents, who said that governments spend too much on homeless people, that homeless people have chosen their situation and that they can continue to participate in life despite their homelessness. In Germany, public attitudes towards the homeless deteriorated in the 2000s: about one-third were in favour of removing homeless people from public places in 2011 ([531], p. 39). The fact that a fairly large part of the general public thinks negatively of the homeless fits well with Fiske's model of stereotype content (Sect. 3.2.4, Fig. 3.1): this is a demographic that is attributed with neither warmth nor competence.

7.2.4 EXPERIENCE OF DISCRIMINATION

The exclusion of homeless people has a long history. During the Nazi era, 'asocials'—among them homeless people—were marked with a black triangle in camps and were murdered in large numbers from 1942 onwards. In the German Democratic Republic (GDR), 'asocial behaviour' was punishable until 1990 (§ 249 StGB, the German Criminal Code). For the West German 'Psychiatrie-Enquete' and the subsequent reforms of the 1970s, the topic held a lot of significance (Sect. 2.1.3). Long-term patients released from the psychiatric hospitals needed other forms of housing. All of a sudden, housing became an important part of (social) psychiatry. The transfer to 'normal' housing conditions was partially successful, with the support of and through the expansion of outpatient care. Others after being released from the hospitals were transferred to nursing homes, replacing one institution with another. The fragmentation of the German healthcare system (outpatient/inpatient; different responsibilities of service providers and cost bearers; Sect. 7.3.3) contributed to this so-called reinstitutionalisation.

Many homeless people, regardless of mental illness, still experience everyday discrimination today: 'the public spit on homeless people' ([532], p. 157). Stigma is a consequence of homelessness, poverty, mental illness or substance abuse—or it is due to the combination of them (Sect. 3.1.8). Areas where unfair treatment is particularly common include employment and housing access, as well as dealing with the police and the healthcare system. The stigma of mental illness exacerbates experiences of discrimination in all of these spaces, which is why many sufferers reject the label of a psychiatric diagnosis. Self-stigma and shame are common obstacles on the path to treatment and recovery [533].

7.2.5 PROBLEMS IN THE SUPPORT SYSTEM

Providing support and treatment for homeless people is difficult for several reasons [534]; there are complex social, physical and psychological problems involved. The various support providers tend not to work together, and there is a lack of integrated care from a single source. Homeless people often end up in accident and emergency (A&E) departments where they are not offered adequate, long-term, coordinated care. And many homeless people have negative experiences in health and social care [535]: the staff in treatment and support facilities are often hostile and prejudiced, the rules are rigid and access to help is often denied. A study in 14 European capitals has shown that almost a quarter of the services specifically targeted at homeless people did not include aid to people with substance use problems [536]. This is a bizarre situation given the frequency of alcohol and drug abuse amongst homeless people. Additionally, only a minority of the services offered did reach-outs (i.e. went to homeless people on the street or in emergency accommodation), there were very few personnel in these services that were qualified in mental healthcare and few services offered addiction treatment. Integrated care combining general medical, psychiatric and social services is possible and effective—for the physical and mental health of those affected and for a way out of homelessness [534].

Apart from the service structure, many homeless people have difficulty gaining trust in care providers and institutions. This is understandable given their many experiences of discrimination: 'The most hurtful thing that I've been through with mental illness is the stigma that because it happens to be an emotional disability, they write you off completely … I didn't have a voice. I was seen immediately as incompetent because I had a mental illness' ([537], p. 1318). To rebuild trust and prevent stigma in the healthcare system or when dealing with authorities, *peer navigators* (i.e. people with their own experiences of homelessness and mental illness) could be helpful (Sect. 7.3.4, 'Peer Support, Trialogue' [538]).

While commenting on German legislation in the area of SGB XII (social care law, Sect. 7.3.3), Hans Joachim Salize has pointed out obstacles to access for homeless people with mental illness [488]. The so-called *integration support* (Eingliederungshilfe, § 53 SGB XII) regulates social-psychiatric and rehabilitative services for people with mental illness. Alternatively, there is *support for overcoming particular social difficulties* (Hilfen zur Überwindung besonderer sozialer Schwierigkeiten, § 67 SGB XII). Homeless people who benefit from the latter cannot simultaneously receive integration support. This division acts 'as a de facto obstacle in accessing mental healthcare for homeless mentally ill people' ([488], p. 8)—an example of structural discrimination against one of the most vulnerable groups in our society. In light of the healthcare system's fragmentation, one of the numerous recommendations given in the aforementioned study by the Federal Ministry of Labour and Social Affairs [523] is the strengthening of outreach community psychiatric services that can offer medical and psychiatric–psychosocial care from a single source. This is not an issue of 'psychiatrising' the homeless but rather of not withholding help from those who need and want it.

Finally, there is a lack of prevention [539]. There are possibilities for primary prevention (i.e. preventing the onset and occurrence of homelessness), in particular through better availability of affordable housing. Secondary or indicated prevention is necessary shortly after the start of homelessness or when there is an immediate threat of homelessness. Programmes that undertake this approach are those that take care of people upon release from prison or the hospital (so-called critical time interventions) and those who are already mentally ill and on the verge of homelessness. Hans Joachim Salize successfully implemented such a programme in Baden [540]. Additionally, as far as the prevention of homelessness is concerned, the research field of *Urban Mental Health* (i.e. urban planning in relation to mental health) has recently attracted increasing attention [541].

7.2.6 HOUSING FIRST

What can be done when homelessness occurs? Despite all the difficulties mentioned, there is no reason to feel resignation. Similar to work rehabilitation (Sect. 7.1.2), there are two contrasting models for ending homelessness. In the traditional phased model, homeless people must first prove their worth in tightly controlled forms of housing with obligatory treatment participation, drug abstinence, etc. before they can move into more independent forms of housing. Comparable to the work rehabilitation approach of *first train, then place*, they are supposed to practice living, as it were, before they are allowed to live more independently.

The opposing and more recent approach of work rehabilitation is called *first place, then train* (Sect. 7.1.2, 'Supported Employment'), and in the housing sector, the same principle is *Supported Housing* or *Housing First*. Like Sam Tsemberis has said, 'Housing First ends homelessness. It's that simple.' In the 1990s, Tsemberis built a programme in New York City that is now internationally known as Housing First. Previously homeless participants can become direct tenants on the free housing market (e.g. through rent subsidies) without having to go through phased forms of assisted living. The tenancy agreements are meant to be unlimited and applicable to single flats in preferably 'normal' living environments to prevent ghettoisation of previously homeless mentally ill people [542].

Housing First is based on certain fundamental values: everyone has a right to housing (Article 19 UN-CRPD). To be offered housing should not require treatment participation or abstinence from drugs. People must have the choice to live in an independent flat (rather than in a homeless shelter or assisted living facility). An unconditional offer of housing allows for a break in the vicious cycle of homelessness and physical, mental and social emergencies (i.e. not having to worry about a place to live allows people the time to deal with their problems). Support should be actively offered in the form of case management or outreach psychiatric–psychotherapeutic treatment. It is up to the person concerned to decide whether to take part in treatment, and refusal will not result in the loss of the flat.

How does Housing First work for mentally ill homeless people? The overwhelming majority want to live independently [543]. Housing First enables this choice and self-determination. Meta-analyses show that the primary goal of independent living can be achieved through the intervention: the vast majority of participants are no longer homeless as a result of Housing First [544]. In one large Canadian study, the intervention effectively reduced homelessness for about 5 years [545]. Its effects on quality of life and mental health were less clear but tended to be positive.

Is investment in Housing First worthwhile? Through Housing First, costs in other areas decrease considerably, in part because of the reduction in A&E visits and hospital admissions [546]. The cost of the programme and the cost savings made in other areas are dependent on the local conditions, such as rental prices and the other offers homeless people are receiving (i.e. what Housing First can be compared with). According to different studies, Housing First seems to provide minimal overall savings but is a more efficient use of resources than conventional models [544].

As with finding work, there is no silver bullet for homelessness. Housing First does not help everyone, and not all homeless people—including those with severe mental illness—can and want to participate. To be effective, Housing First should be offered primarily to those for whom no other offer is appropriate (e.g. due to the severity of their mental illness). Housing First takes into account some of the points in the UN-CRPD (Sect. 7.5.2); namely, the right to choose one's own form of housing and the right to autonomy [544]—these values should be enough to popularise and disseminate this approach. The fact that Housing First is not offered outside some model projects in Germany is therefore problematic and contradicts the recommendations of the guidelines for psychosocial interventions [66]. As in the field of work rehabilitation (Sect. 7.1.2), paternalistic models tend to persist even though they are less effective and less appreciated by participants. It is time to practice what is often invoked in political speeches and to implement care that is directed towards the individual and his or her freedom of choice.

7.3 Healthcare System

Many people with mental illness seek help from the healthcare system, especially in acute phases of their illness and crisis situations. In my experience, they are typically well-looked-after; on the whole, most professionals and institutions do good work in good faith and often under very difficult conditions. Despite all of the weaknesses, inefficiencies and fragmentation in the health services of the German-speaking countries described in Section 7.3.3 ('Fragmentation'), the systems can often be effective. When a desperate person turns up to a psychiatric hospital late at night, his admittance is usually feasible. This type of ready access is crucial, but in many other countries it is not a routine matter [547].

Regardless, prejudice and discrimination have an impact within the healthcare system—through the behaviour of individuals and in the way the system is organised and operates. This is clearly problematic: people seeking help tend to be especially vulnerable to stigma and discrimination, and healthcare systems in particular should be free of prejudice towards those seeking help. As Stephen Hinshaw said ([548], p. 384):

> *Indeed, even a small amount of stigma among professionals will translate into many thousands of negative social interactions in any given year, with the potential for long-term damage to morale and the promotion of stigma by the very personnel entrusted with helping those with mental illness.*

A look at the healthcare system makes it clear that stigma is not an abstract problem, a little blemish or an awkward interaction between individuals. To put it bluntly, stigma can be a matter of life and death and discrimination can be fatal. People with severe mental illness die on average 10 to 20 years earlier than members of the general public [549]. This reduced life expectancy has various causes, in particular infections and cardiovascular and respiratory diseases—all of which are more common and more serious among people with mental illness. Additionally, psychotropic medication can lead to weight gain, which increases the risk of physical illnesses; many service users also smoke. But stigma also contributes to inadequate care and early death at the systemic and individual levels [549].

Inequality and stigma in care can be so detrimental and pronounced for people with mental illness that the *Lancet*, a leading scientific journal, has soberly written of it as a *health crisis*: 'Stigma not only drives this inequality, but also silences our outrage' [550]. People with severe mental illness in particular are socially marginalised and stigmatised many times over because they are often affected by poverty or unemployment in addition to their illness (Sect. 5.5). But they lack a strong lobbying or advocacy group to fight for them with righteous anger. Imagine that some of the care shortages described in Section 7.3 affect children with cancer—a public outcry would (rightly) be the result. Recently, there has been lively debate in Germany about liposuction reimbursement for overweight people even though there is no evidence that the procedure is effective. Everyone, whether they have cancer or are overweight, deserves and needs good treatment. But I wish the often precarious care situation of people with mental illness could receive even half as much attention as other health issues—especially because the many people who are affected often have fewer resources to find points of contact in the maze of the care system. There is also clear evidence of many interventions' effectiveness in the field of mental illness, yet few are made available.

For a better overview, two levels of the healthcare system are differentiated:
1. the individual level (i.e. those patients and professionals who may experience or endorse prejudice or discrimination) (Sect. 7.3.1),
2. the care system level, where structural discrimination against people with mental illness occurs in some areas (Sect. 7.3.3).

Antistigma interventions are described for both levels (Sects. 7.3.2, 7.3.4). Here, only interventions within the healthcare system are discussed; broader antistigma interventions follow from Chapter 8 onwards. The issue of stigma as a barrier to seeking help and treatment participation, which leads to people not being treated at all, has been discussed previously (Sect. 5.1.7). This so-called treatment gap also affects the health services (e.g. support is sought too late or terminated prematurely).

7.3.1 STIGMA IN THE HEALTHCARE SYSTEM AT THE INDIVIDUAL LEVEL

Even in our digital age, whether in a doctor's office or a hospital, in an outpatient clinic or during a home visit, most of the work in the healthcare system remains interpersonal. Stigma can impede or complicate successful encounters when professionals are prejudiced, when patients experience or fear discrimination, or when they suffer from self-stigma and shame [551].

Attitudes of Professionals

For people with mental illness, family doctors or general practitioners (GPs) are often the first point of contact. Unfortunately, a systematic review has shown that GPs often hold negative attitudes, especially towards people with schizophrenia [552]. The GPs were found to be more prejudiced than other healthcare professionals and the general public. Many were pessimistic about patients' chances of recovery and the course of the illness. The GPs were often poorly trained in treatment of depression, for example, and less knowledge was associated with more negative attitudes. Furthermore, the less GPs could imagine seeking help for their own psychological problems, the more prejudiced they were (see later in this section). The prejudice of doctors ultimately affects treatment: various studies show that being more strongly prejudiced is associated with less somatic treatment (e.g. fewer weight reduction programmes being offered) [553].

A study of more than 100,000 patients with acute myocardial infarction in the United States found that those who also suffered from mental illness were examined and treated with a cardiac catheter much less often than patients without a mental illness [554]; patients with myocardial infarction and schizophrenia received an examination less than half as often. This discrepancy could not be explained by the severity of the heart disease. One may ask why people who are suffering from a life-threatening physical disease and mental illness are treated worse in an emergency situation. One possible explanation is that physical symptoms are mistakenly perceived as signs of mental illness. This misjudgement is known as *diagnostic overshadowing*: professionals may not take a clear diagnostic view and will misinterpret, for example, the tachycardia of an acute heart disease as a symptom of the known mental illness. According to one young doctor: 'Once you have been labelled as having a psychiatric illness, it's very difficult to put that label to one side and to try essentially to deal with what you have in front of you' ([555], p. 259).

Are psychiatric professionals also prejudiced towards their patients? Though different studies have yielded very different results, this does unfortunately seem to occur [556]. In one Swiss survey with more than 1000 professionals, mainly psychiatric nurses and psychiatrists, professional prejudices were more pronounced than those of the general public [557]. However, professionals tended to advocate for fewer restrictions on people with mental illness (e.g. the withdrawal of the driving licence or the right to vote) than the general public (Sect. 7.5.4). Among professionals and compared with other mental disorders, schizophrenia is one of the most stigmatised conditions [558].

It is not entirely clear why even those working in psychiatry have prejudices. One possible reason is that over the years they repeatedly encounter their patients in acute crises, in which unpredictable behaviour or violence can occur (whereby professionals can suffer from and also exercise violence [158]). Additionally, due to the revolving door syndrome, these practitioners often see service users with particularly severe illnesses. It is thereby easy to overlook the fact that most patients never enter a hospital, and those who do spend most of their time elsewhere and get along well otherwise. All of this may promote prejudice and therapeutic pessimism.

These results are relevant for antistigma interventions for two reasons:
1. They show that the transfer of knowledge (Sect. 8.1) about mental illness alone is not enough to reduce stigma (otherwise professionals would be much less prejudiced than the general public).
2. Not every type of contact between people with mental illness and others reduces prejudice; rather the type of contact and good environmental conditions are key (Sect. 8.4.3).

Experiences of Patients

Fortunately, many patients in the psychiatric–psychotherapeutic healthcare system have positive experiences. That this is not always the case, however, is dependent on many different reasons including the treatment context and people involved. People with serious mental disorders or in suicidal crises are often worried about being admitted to and forced to stay in a psychiatric hospital against their will by professionals. If there is no sufficiently intensive outpatient treatment available (Sect. 7.3.3), and the situation becomes more acute, hospital admission may be necessary. And if that experience goes badly, it can be perceived as violent or even humiliating. As a result, service users can be really frightened of hospitals and may ultimately receive treatment they do not want—an unfortunate situation for all involved [559].

Notwithstanding these reasons, both outpatients and inpatients experience being treated as less than human and reduced to an 'illness' time and again: 'I got a new psychiatrist who was absolutely brilliant … he didn't talk to me as if I was somebody with an illness; he talked to me as if I was a person' ([559], p. 1083). Categorising people as *mentally ill* often seems to dominate the perceptions and behaviours of professionals (Sect. 3.2.1). In the International Study of Discrimination and Stigma Outcomes (INDIGO) study conducted by Graham Thornicroft and colleagues, nearly 800 people with schizophrenia from 27 countries around the world reported experiences of discrimination in their respective healthcare systems [560]. One in six had experienced discrimination in somatic medicine, and more than one in three had experienced discrimination in psychiatric care. Experiences of discrimination against women in the healthcare system with regard to family planning, pregnancy and childbirth (e.g. statements made by doctors that they should not have children) were found to be similarly frequent.

Interactions Between Patients and Professionals

All interactions and treatments are different, and generalisations are not always useful. Contact between healthcare professionals and their patients is often positive. But we can see that there are common problems related to stigma. For example, professionals can be very focused on diagnoses, which are necessary for health insurance reimbursements as well as other cost bearers. But this fixation leads to patients being labelled diagnostically more often than would be necessary and helpful. Patients continue to report that they are treated by professionals as though they are ignorant children, a behaviour professionals in turn justify with the best of intentions (cf. benevolent sexism, Sect. 3.2.4, 'Content Dimensions'). Yet patients find such behaviour condescending; it can hinder their self-confidence and their active participation in treatment. Studies have found that patients suffer more from self-stigma and loss of empowerment when they perceive stigmatising attitudes from their caregivers [200].

In the past, a professional would make decisions about a patient's course of treatment (e.g. psychiatric medication) and only then would inform the patient, if ever. Today, there is the dominant model of *Shared Decision-Making*. Professional and patient discuss the goals of the treatment, as well as possible ways of achieving them, together and on equal terms. The decisions are made jointly, such that treatment often becomes a negotiation. This has two advantages:

1. This dynamic reduces the power gap between professionals and patients, which is particularly noticeable in hospitals (regarding power and discrimination, see Sect. 3.1.4).
2. The probability of agreeing on a form of treatment or medication dose that feels acceptable to the patient in the long term, and which is maintained after discharge, increases with this model.

In my experience, one of the many advantages of outpatient treatment is that such negotiations can take place on equal terms—quite literally when sitting on a couch in a living room—which is much easier for both sides (Sect. 7.3.3). Interventions that specifically promote joint decision-making strengthen the empowerment of patients, such as those with psychoses [561]. The more patients in psychiatric treatment are involved in shared decision-making, the less they suffer from self-stigma [562].

Professionals With Mental Illness

Doctors, nursing staff and psychologists can also become mentally ill—a truism that strangely remains taboo in the healthcare system. Professionals often work under the impression that *they*, the mentally ill, are completely different and separate from *us*, the healthy ones. Yet this notion has little grounding in reality. In German-speaking countries, Wolfgang Schmidbauer pointed out the psychological strain and risks for *helpless helpers* as early as the 1970s [563]. In medical school, many facts are taught, but how to deal with one's own misery is neglected: 'Yes, well you don't get ill, do you? … We see it as a sign of weakness … I think it's just part of the sort of macho thing which is first drummed into you at medical school … if you can't take the heat, get out of the kitchen' ([564], p. 5).

A sad consequence of this taboo and concealment of personal mental distress is that suicide rates amongst doctors, especially female ones, are significantly higher than in the general public [565]. Psychiatrists are also particularly at risk [566]. In England, almost two-thirds of a large number of clinical psychologists interviewed for a study reported their own experiences of mental illness, particularly anxiety and depression [567]. I am not aware of any evidence that demonstrates this frequency as being much lower in other related professions (e.g. psychiatric nurses or psychiatrists) or in other countries. Of almost 1500 English GPs and psychiatrists, nearly half have reported having depression themselves [568]. Many had not sought help, in particular because they were worried that this might make their illness known amongst colleagues. This is consistent with the gloomy finding that one of the groups most deterred from seeking help due to stigma is that of healthcare professionals (Sect. 5.1.7).

Most of the English psychologists mentioned kept their history of mental illness hidden at work, usually out of shame or fear of professional consequences. Doctors who are abusing or dependent on drugs or alcohol face particularly difficult issues. Due to the stigma of addiction (Sect. 5.4.7), the number of unreported cases amongst healthcare professionals is likely to be high, with an estimated frequency of up to 10% [569]. Self-medication is one way into addiction for doctors, who can access prescriptions more easily and may opt to treat themselves (e.g. with painkillers). The consequences, both for them and their patients, can be very serious. Shame and fear of stigma are amongst the most prevalent reasons why doctors refuse to accept the role of patient and do not seek help for their own addictions [566, 569].

Are Psychiatrists Stigmatised?

A former colleague of mine, now well known in his field, once told me that the worst thing about being a psychiatrist is that, time and again, you are mistaken for a psychologist (and thereby not considered a medical doctor). I initially assumed he was joking, but he wasn't. Being concerned about one's own status is not exactly alien to psychiatrists (or to other doctors). Some of my colleagues take it one step further and consider psychiatrists to be *stigmatised;* they see the *image* of psychiatrists and their profession as under threat [570]. The World Psychiatric Association even founded a task force to combat this suspected stigma. There are two issues here that must be teased out. First, the subject of psychiatry must be differentiated from psychiatric institutions (i.e. large inpatient psychiatric hospitals). Second, the question as to whether there is any truth to the lamented stigmatisation of psychiatrists should (and can) be answered conceptually and empirically.

As far as psychiatry is concerned, negative opinions likely reinforce the challenge of enticing prospective doctors and other professionals towards the field of mental healthcare. In this respect, efforts by professional associations to improve the image of the field and attract more people to it are understandable [570]. However, the fact that cardiology or paediatrics are more popular specialties is not a sign of psychiatry's stigma. The separate issue of stigma in relation to psychiatric hospitals as institutions is discussed in Section 7.3.3.

The assumption that psychiatrists are stigmatised is based on a conceptual misunderstanding. Stigma is an umbrella term for the concurrence of negative stereotypes, prejudice and discrimination towards a group; the prerequisite for stigma is a power difference that disadvantages the stigmatised group (Sects. 3.1.3, 3.1.4). There are undoubtedly stereotypes about psychiatrists (e.g. that they themselves are crazy). These are also prevalent in the media (Sect. 7.4.2). But unlike for socially marginalised groups, such as people with severe mental illness, these stereotypes do not result in discrimination. I do not know any psychiatrist who has difficulty in finding work or housing. Patients may find psychiatrists strange and express prejudices, but they lack the social power to discriminate against psychiatrists even if they want to (Sect. 3.1.4 [77]). It is therefore astonishing that some psychiatrists address the question of their own alleged stigmatisation and bother to conduct surveys on this topic. It would be far more helpful to use their positions of power to aid and bring justice to their patients and increase their patients' social inclusion.

There is also a lack of empirical evidence that psychiatrists and their work are undervalued or even stigmatised in the eyes of the public. A meta-analysis by Matthias Angermeyer and Georg Schomerus of over 160 studies from four continents examined whether members of the general public recommend that people with depression or schizophrenia consult a psychiatrist [571]. An overwhelming majority recommended the psychiatrist, and the percentage has increased in recent decades. This finding is incompatible with the idea that there is a strong distrust of or disrespect for psychiatrists (let alone discrimination).

7.3.2 ANTISTIGMA INTERVENTIONS FOR PROFESSIONALS

Prejudiced healthcare professionals are a serious yet avoidable obstacle when it comes to contact between professionals and patients (and thereby good treatment). But which interventions reduce prejudice amongst professionals? Most approaches combine education with direct contact (on education and contact as antistigma strategies, see Sects. 8.1, 8.4). The Canadian antistigma campaign *Opening Minds* (Sect. 12.1 [572]) has chosen the reduction of prejudice among healthcare professionals as one of its priorities and outlines four core elements of effective interventions:

1. Professionals should internalise a recovery attitude (i.e. work towards the recovery of their patients), giving hope for improvement. Therapeutic pessimism should be avoided; it leads to the devaluation of their 'hopeless' patients as well as their own work.
2. Professionals should see the person first and then the illness. They should thereby not speak of 'the schizophrenic in room 20', but instead of 'Mr Smith, the tax counsellor with four children and schizophrenia' (Sect. 1.2).
3. Skills deficits amongst professionals should be addressed, as they reinforce the consequences of prejudice and can lead to further fear, insecurity and avoidance.

4. Professionals should reflect critically on their own prejudices or reservations, including the extent to which they have developed a distorted picture of their patients through their work (e.g. with seriously ill patients in crisis situations) [158].

In addition to these core issues, successful interventions with professionals have three prerequisites—especially in hospitals [572]: First, hospitals are hierarchical structures, and the antistigma programme must therefore be actively promoted by the management. Second, long-term programmes are necessary; flash-in-the-pan measures cannot change a culture (or invent one). Finally, the role of peers is key, as they can talk about their experiences when meeting with professionals and thus facilitate contact on equal terms (Sect. 8.4.3).

A number of studies have shown that antistigma work with healthcare students and professionals can be successful. In the Czech Republic, Petr Winkler has compared the effectiveness of different approaches in reducing nursing students' prejudices against people with mental illness [573]. One intervention consisted of a seminar along the lines of the programme *Irrsinnig Menschlich* (Madly Human) developed in Leipzig, which combines education and contact (Sect. 8.4.5). Another consisted of short videos. Although the seminar option had a stronger and longer-lasting antistigma effect, the videos are easy and inexpensive to distribute; they are also a possible way forward. An antistigma programme for medical students that consists of contact, information, and role-play exercises is currently being evaluated internationally by Claire Henderson and her colleagues in the INDIGO network [574].

Matthew Lebowitz has studied the effectivity of an antistigma intervention amongst mental healthcare professionals that highlights two particular foci [575]: the character and identity of the patient (i.e. the person behind the illness) and the patient's decision-making abilities. This kind of approach counters that of one-sided biological illness models, through which the illness is seen as an expression of defective genes or brain mechanics (and in extreme cases can lead to the dehumanisation of those affected and thus increase stigma) (Sect. 5.1.2). The intervention studied by Lebowitz, on the other hand, emphasises personhood. Despite its brevity, it proved to be effective, and the professionals' desire for social distance from those affected decreased.

Another approach is to break down the perceived separation between *us professionals* and *the ill* by emphasising the illness/wellness continuum along which everybody lives (Sect. 8.1.4). Whether this approach reduces stigma among professionals is an open question. One RCT has found that such an intervention for professionals reinforced this concept of the continuum but did not actually reduce prejudice [576].

The association *Blaupause*, also known in English as *Blueprint—Initiative for Mental Health in Healthcare* (https://blaupause-gesundheit.de), was recently founded by young people in Germany. Through this platform, prospective and current professionals actively try to break the taboos of mental illness in the healthcare system. They also work towards the prevention of mental illness and increase in accessible services. Blueprint allows for an exchange of information between participants regarding these goals. The German Society for Bipolar Disorders (https://dgbs.de) also has a section for professionals with bipolar disorder that deals particularly with stigma management.

7.3.3 STRUCTURAL DISCRIMINATION IN THE HEALTHCARE SYSTEM

Are people with mental illness structurally discriminated against in the health and social care system? The answer would be an obvious yes if they were explicitly, systematically disadvantaged in comparison to people with physical illnesses. Yet the reality is more complex: structural discrimination takes place both intentionally and unintentionally, and even when individuals are not behaving in a discriminatory manner (Sect. 3.1.5). This section therefore addresses the level of the system rather than the actions of individuals (Sect. 7.3.1).

There are undoubtable shortcomings in the ways physically ill people are treated. However, as is argued later in this section, structural discrimination against people with mental illness is uniquely significant for two reasons:

1. The quality of the fragmented mental healthcare system is lower than that of the somatic healthcare system.
2. People with severe mental illness are more affected by the shortcomings of their healthcare system and have fewer resources than physically ill people to cope with the maze of the system.

More than physical illness, mental illness leads to impairments in the areas of work, housing and social relationships. The integration of health and social care systems could therefore be tremendously helpful, but it rarely takes place [488].

Fragmentation, Wrong Incentives, Interfaces

The mental healthcare system in Germany, as in many countries, is fragmented and broken up into various parts. There are both psychiatric and psychosomatic (i.e. a branch of psychodynamically oriented mental healthcare services for nonsevere mental disorders in Germany that parallels the psychiatric care system) hospitals; day clinics and outpatient clinics; psychiatrists in private practice, neurologists, psychosomatic doctors and psychotherapists; GPs who provide a large amount of primary mental healthcare; social psychiatric services and psychiatric residential homes; workshops for people with psychiatric disabilities and day care centres; family care, assisted living, outpatient sociotherapy, and medical and vocational rehabilitation services; and advice centres for a wide range of social services. The list goes on. In all of these contexts, professionals work with completely different orientations and methods: from the psychoanalytical couch to psychotropic drugs, electroconvulsive therapy and online therapy—everything can be found, although for some approaches there is little proof of their effectiveness.

I have been working in psychiatry for about 20 years, primarily with a social psychiatric orientation, but I still feel unfamiliar with the German healthcare system. How are people (who when in crisis can hardly leave their homes) supposed to cope, let alone spend months looking for the right point of contact? This bizarre fragmentation is itself a structural barrier and disadvantage to those who need help most. Precisely tailored help often cannot be found. It becomes even more bizarre when one considers how often the priority of patient-centred care is laid claim to in political speeches. The opposite is in fact the case: the many subsystems of the healthcare system are run in a largely uncoordinated fashion alongside one another. All of them insist on their rights and privileges. Attempts to integrate and improve care that could save lives and improve quality of life meet regularly with angry opposition from stakeholders who fear the loss of their influence and income. This is obviously not admitted to, but the status quo is praised, and threatening innovations are torpedoed with sometimes bizarre arguments (for an example, see the end of Sect. 7.3.4 'Strengthening Outpatient Care').

The fragmentation of care in Germany has worsened because parts of the care system are financed separately, and access rights, areas of responsibility and scope of benefits are regulated differently—including in different social security codes (SGB). There are inpatient and day care treatments in hospitals according to SGB V, outpatient treatment (e.g. in doctors' practices) (SGB V), health assistance (SGB XII), support for mentally ill unemployed people through employment agencies (SGB III) or job centres (SGB II), integration and participation benefits (SGB IX), child and youth welfare (SGB VIII), care services (SGB XI) and rehabilitation benefits of the pension insurance (SGB VI).

The fragmentation of the cost bearers leads to paradoxical incentives. Among other examples, psychiatric hospitals are not interested in providing less inpatient treatment for fear of losing money. Conversely, outpatient psychiatrists have no incentive to provide intensive outpatient treatment; there is no advantage for them to avoid sending patients into hospital treatment.

Statutory health insurance, on the other hand, saves money by letting people with mental illness finish their working lives and retire early. There is therefore little incentive for health insurers to invest preventively in maintaining employability—one reason for the low proportion of people with mental illness in the labour market (Sect. 7.1).

One unfortunate consequence of this fragmentation is that people with mental illness do not experience continuity in treatment from one provider [488]. Instead, they migrate from one part of the care system to another—from inpatient to outpatient, rehabilitation, complementary, and onwards. The left hand often does not know what the right hand is doing—coordination is costly and tends to be inadequate. After discharge from the hospital, information such as medication changes can be lost in the transition to outpatient treatment. This often leads to patients' discontinuation of treatment, and they 'disappear'. This is unfortunate; the transition from psychiatric inpatient to subsequent outpatient treatment is a particularly critical phase during which relapses and suicides are more frequent [577].

The fragmentation of the healthcare system affects people with mental disorders more severely than those with physical illnesses. Mental healthcare services specifically tend to be more fragmented. Yet personal, trusting, and stable relationships with caregivers are even more crucial to a psychiatric treatment's success than in somatic medicine. And although the integration of health and social care is necessary for coping with the complex psychosocial consequences of mental illness (particularly in relation to housing, work and the social environment), there remains a lack of coordination between care providers and a lack of navigators for service users (for peer navigators, see Sect. 7.3.4, 'Peer Support, Trialogue').

The problems outlined here are well known. Ingmar Steinhart and Günther Wienberg have pointed out that in Germany, there is a huge gap between inpatient and outpatient psychiatric care when it comes to financing by the statutory health insurance system ([578], p. 25). The treatment costs in a psychiatric hospital equal approximately 250 euros per day. Outpatient psychiatrists in their independent practices, on the other hand, receive a flat rate per quarter with an equivalent of less than 1 euro per day—regardless of whether they see the patient once or several times in that quarter. With several appointments per quarter, the flat rate very quickly no longer covers costs. This financing mechanism contributes to severely ill patients being admitted to hospital much more quickly than would be necessary with good outpatient care—even if the costs of hospital treatment are many times higher. These structures are not only inflexible and harmful to service users, they are also not cost-effective. This is one of many examples where care is not directed at the needs of patients but simply follows its own rules. This problem could be solved by billing outpatient psychiatrists according to their time, as is the case in Switzerland. In this way, given more time to spend with patients, practitioners could also accompany people in acute crises in an economic manner.

Lack of Psychosocial Interventions

Psychosocial interventions aim to make it easier for people with severe mental illness in particular to live in their social environment and participate in social life. Important areas of focus here include housing, work, and education. The German Association for Psychiatry, Psychotherapy and Psychosomatics (DGPPN, see 'Glossary') guidelines provide an impressive overview of the effectiveness of a wide range of such psychosocial interventions [66]. Despite this, many of these interventions are unfortunately not (or rarely) available to the public. Some examples have already been mentioned in other sections of this chapter: in the area of Supported Employment, especially in the form of IPS (Sect. 7.1.2, 'Supported Employment'), or in relation to Housing First (Sect. 7.2.6). A few further examples are briefly mentioned here (details in [66]):

- According to SGB V, *outpatient sociotherapy* has been a service since 2002. Psychiatrists or neurologists in private practice can prescribe sociotherapy, such that social workers or psychiatric nursing staff accompany patients, coordinate different care services, and therefore take on a kind of case management for the often complex treatment of people with severe mental illness. Given the high degree of fragmentation between support systems, such coordination would be urgently helpful. But outpatient sociotherapy has a niche existence and is hardly ever offered, in particular due to insufficient funding and excessive bureaucratic requirements. This attempt to improve outpatient care might as well be considered a failure, shredded by the usual conflicts of interest between social service authorities, health insurance companies and healthcare providers [579]. There is currently a lack of political will to implement complex outpatient treatment.

■ As far as *health promotion* is concerned, many people with mental illness suffer from the consequences of being overweight, sedentary, or smoking—major reasons for their reduced life expectancy (Sect. 7.3.1). Effective programmes in this field, including nutritional advice, sports activities, and giving up smoking [66], are not systematically implemented in the healthcare system.

■ Schizophrenic disorders begin in young adulthood, which is a primary reason why family members are especially affected by the diagnosis (Sect. 5.6). Families, however, can be an important support for those who are ill (Sect. 6.2). The effectiveness of *family interventions* for people with schizophrenia and their relatives is well-documented: symptoms tend to abate, there is less need for repeated hospital admissions, and the burden on family members is reduced. The current DGPPN guideline therefore strongly recommends family interventions: at a minimum, they should carry on for several months and comprise at least 10 sessions [580]. And yet, these programs are seldom provided in Germany. This is incomprehensible, especially since this gap in provision puts patients, relatives and the wider care system at a disadvantage.

Conclusion

These gaps in care highlight the structural discrimination faced by people with mental illness compared with those with physical illnesses. But they particularly disadvantage those with severe mental illness. These include all those whose illness is long-lasting and leads to disability, including in the areas of work, housing and social participation. It is precisely these patients who need integrated care through psychosocial interventions in the outpatient sector.

Somatic Care

The majority of available studies show that the care that people with mental illness receive for their physical complaints is worse than for those who are only physically ill. This concerns a wide array of issues, spanning from cardiovascular disease to diabetes, cancer and infection [581]. The causes of this poorer care are complex. As previously mentioned, the attitudes of individuals (practitioners as well as their patients) are likely to play a role (Sect. 7.3.1), and early, unbiased contact and diagnosis are made even more inaccessible. A study of more than 300,000 cases of patients who had had a stroke in the United States showed that the approximately 40,000 patients who also suffered from mental illness were significantly less likely to receive intravenous therapy to dissolve the blood clot (thrombolysis) than those without mental illness [582]. Various explanations for this poorer quality of treatment are possible and are directly or indirectly related to stigma and social isolation:

■ People with mental illness have fewer social contacts and support and live alone more often; on average, they reach A&E later following a stroke, and it is often already too late for thrombolysis.

■ Prejudice can influence diagnostic and therapeutic decisions by doctors.

- Patient information regarding immediate medical history is crucial, and doctors often consider psychiatric patients to have little credibility and do not take them seriously.
- The neurological symptoms of a stroke, which are not always easy to classify, can be misinterpreted as 'psychological' (Sect. 7.3.1, 'Attitudes of Professionals': diagnostic overshadowing).

These are all examples of how diverse and—taking everything into account—deadly stigma can be. The problem cannot be solved by focusing on just one aspect.

Other structural factors worsen the somatic care of people with mental illness. Psychiatric and somatic hospitals are often located in separate buildings (see the next subsection); it can be challenging to persuade colleagues dealing with somatic illnesses to visit and advise the psychiatric ward. Psychiatric liaison services, in which mental healthcare professionals work and learn in a team alongside somatic doctors, are rare.

Architecture

In the 19th century, a large number of psychiatric institutions were built and tended to be placed far away from city centres. At the time, this was done with the intention of reducing the high number of patients who were being incorrectly placed in prisons and other institutions. Psychiatrists also hoped that these isolated locations would bring peace and healing to the inmates. People were often locked up in these institutions for many years against their will. In the 20th century, Erving Goffman described them as *total institutions*, wherein inmates were at their mercy and painfully aware of the social exclusion caused by the *madhouse* [33]. In a poem by Heinrich Hoffmann, a Frankfurt psychiatrist of the 19th century and author of the *Struwwelpeter*, the madman in the madhouse says: 'I too have friends, honest friends / But they shy away from this place / They will lament me, cry for me / Then forget; this is where the loyalty ends.' The stay in the institution meant a social demise: 'A living death so hideously painful' ([583], p. 226).

As early as the end of the 19th century, and partly in response to public criticism of the conditions in mental institutions, there were attempts to improve the image of psychiatry. (The concern of today's psychiatrists for their reputation is therefore not new; see Sect. 7.3.1; [35], pp. 184 ff.) Lunatic asylums were renamed psychiatric clinics or mental hospitals, and departments for less seriously ill middle-class self-paying patients were established.

Many of the grievances only hinted at here fortunately belong to the past. Some of the aforementioned countryside institutions continue to exist on a smaller scale as monuments to the former physical segregation. It was a declared goal of the 1975 West German Psychiatrie-Enquete (Sect. 2.1.3) to integrate psychiatry into somatic medicine by opening psychiatric departments in general hospitals and to align the quality of care for the mentally ill with that of the physically ill. By treating people with somatic and mental disorders in one hospital, with one entrance and under one roof, there was a hope that the exclusion and stigma of mental illness would be reduced. But this integration was only partially successful. There were also reform efforts in the GDR (Sect. 2.1.3) that led to structural improvements in some areas, such as in Leipzig's social psychiatry.

Even though these large institutions are part of history, the stigma of mental illness today leads to resistance against the opening of even small psychiatric institutions in city districts. The phenomenon is called *Not in my backyard* (NIMBY). This is often rooted in the fears of local residents that people with mental illness are too dangerous to live in their communities. Architect Evangelia Chrysikou has studied the consequences of this phenomenon for small psychiatric institutions in a London district [584], comparing them with somatic healthcare buildings. Two things stood out. First, psychiatric institutions were remote and more difficult to get to (e.g. more distant from tube stations). Second, they were less visible from public spaces (i.e. the street or public squares), as though they wanted to hide. Chrysikou understands this *social invisibility* as a consequence of the stigma of mental illness, which perpetuates the structural and social exclusion of people with mental illness.

Architecture also plays a major role in the outer and interior design of psychiatric hospitals. Whereas in the past the focus was on aspects of security and surveillance—due to dominant stereotypes of dangerousness and in the tradition of institutional psychiatry (panopticon; Sect. 2.1.3)—modern architecture of psychiatric hospitals often attempts to promote and aid recovery vis-à-vis interior design: its façade, corridors, wards, and outpatient clinics. This is a fertile new field of research; keywords are *therapeutic architecture* and *evidence-based design* [584]. Redesigns of existing hospitals in this sense appear to have positive effects on patients and staff [585]. The participation of people with mental illness in the planning process is helpful (co-design [586]).

7.3.4 INITIATIVES AGAINST STRUCTURAL DISCRIMINATION IN THE HEALTHCARE SYSTEM

As outlined in the section on stigma and discrimination in the healthcare system (Sect. 7.3.3), interventions aimed only at individuals (e.g. professionals) will not be enough to rectify structural deficiencies (Sect. 7.3.2). This section therefore describes interventions that aim to reduce structural disadvantages faced by people with mental illness in the healthcare system. Other interventions, for example for the general public or specific target groups outside the health sector, are discussed from Chapter 8 onwards.

There is a lot that needs to be done in this area. At the suggestion of the Friedrich-Ebert-Foundation, a thought-provoking position paper by Elke Prestin and her colleagues described the need for actions to reform psychosocial care [587]. Some of the problems and solutions they wrote about are dealt with in the following section; others are discussed in the sections on housing and work (Sects. 7.1, 7.2). It should also be mentioned that good healthcare requires coordination between somatic and psychiatric professionals (Sect. 7.3.3). This is one way to extend the reduced life expectancy of people with severe mental illness [588].

Strengthening Outpatient Care

An obvious solution to the fragmentation of the mental healthcare system (Sect. 7.3.3) is to increase support for outpatient care, giving it control and oversight functions. The aim would be to create teams that are willing and able to provide a sufficient level of outpatient care, including for people with severe mental illness and complex needs, and to efficiently coordinate the various forms of assistance. This objective has been repeatedly formulated in recent years. Ingmar Steinhart and Günther Wienberg have outlined a complete model of primarily outpatient-based care called 'all-round outpatient care' [578]. It is important that outpatient care is outreach based, such that if a person with a severe anxiety disorder can no longer leave their home, the mobile treatment team can go directly to them and thereby avoid hospitalisation. This possibility should be available around the clock.

There are three significant types of team-based outpatient treatment that originate from Anglo-American countries and that have proven effective [66]. They are also recommended for German-speaking countries and are briefly outlined here (Fig. 7.1):

1. *Home Treatment*: a team of nurses, doctors, and social workers comes to visit several times a week to treat people in an acute episode. A typical example is that of a mother who becomes severely depressed after giving birth and is treated at home for an initial 2 months (and then returns to less frequent outpatient care).

2. *Assertive Community Treatment* (ACT) was created in the 1980s in the United States to provide good long-term outpatient care for patients released from institutions. With ACT, people with serious mental illness are cared for at home on a long-term basis, often for many years.

3. *Community Mental Health Teams (CMHT)*, which are particularly widespread in Great Britain, provide outpatient care locally. They share similarities with the psychiatric outpatient departments of German psychiatric hospitals (Psychiatrische Institutsambulanzen).

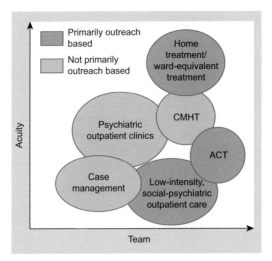

Fig. 7.1   Outpatient community mental health services according to their level of teamwork and the acuity of illness; CMHT and ACT stand for Community Mental Health Teams and Assertive Community Treatment. (Based on Gühne U, Weinmann S, et al. (DGPPN). *S3-Leitlinie Psychosoziale Therapien bei schweren psychischen Erkrankungen.* 2nd ed. Springer; 2019; Becker T, Hoffmann H, Puschner B, Weinmann S. *Versorgungsmodelle in Psychiatrie und Psychotherapie, 1. Auflage 2008.* Kohlhammer GmbH. Courtesy of Heike Hübner, Berlin.)

To date, apart from some psychiatric hospital outpatient clinics and individual model projects, these three intensive outpatient treatment options are hard to find in Germany. For the last few years, I have had the good fortune of working at the Günzburg District Hospital in a home-treatment team that was founded there some 15 years ago by Thomas Becker and his colleagues. I've learned first-hand that with a multiprofessional team, even seriously and acutely ill people can be well-cared-for at home. For many, this service is the only possibility—not all service users want or are able to receive psychiatric inpatient care (e.g. because they have small children at home). But in Germany, such teams are few and far between.

Why is this the case? An example of legislation that was designed to significantly improve outpatient mental healthcare in Germany is helpful here. The details illustrate how difficult it is to achieve improvement. At the end of 2016, the law on the further development of care and remuneration for psychiatric and psychosomatic services (PsychVVG) was passed. For the first time, the *PsychVVG* made it possible for psychiatric hospitals to provide acute intensive outpatient treatment based on the model of home treatment. In legal terms, this form of treatment is called '*stationsäquivalente Behandlung*' (StäB; treatment equivalent to hospital care). This treatment was intended to overcome the divide between outpatient and inpatient treatment, one of many sector boundaries in the German health and social care system. However, what seemed to be a major step forward was largely ruined by its rigid implementation and financing conditions. In home treatment, for example, a basic requirement is flexibility and the ability to adapt to the condition and needs of the patient—being patient-oriented should be a matter of course. If a person with psychosis requires home visits but cannot cope with more than three a week, I do not go to him more than three times a week. In contrast to this patient-oriented approach, StäB requires that every patient be seen daily, seven home visits per week—otherwise the health insurance companies do not cover the costs. Many of the patients we have treated in home treatment have relayed that they certainly would not want to be treated by StäB under these conditions. I can understand that even in a crisis, having professionals in one's living room every day would feel unnecessary or too much.

The reasons for this absurd regulation are not clear. Perhaps various stakeholders (e.g. health insurance companies) have insisted on rigid regulations (e.g. seven visits per week) that make StäB treatment impractical and hinder its implementation. It would not be the first example of how complex outpatient treatment is in fact circumvented due to its design and system of reimbursement (on outpatient sociotherapy, see Sect. 7.3.3). The negative consequences of this rigid StäB requirement are numerous:

- With daily compulsory visits, even a large StäB team can only treat a few patients. The cost efficiency is low and undersupply persists (especially in rural areas).
- Smaller psychiatric hospitals in particular can barely set up StäB teams. They simply do not have enough staff.
- It is unethical not to leave the choice of treatment frequency to the patient. Patients who do not want daily visits are otherwise excluded from intense outpatient care.

All of this is a sad lesson in how a good idea for reform can fail for the most part in execution. Furthermore, StäB was introduced as an isolated innovation in the complicated maze of the care system and, as yet another new component, is likely to further increase complexity and interface problems.

In recent years, I have come across bizarre arguments about home treatment and StäB. At a conference in the run-up to the PsychVVG, an influential representative of outpatient psychiatrists in independent practice said in his lecture that people with serious mental illness did not want to be visited at home. Home treatment and StäB should therefore be rejected (irrespective of the frequency of home visits, which was not discussed at the time). This line of reasoning is not only factually incorrect—many patients highly appreciate the possibility of home treatment, as numerous quantitative and qualitative studies have shown—but is also profoundly cynical. The argument rejects reform while pretending to consider the will of the patients. The truth is that it is about defending these providers' own sinecures—in this case, keeping hospitals away from outpatient care. But this is not discussed openly. When I asked that representative on what he based his claim (that patients dislike home visits), he simply replied: 'I have experience.' Everyone likes to talk about evidence, guidelines, medical ethics, patient orientation and participation. But when it comes to the self-interest of professionals, institutions or cost bearers, the discussion drops to this level and prevents the implementation of effective help for the seriously ill.

Integrated Care and Regional Budget

There are various models of integrated care for people with mental illness. Their approaches primarily aim to bridge the gap between different parts of the healthcare and social service systems. In Germany, they are regulated in SGB V as selective contracts of individual health insurance companies (§ 140a) or as model projects (§ 64b). They are, unsurprisingly, only available to members of the participating health insurance company or to people in the catchment area of the model project. These approaches therefore have the undesirable side effect of making the fragmented care system even more confusing. Nevertheless, they show what is possible through integrated care. One example is the Hamburg model, RECOVER, which strengthens outpatient services, follows a graduated procedure depending upon severity, and includes family doctors, psychotherapists and eMental Health (i.e. digital assistance) (https://recover-hamburg.de).

With a regional budget, a psychiatric hospital responsible for a particular area no longer receives money for its inpatient treatment. Instead, the hospital and cost bearers agree to a fixed budget, the regional budget. Based on this amount, the hospital can freely choose the type of patient care available: inpatient, day clinic, outpatient, home visits, etc. Experience with this approach to date is positive and shows that the proportion of outpatient treatments increases with a regional budget [589]. However, this model does not include outpatient psychiatrists and psychotherapists in their independent practices. It is therefore rather a regional hospital budget (and only inclusive to this extent).

Thoughtful stakeholders therefore call for structural, regulatory changes that go beyond individual projects to achieve fundamental improvements, overcome fragmentation and implement integrated care [587]. Some of their statements suggest quiet resignation to the sustained blocking of cross-sectoral care by various interest groups: 'The legislator must make the framework conditions mandatory, as partial interests usually prevail' (Iris Hauth, DGPPN president 2015–16, *Deutsches Ärzteblatt*, 6 Aug. 2018).

Prevention

There are four simple reasons for the prevention of mental illness:

- First, mental illness is common and can cause a great deal of suffering to individuals and their environments, as well as high societal costs.
- Second, as with physical illness, it is better to prevent the occurrence of illness than to act only after the onset of illness.
- Third, mental disorders start early: about half of them by the age of 15 and three-quarters by age 25. Successful prevention thus ensures decades of preserved health, social participation, ability to work, etc.
- Fourth, the success rate of mental healthcare is limited. This is shown by model calculations using depression as an example: even if all depressive patients could participate in evidence-based treatment, their burden of illness would only be reduced by about one-third [590]. The remaining two-thirds can only be tackled preventively. In reality, prevention is even more important because only a minority of people with mental illness receive effective treatment, in part because of fear of stigma and labelling, self-stigma and shame, and in part because of the structures of the care system (Sects. 5.1.7, 7.3.1).

In the realm of physical illnesses, the concept of prevention is well established. For smoking or HIV, a broad social awareness and a change in values towards prevention has occurred. In comparison, the prevention of mental illness is neglected—not only, but also in the work of the BZgA ('Glossary', Sect. 5.2.3). Three approaches to prevention can be differentiated:

- *General or primary prevention* is aimed at the general public to reduce newly occurring illnesses. One example from the somatic field is vaccination against infectious illnesses; an example from the mental health field is action against child abuse to reduce emerging mental illness as a result of violence.
- *Secondary or indicated prevention* is aimed at people who already show possible early symptoms or warning signs or who have an increased risk of becoming ill. One example from the field of somatic medicine is cancer screening (e.g. mammograms); in the field of mental illness, examples include screening programmes for suicidal behaviour, programmes for young people at risk of psychosis (Sect. 5.3) and programmes for children of mentally ill parents.
- *Tertiary prevention* is about preventing relapses in people who have a history of mental illness.

The stigma of mental illness is one reason why mental health prevention is neglected [591]. Public stigma and structural discrimination lead to a lack of prioritisation of mental health in the broader field of prevention policies and, as a result, prevention is not funded or implemented. On the other hand, public stigma and self-stigma/shame make it difficult to participate in prevention measures when they are available. This is comparable to stigma as an obstacle to seeking help (Sect. 5.1.7).

What is the basic principle of prevention work? It is focused on practising behaviour that maintains and promotes mental health. This is why we also speak in terms of *behavioural vaccination* [592]. A long-time example of preventive behavioural practice is wearing a seat belt when driving a car. If this behaviour becomes normalised and instinctive, it saves the lives and well-being of countless drivers and passengers. As with vaccination against viruses, repetition also improves the effects of behavioural vaccination. Similarly, information and training programmes of all kinds can help to strengthen mental health and improve the management of stress.

Does prevention work? And if so, how? It is helpful to outline here an example of a well-known prevention programme, *Triple P* (*Positive Parenting Programme*; https://triplep.net/glo-en/home/). The programme aims to improve parenting behaviours. Originally developed in Australia, it is now used all over the world and has been widely studied. Triple P can be offered in a variety of contexts and consists of information on education, counselling, and individual and group training (as needed). It can therefore be used as a primary (e.g. as an information campaign for the general public) or secondary prevention measure (e.g. for parents with specific problems).

STUDY

Triple P not only reduces psychological stress and behavioural problems of children and parents but also lowers child abuse rates. In a US study, a lottery was used to determine whether Triple P would be offered in various counties across one state; the programme was implemented in 9 of 18 counties [593]. The intervention involved training professionals in the health, social and educational sectors to use the Triple P programme in their support of parents. Compared with counties without Triple P, the programme reduced the number of documented cases of child abuse, foster care placements and child abuse injuries confirmed in hospitals.

Violence against children is so horrific that this finding alone underscores the importance of wide-ranging prevention in this area: longitudinal studies show that children who have suffered violence, abuse or neglect are later found to have a much higher incidence of various mental disorders and poor social outcomes, including addiction, being overweight, failing in education and work and contact with the judicial system (as they more frequently became offenders themselves) [594]. Triple P is thus an example of a 'good parenting' programme that works on multiple levels and is cost-effective. On average across various programmes of this kind, it costs approximately 2500 US dollars to improve the behaviour of a child with behavioural problems. However, this amount is often outweighed by savings in other areas (more on this later in this section [595]).

What about the *prevention of depression*, one of our most common mental disorders? Studies on secondary (indicated) prevention have so far only shown a small to medium effect. Researchers in this field therefore tend to ask for two things to improve preventions of depression [596]:

1. Interventions should focus on risk groups, such as parents with problematic parenting behaviours (poor parenting) and children with difficulties in emotional or behavioural regulation.

2. Prevention programmes should be grounded in social policy (e.g. in administration, child-care and education systems). Attitudes must change in society such that mental health prevention becomes a recognised goal, as has been the case with smoking.

Should society invest in the prevention of mental illness? Besides an ethical obligation to prevent avoidable suffering, there are strong arguments for doing so. Health researcher David McDaid has made an economic argument for the prevention of mental illness based on experimental research, large observational studies and model calculations (Sect. 2.2.4) [53]. According to his studies, the costs of prevention are more than offset by future savings. It is first crucial to recognise that prevention work, especially with young people, can provide benefits for decades. Second, the benefits of mental health prevention are by no means limited to the healthcare system; prevention can lead to savings in education, training, employment, welfare and the justice system. Taking all of these areas into account, every euro invested in the coming decades on prevention programmes for parents of small children could generate a return on investment of around 5 to 10 euros. It is a strange irony that our societies that tout certain economic priorities have not already implemented such prevention programmes. There are particularly good economic arguments for prevention in the areas of mothers/infants, children and adolescents (Sect. 2.2.4), work, suicidality and healthy ageing [53].

Hans Joachim Salize once pointed out to me that preventive risk warnings are unequally distributed in society. Every electrical appliance, no matter how harmless, needs an electrical certificate or proof of its carbon emission or energy balance. Apart from addiction warnings on certain substances, the same cannot be said for psychological risks. Let us assume that a flat is located in a high-density area on a narrow, busy street without sufficient sound and heat insulation and without green public spaces nearby. Due to the increased chance of mental illness from growing up and living in such environments [541], a label—comparable to a car's emissions certificate—could be useful to indicate stress as a risk for residents of this flat. It might even encourage property developers, landlords and urban planners to take action.

The German federal budget for 2020 (before the supplementary budget adopted in March 2020 due to the coronavirus pandemic) was around 360 billion euros. Forty percent of this (around 150 billion euros) was earmarked for employment and social affairs, not including employers' and employees' social security contributions. Given this budget allocation and the long-term consequences of mental illness for social systems and employment, the lack of comprehensive prevention programmes for maintaining mental health is a bizarre malfunction. Money is (rightly) spent on social welfare, but this is done decades too late when taking the whole life course into account. The promotion of mental health amongst children and young people today must be seen as an economic and ethical imperative, so that fewer of them will be the unemployed, sick, early retirees of tomorrow.

One would think that the proven effectiveness of prevention measures would facilitate their implementation. But the opposite seems to be the case. In terms of funding, accountability, and entry rules, the systems of healthcare, education, employment, welfare and justice are so divided that a coordinated approach and joint budget for prevention rarely succeeds. The various systems wherein a positive effect is evident are not even taken note of, let alone acted upon. Who can motivate a health insurance company to invest in the prevention of mental disorders in mothers and infants if many of the savings only become apparent decades later (e.g. in the school system and labour market)? (On the problem of diagonal accounting, see Sect. 2.2.4, forecasting and policy response.) As in the health and social care systems (Sect. 7.3.3), there is no single, central provider of preventive programmes. The German Prevention Act, which has been in place since 2016, has yet to noticeably contribute to improving prevention. Fragmentation is more likely to hamper prevention of mental illness compared with that of physical illness because the causes and consequences of mental illness are more complex.

Conclusion

Antistigma work (Ch. 8 ff.) can be regarded as secondary prevention. A reduction in public stigma would make it easier for people in crisis to seek help because they would not be as deterred by fear of stigma (Sect. 5.1.7). When public attitudes improve, self-stigma and shame also decrease as results of social prejudice. Without self-stigma, the search for help (e.g. from friends or the family doctor) is made easier, and the burden of shame falls away.

Peer Support, Trialogue

The traditional concept of mental healthcare has placed healthy professionals on one side of the desk and sick patients on the other. Anyone who has ever heard how (some) professionals in psychiatry or psychotherapy talk about their patients is aware of this separation between them and us (Sect. 3.1.4). But it's nonsense, and not only because there are professionals who have mental illness (Sect. 7.3.1) and service users who used to be healthcare professionals (Sect. 6.1). But all people live on the continuum between complete mental health and severe mental illness in a constant state of flux that depends on one's social situation and living conditions (Sect. 1.6). One approach to overcoming this supposed division is to involve people with lived experience (of mental illness) in our care and support systems. They are experts not through training but by experience and therefore need to be seen as peers ('Glossary'). Peers have experience in coping with illness and in personal recovery.

Anyone who has gained a qualification or undergone further training as a peer is also called a peer support worker. When training to be a peer support worker, participants reflect on their backgrounds and experiences and develop ways to use them in their help of others. In German-speaking countries, the established form of training to become a peer support worker consists of 12 modules and two internships (https://ex-in.de). The topics of the modules are varied and include the basic principles of peer work: recovery, empowerment, social participation and salutogenesis (i.e. looking at recovery rather than at deficits and symptoms). Another topic is how peers can accompany and support others with mental illness. An impetus for the development and establishment of peer support in Germany has been the *Trialogue*, an exchange and equal cooperation of service users, relatives and professionals in different contexts [460]. Among others, it was established and is maintained in Hamburg by Thomas Bock and colleagues. The programme was inspired by Dorothea Buck (1917-2019 [597]), a sculptor, author and victim of forced sterilisation and psychiatry in the Nazi era (Sect. 2.1.2): 'If the professionals speak to us at eye level, they at least do not kill us anymore' ([598], p. 25).

In *peer work*, the experience of illness is also seen as an opportunity for enrichment and new insights, despite the suffering associated with it. Mental illness is a deeply human experience. Peer work in clinical environments, social institutions or counselling centres can be particularly valuable for patients and clients. Those seeking advice can meet people who are peers and have experienced and overcome similar crises themselves. This allows for an equal exchange and increases the credibility of the peers (compared with professionals, for example). Increased social contact between people with lived experience of mental illness counteracts widespread social isolation. At the same time, peers can provide hope and serve as role models for those in crisis: 'He has overcome his illness and can work here as a peer. Then I might as well do it too.' I was unfamiliar with peer support back in 2000, when I was working with Pat Corrigan at his psychiatric rehabilitation centre in Chicago. I met a former rabbi with bipolar disorder who was working as a peer there, and I remember the gleam of hope in the eyes of the often seriously ill patients when they talked to him. In him, they could envisage a life after and with the illness.

Does peer support work? There are several reasons why this is not an easy question to answer empirically. First, it is a new field of research with very little robust data. Second, peer support takes on very different forms, including peer-led group programmes, peer-to-peer support and peer-led counselling or treatment facilities [599]. A meta-analysis of 23 studies has evidenced that peer-led group interventions improve empowerment [600]. But good-quality studies are rare. In one large English RCT, one-to-one peer support to promote recovery reduced the number of admissions to psychiatric hospitals [601]. However, a different overview of peer support for people with severe mental illness was unable to provide clear evidence for or against its benefits due to a lack of strong studies [602]. Peer support seems to work best in the area of self-management on specific challenges like strengthening problem-solving skills and self-efficacy. *Peer navigators* also seem to have a positive effect alongside GPs or in health-promoting activities [603].

Despite patchy data, peer support is likely to be an important component of future support for people with mental illness. The reasons are manifold. First, the idea has long proved itself as reliable and is rooted in the self-help movement. Second, professionals are (or should be) increasingly aware that standard deficit- and symptom-oriented treatments lack essential features for service users, such as hope, recovery orientation and human contact. Third, peers bring a new perspective that is refreshingly different from those of professionals. The two are not mutually exclusive and can complement one another. Many professionals react to peer support with reservations, often making it more difficult to implement. This difficulty is not due to peer support in principle but rather is because of the usual vested interests, prejudices and resistance to change within our institutions. Hospitals and other organisations should be open to the new experiences that peer support brings. It will not succeed otherwise [604]. And it is not enough to simply employ peers and let them get on with their work without systemic support—prejudices and assumptions of their failure would inevitably be confirmed.

As with any new approach, it is important to consider what the aim is and what the peer work should essentially consist of. These types of goals are not always clear—and could also explain the inconsistent data mentioned earlier. Some professionals say that peers should lead psychoeducation groups, sharing the information as written by professionals. This strategy is not particularly convincing. Peers can only make a valuable contribution if they are able to bring their own experiences as peers to the table. They can of course lead groups—alone or together, and on an equal footing with professionals. When they do, the dynamics and the contents of the group change. This does not mean that a peer should be treated as some kind of unskilled worker in the mental healthcare system. There is a risk worth noting that peers will be hired as low-paid replacements for expensive professionals [224], especially when the latter are scarce in the labour market. But peers can and should fulfil a new role in the support system [605]. They can offer a balanced relationship to service users without focusing solely on symptom relief. This would emphasise the value of social contacts that people can continue to enjoy even after cessation of treatment. And a peer support focus could help to improve the bureaucratic culture of treatment institutions and lessen the competitive feelings of professionals.

Conclusion

Peer support is something that can only be provided by peers, not professionals. When this work is done by people in the capacity of being peers, it is like a well-needed and practical breath of fresh air [220]. The role of peers is also crucial to antistigma work: they must lead and thereby make credible antistigma programmes (Sect. 12.4). An example of a peer-led group programme on stigma management is *Honest, Open, Proud* (Sect. 9.2).

A consideration of the social aspects of peer support should also take into account its historical roots. Similar to the recovery movement (Sect. 5.1.6), peer support emerged in the 1970s in the context of the civil rights movement and social reforms for equal rights of marginalised groups, including ethnic minorities, ex-patients and psychiatric survivors. For decades, peer work was not part of psychiatry—on the contrary, it challenged its institutional practices. Only recently have attempts been made to integrate peer work into psychiatry. This offers opportunities as well as risks. Stigma is based on power (Sect. 3.1.4), and peers can be appropriated and dominated by professionals in institutions. For these reasons, an independent, socially oriented role that is not limited to symptom management or psychoeducation is crucial [220]. For the *Hearing Voices Movement*, an example of peer support outside of psychiatry, see Section 8.1.4 ('Continuum?').

Avoidance of Coercion and Violence

In most countries, people with mental illness can be brought to a psychiatric hospital against their will. This is only possible if they are a considerable danger to themselves (e.g. suicidality) or others. In Germany, the regulations regarding forced hospital admission are confusingly regulated into 16 individual state laws, the PsychKHGs ('Glossary'). Since 2011, in response to decisions of the Federal Constitutional Court and to the UN-CRPD (Sect. 7.5.2 [606]), all of these laws have been in an amendment phase. What they hold in common is that in emergencies, hospital admissions can be made by the police or by regulatory authorities such as the district office, but that the involuntary stay in the psychiatric hospital must be reviewed and approved by a judge. In addition, legal guardians can apply to the court under civil law for hospital admission.

Despite increased clarity in recent years and the necessity for court orders, this issue remains controversial. Many people with mental illness reject forced admissions on principle. It is undeniable that coercion is a serious interference when it comes to self-determination. However, people in mental crises are not always able to make decisions based on the situation at hand. Should I want to kill myself in some future episode of serious mental illness, I would hope that someone would stop me, and by force if necessary. From my point of view, this other person would not only have the right but the duty to hold me back. I have thought this ever since, as a young doctor, I met a young mother shortly after her serious suicide attempt; she was glad to have survived and to be able to live with her children. But there are very different, respectable views on this topic among service users as well as psychiatrists and ethicists. A pragmatic problem is that involuntary hospitalisations do not reliably prevent suicides in the short term or in the long term [607].

Despite all of the justified criticism of psychiatry, this field is uniquely confronted with societal demands that are difficult to reconcile. Suppose a man with acute psychosis walks on a city street screaming and behaving aggressively. The police take him to a psychiatric hospital because they perceive him as mentally ill rather than as a delinquent. For psychiatry, this presents the dual societal task of not only helping the man but also being involved in the prevention of danger. A person who is aggressive in this situation will not always become calm at the very moment the police officers leave the hospital. Anyone who resolutely rejects violence, even if the man throws a chair at staff or fellow patients, should reconsider the aforementioned mandate to psychiatry, take note of the risks for fellow patients and those working in psychiatry, and name constructive alternatives. The advice given by antipsychiatry was to simply put such a man in prison. Although that line of thinking is consistent with the rejection of psychiatry, it raises other questions about whether and how the man would receive help if imprisoned and whether he would suffer less fear and violence there.

Additionally, with regard to dealing with the risk of suicide, societal attitudes seem to be contradictory. If a woman expresses suicidal intentions and is taken to a psychiatric hospital by police at night against her will, I as a psychiatrist have two options when I see her the next morning and she refuses to stay in the hospital: I can let her go, or I can apply to the court to continue her stay in the hospital against her will. If in the first scenario she subsequently kills herself, I would be accused by relatives or lawyers of irresponsibly violating my duty to help ('she was ill and did not know what she was doing'). In the second scenario, I would be accused of violence and unlawful detention (possibly by the same people: 'she knows very well what she is doing, and the choice is hers').

What does the societal ambivalence outlined here have to do with stigma?
1. This is ultimately about the consequences of labelling people as mentally ill and the question of who takes responsibility for people in acute crises.
2. Stigma is based on power, and many service users accuse psychiatry of an abuse of power (including scenarios like the ones just mentioned). The fact that power is exercised is beyond question.
3. Involuntary admissions usually come at the end of a long chain of escalation during which no adequate outpatient help was available. This deplorable state of affairs is a consequence of the fragmentation and underfunding of the mental healthcare system (Sect. 7.3.3).
4. The handling of risks is an important topic within recovery. Among other things, recovery means overcoming the harmful consequences of stigma (Sect. 5.1.6) and requires taking

more responsibility for oneself. This responsibility entails risks. People (with and without mental illness) have the right to make mistakes. If the self-determination of people with mental illness is (rightly) to be supported, this includes greater tolerance for the fact that recovery is nonlinear and can be risky. Dealing with risks in individual cases will remain difficult (see the aforementioned allegations).

For the time being, we will have to live and work with this tension between freedom and personal responsibility (whenever possible) on one hand, and power and assumption of responsibility for others (temporarily, in an emergency) on the other. This does not mean to suggest that psychiatry is faultless—there is much to improve. But the problem goes far beyond psychiatry: it is about societal attitudes, and there will rarely be simple solutions. Lashing out at psychiatry or the police tends to be unhelpful (and makes creating partnerships all the more challenging). Unfortunately, I have yet to find a reasonable public discussion on this topic. Instead, sensational media reports dominate discourse and highlight individual cases where risk assessments retrospectively appear to have failed (i.e. people died or were unlawfully detained).

That said, more can and must be done to reduce the number of involuntary admissions and mitigate their consequences. Comparing cases between countries, the frequency varies [608]: per 100,000 inhabitants, about 280 people are involuntarily admitted in Austria per year, about 170 in Germany, about 130 in Switzerland, about 115 in England, but only about 15 in Italy. Such differences, even between individual hospitals, are difficult to justify objectively. It is clear that many service users experience coercion as stigmatising and humiliating, and that these experiences have long-term consequences. In a follow-up study, a greater feeling of shame due to the coercion experienced during hospital admission was associated with more self-stigma and less empowerment even 1 year later [199].

Adequate Staffing Levels

Good care only succeeds when there is enough staff that has time to listen and converse. The aforementioned PsychVVG of 2016 therefore contained a mandate for the Federal Joint Committee (G-BA, Gemeinsamer Bundesausschuss), the highest body of self-administration in the German healthcare system, to present guidelines for staffing in hospitals for psychiatry, psychosomatics, and child and adolescent psychiatry by 2019. The G-BA represents health insurance funds, GPs and other outpatient doctors and hospitals. However, the study it commissioned in 2016 to assess staffing requirements was later rejected by the G-BA in 2019 due to methodological problems—a thoroughly Kafkaesque situation. As a result, at the end of 2019, and without any empirical basis, the (very dated) psychiatric staffing level plan of 1991 was by and large updated as a minimum standard. At the same time, the documentation requirements for hospitals were further increased.

The hoped-for adaptation of staffing levels to current standards of good care failed to materialise. Today, due to higher-quality requirements and an increase in therapeutic knowledge compared with 1991, the following are necessary in the clinic: differentiated somatic and psychological diagnostics, patient education, shared decision-making, intensive individual and group psychotherapy, cooperation with social services, planning of treatment after discharge, discussions with relatives, supervision, case planning and team coordination—not to mention the documentation requirements that have spun out of control. If all of this is neglected due to a lack of personnel, there is a risk of relapse into custodial psychiatry. Unfortunately, most of these requirements tend to be neglected, in particular because documentation comes first—not only for legal reasons but also because health insurance companies do not pay without the paperwork. So doctors, psychologists, nurses, social workers, occupational therapists and many others sit at their computers and spend a good part of their working day typing out reports instead of talking to patients. Wasting precious time on excessive documentation is getting worse year by year, and there is no sign of any counteraction.

Conclusion

Continued understaffing is an obstacle to overcoming many of the aforementioned problems (Sects. 7.3.1, 7.3.3). If patients are not properly engaged with, then self-determination, orientation towards recovery, and hope will not flourish. Is this a case of structural discrimination against psychiatric compared with somatic patients? Yes. People with mental illness are in a unique situation: their treatment will hardly succeed without the time and attention of their healthcare staff. If need be, a broken leg heals without conversation. But the mind and soul cannot. Political persuasion is needed to create the conditions for good and equal care for people with mental illness.

7.4 The Media

For most people, hardly a day goes by without taking in information, opinions, pictures, films or texts from the media. Whether we welcome it or not, the media is everywhere (and this is even more true when considering the expanse of the internet). People with mental illness are frequently featured in the media, and both stigmatising and positive portrayals abound [609, 610]. In this section, common stereotypes about people with mental disorders that appear in the media are outlined first (Sect. 7.4.1), and specific types of media that engage with these stereotypes are then presented (Sect. 7.4.2). This is followed by discussions on the role of (dis)information in the media (Sect. 7.4.3), why the media is important for maintaining and reducing stigma (Sect. 7.4.4), and the issue of suicide (Sect. 7.4.5). After examining possible motives for stigmatising media content (Sect. 7.4.6), antistigma interventions in the media sector are presented (Sect. 7.4.7). On antistigma interventions in general, see Chapter 8.

7.4.1 STEREOTYPES

Three common stereotypes about people with mental illness appear repeatedly in the media: dangerousness, comic effect and how the ill are different (Sect. 3.1.4).

Dangerousness

Dangerous lunatics and psycho killers have long haunted various media genres. As far back as Fritz Lang's 1922 film *Dr. Mabuse, the Gambler*, we see the ingenious criminal descend into madness by the end; as a psychoanalyst he uses his hypnotic arts destructively, and in a later Mabuse film he controls the criminal activity as an inmate from inside a psychiatric ward. Equally famous is Alfred Hitchcock's *Psycho* of 1960, in which the murder motif of the mentally ill perpetrator is psychoanalytically interpreted in the context of the relationship with his mother.

In these films, and widespread in news as well as in fictional media, is a narrative that the subject presented by people with mental illness is one of mortal danger. This stereotype of the danger that is posed is greatly exaggerated (Sect. 3.2.4, 'Do Stereotypes Contain a Kernel of Truth?'), yet it has a particularly negative effect when applied to individuals in a generalised way. For the media, the same old story can be told in many different ways: from one end, the portrayed dangers that people with mental illness pose in fictional media such as film and literature have come to be regarded as universally valid and typical. From the other end, one-off news stories about rare, sensational crimes committed by people with mental disorders contribute to the stereotype, as they are often luridly embellished and very memorable (Sect. 3.2.5, 'Illusory Correlation').

There have been studies conducted on how often people with mental illness were portrayed as dangerous on television: about three-quarters were violent, and more than one in five had killed someone. Even for women, who are hardly ever presented as violent, these rates were similarly high if they had a mental illness [611]. The perpetrators or suspects in German television crime series are often mentally ill [612].

Comic Effect

Mental illness is often presented as bizarre or ridiculous. This ties in with the content of stereotypes discussed previously, which can ambivalently combine warmth and incompetence (i.e. positive and negative aspects) (Sect. 3.2.4, 'Content Dimensions of Stereotypes'). These stereotypes lead to people with mental illness being portrayed as childish, foolish, or helpless to evoke amusement in the viewer or reader. Examples of films in which mental illness provides amusement can be found in Section 7.4.2 ('Film and Television'). This type of humour can also be found on social media and websites with collections of jokes: 'Hello and welcome to our hotline for people with mental health problems. If you suffer from obsessive-compulsive disorder, then please keep pressing 1. […] If you are schizophrenic, listen very carefully. A small, clear voice will whisper to you which number you have to press'.

Although many may find this funny, or think it harmless, or dismiss this as an issue of political correctness, such jokes are often perceived as disrespectful and hurtful by people with mental illness and their relatives. Even further, there are three problems raised by jokes about people with mental illness. First, these illnesses can cause so much suffering that they are hardly suitable to joke about. Second, it is doubtful whether jokes about other groups, such as ethnic minorities, would be similarly accepted. Finally, humour that makes fun of others can certainly have a useful corrective function in a social context. But this is true when it is directed against powerful people (e.g. in political satire). People with mental illness are not a powerful social group and humour about them tends to punch down, not up. The imbalance of power disadvantaging the stigmatised group is a prerequisite for stigma (Sect. 3.1.4).

Differentness

The idea that they or the mentally ill are different from us healthy people is, as described in previous sections on stigma models and categorisation (Sects. 3.1, 3.2), a precondition for stigma. In the media, this can lead to people with mental illness being portrayed as bizarre and conspicuous; their otherness is easily recognisable. One example is the actor Peter Lorre, whose striking appearance and large, protruding eyes predestined him for the role of the dangerous lunatic in Fritz Lang's *M* (1931)—he was 'obviously almost mad' ([609], p. 37; Fig. 7.2).

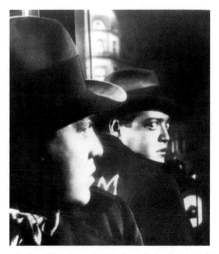

Fig. 7.2 Peter Lorre in *M*, 1931. (From Moviestore Collection Ltd, Alamy stock photos.)

Today's media professionals and advertising experts also rely on the cliché of obvious different-ness: in 2013, British supermarkets were selling a *'mental patient costume'*, a blood-stained monster outfit with a hatchet, for Halloween. The sale of the costume was stopped after pro-tests (Sect. 8.3). This stereotype can be so extreme that certain films (e.g. *Halloween II* [1981]) describe a mentally ill murderer as 'it', 'some kind of animal' and not 'even remotely human' ([609], p. 45). The consequences are obvious: these beings, who are no longer human, deserve every conceivable form of exclusion (Sects. 2.1.2, 3.1.3).

The contrast between such media representations and reality could not be greater. First, men-tal illness is not usually easily identifiable. Peter Lorre's big eyes tell us little about his state of mind. This is another reason why deciding whether to disclose one's own mental illness can be challenging (Sects. 5.1.4, 9.2). Second, all people, whether they have mental illness or not, are first and foremost *people* and connected by this commonality. No one should be defined by their illness alone or is fundamentally *different* because of it.

7.4.2 TYPES OF MEDIA

Film and Television

While older films have already been discussed in Section 7.4.1, negative stereotypes of those with mental illness have extended well into modern cinema. In Steven Spielberg's successful animated series for children from the 1990s, *Tiny Toon Adventures*, the episode 'How I Spent My Vacation' depicts the following scene: a family is out and about together, driving in their car. They hear on the radio a warning of a 'psychotic killer' who has escaped from a nearby maximum-security prison. This person just so happens to be the hitchhiker who the family has picked up—he is described as a raving lunatic. Of course, soon afterwards, he grabs a chainsaw and wants to dis-member the children of the family [609]. When children are fed such information (or worse), it is unsurprising that such a threatening stereotype thrives in our society. It is even more cultivated in films for adults: a study of films about people with psychosis showed that almost 80% depicted murderous lunatics, and almost two-thirds of the films contained disinformation about schizo-phrenia being a split personality; straitjackets were also commonly used as a prop [613].

Professional treatment of mental disorders is also a common subject of films; the tonal spectrum is wide but tends to lean negative. It ranges from psychiatrists who are themselves psychopathic serial killers (*The Silence of the Lambs*, 1991) to Miloš Forman's famous *One Flew Over the Cuckoo's Nest* (1975), in which the so-called treatment in a psychiatric hospital consists of violence and repression, including lobotomy (Sect. 5.1.2). There are also more positive portrayals, such as that of Robin Williams (who died by suicide in 2014) as a sensitive psychotherapist in *Good Will Hunting* (1997).

Another film motif is that of the mentally ill genius, known for example from the film about mathematician and Nobel Prize winner John Nash (1928–2015), who had schizophrenia (*A Beautiful Mind*, 2001). One of the film's key traits is that the viewer watches life from Nash's perspective, which includes his psychotic symptoms (e.g. hallucinations). *Iris* (2001) is a film about the well-known Irish-English writer Iris Murdoch, her Alzheimer's disease, and the effects it had on her and her husband. Such films align the mentally ill protagonists with many positive things. But this representational approach has also been criticised because most people with mental illness (just like most people without mental illness) are not geniuses or celebrities. The films can thus be misinterpreted to mean that only such exceptional people can be both mentally ill and capable at the same time.

Finally, the stereotype of comedy also exists in film. A well-known example is *Arsenic and Old Lace* (1941), in which the harmless nephew of the murderous protagonists thinks he is US President Teddy Roosevelt. Here, illness and murders are staged as a funny farce. Numerous newer films also vary the comedy motif, such as Robert de Niro as a mafia boss with panic attacks in *Analyze This* from 1999. These depictions hardly do justice for people with mental illness, not only because they are still linked to crime, but also because the mentally ill characters in such films are exposed to ridicule.

Films are incredibly important to the theme of stigma: not only are they enormously popular and reflective of a society's cultural knowledge, but (by combining narrative, image, language, music, and various cinematic stylistic devices) they also strongly influence their viewers both in terms of (dis)information and emotion [614]. Data suggest this connection: in one German study, participants who watched the most television demonstrated the greatest desire for social distance from people with mental illness [615]. Since the study was cross-sectional (i.e. it examined television consumption and attitudes at only one point in time), it cannot prove television as a cause. But this conclusion is consistent with television's reinforcement of prejudices. The same link was found when it came to reading the tabloid press [615].

Newspaper

An evaluation of reputable German-language daily newspapers in the 1990s collected reports on mental illnesses, especially schizophrenia, and forms of their treatment [616]. It turned out that usage of the term schizophrenia to describe an illness was primarily found in local sections of the newspaper and in connection with violent acts. In the arts, sports and politics, however, schizophrenia was used metaphorically to mark something as contradictory or incomprehensible (e.g. a committee or sports club would be called schizophrenic for their actions). Schizophrenia thus seems to be represented in the press as a strange mixture of danger and violence on the one hand and dark incomprehensibility on the other. It is also important to note that mental illnesses are reported less factually and informatively than physical illnesses. Reporting, for example in the context of court proceedings, tends to focus on severely mentally ill persons. This reinforces the impression that there is a difference between the ill and the reader, ignoring the continuum between health and illness [616].

A study of reports regarding depression in daily German newspapers does not come to a more positive conclusion: from 1990 to 2000, the coverage did not improve. Confusing details were given and negative events dominated—mostly about the illness, rarely about the people with the illness. Psychotherapy as a form of treatment was almost nonexistent in these reports [617].

Somewhat more encouraging is a study on the reporting of mental illness in daily Canadian newspapers from 2005 to 2015 [618]. During this time, the Canadian antistigma campaign *Opening Minds*, which includes training and information for journalists and journalism students, launched (Sect. 12.1). Positive reporting increased, and stigmatising reports decreased. However, the topic of danger remained prominent in about half of all articles. Although there is no causative proof that the antistigma campaign changed the coverage, the study shows that such improvements are possible. A similar finding was made in England during the *Time to Change* antistigma campaign there (Sect. 12.1). Overall, positive articles predominated (except in regards to schizophrenia) [619].

The fact that negative reports have consequences has been shown by a study in which young people were asked to read either a report on mental illness and acts of violence or an article with factual information about schizophrenia. Three weeks after reading the report on violence, the readers were about four times as likely to describe people with schizophrenia as dangerous. There was no change in mindset amongst readers of the informational text [620]. The influence of reports regarding singular, negative events does, however, seem to be limited. This was the conclusion of two independent German surveys, wherein members of the general public were interviewed before and after the Germanwings crash in March 2015 [621, 622]. The media reported that the copilot who had caused the crash, killing himself and everybody on board, suffered from depression. But the survey showed very little, if any, deterioration in public attitudes towards people with depression (the survey did not assess attitudes towards pilots with depression specifically).

Social Media

Mental and other illnesses are a frequent social media topic, and stigmatising content has been studied in various ways. One study on psychosis evaluated about 15,000 Twitter messages (tweets) sent on 8 days in 2018 [623]. Tweets on the subject of psychosis were compared with those on other illnesses. Interestingly, the picture was mixed: on one hand, tweets about psychosis tended to be more negative than tweets about other illnesses, and psychosis was often written about pejoratively. On the other hand, medical content in tweets about psychosis was usually correct and contained a wealth of helpful information, particularly about prevention. This demonstrates the risks and opportunities afforded by social media in terms of stigma and education. Social media can be helpful in providing information; about one-third of people with schizophrenia were using these platforms in the early 2010s [624]. Another study examined a similar number of tweets regarding five mental and five physical illnesses. Only for schizophrenia was stigmatisation common (found in almost half of all tweets). One striking discovery was that schizophrenia, obsessive-compulsive disorders and eating disorders in particular were used in an unobjective (i.e. metaphorically) [616] or, as the authors of this study called it, trivialising way [625].

Social media offer people with mental illness the opportunity for exchange and networking. Many people, for example, use YouTube to report on their mental illness. One study examined comments written on YouTube about such videos that had led to exchanges between the publishers and their viewers [626]. Four advantages to these discussions were common: overcoming loneliness and finding new hope, mutual support and encouragement, coping with the illness in everyday life and exchanging experiences on forms of treatment. Interviews show that people with mental illness value being able to overcome isolation online as much as a factual exchange [627]. Professionals sometimes warn that peers are at risk of defining themselves only in terms of their illness through online activities and could neglect the rest of their identity and social environment. Pointing out such risks is justified, but the decision is ultimately up to service users; getting active online often garners positive results [628]. People with psychosis, for example, use social media, and disadvantages are rarely seen in their exchanges—on the contrary, there tends to be a reduction in their sense of social isolation [629].

In spite of all the opportunities that social media presents, disclosure of own experiences with mental illness and the mutual exchanges that follow entail risks: information exchanged online can be incorrect, self-damaging behaviour can be played down or even encouraged in some forums, and very negative comments can be made, including cyberbullying [630]. A further risk is discrimination in the professional or private sphere if one's identity as a person with a mental illness has become apparent online [631]. This risk can be minimised, such as by using Reddit to write about one's illness and using a one-time anonymous account [632]. In general, the opportunities and risks of social media for the mental well-being of young people (whether or not they have a mental health problem) tend to differ between different platforms: for example, in one English study, YouTube scored better overall than Instagram or Snapchat [633]. Given the risks and opportunities of social media, it seems urgent to examine them more in the context of public health [634].

Video Gaming

Some two billion people worldwide spend time playing video games. The majority do not play alone but instead by connecting online with others. It is clear that the portrayal of mental illness in these games influences attitudes in the general public, especially among younger people. One study has therefore investigated how mental disorders, especially psychoses, are represented in 100 commercial games [635]. The theme of danger was found to be prominent and sometimes portrayed in extreme terms. *Slayaway Camp* is about 'a killer puzzle where you control Skullface, a psychotic slasher bent on slaughtering camp counsellors ... this adorable murderer slides around ... decapitating, squashing, and perforating his bloody victims'. The game was rated positively by 96% of the players. In another game, *Wendigo*, psychosis is characterised by violence and an 'insatiable desire to eat human flesh' (quotations in [635]).

As with any medium, video games can be used more positively than in such grotesque caricatures. *Hellblade: Senua's Sacrifice* and *Debris* are examples of games developed with the involvement of mental healthcare professionals and people with mental illness [635]. The developers wanted to make it possible for players to put themselves in the shoes of people with mental illness and thus develop empathy. These games show, amongst other issues, that the symptoms and experience of one's illness do not only have to be felt negatively. Despite these examples, much remains to be done in the realm of the video game industry and its customers. Involving people with mental illness in game development and evaluation is an important first step.

7.4.3 (DIS)INFORMATION IN THE MEDIA

The media can contribute in various ways to information as well as disinformation (in particular by spreading exaggerated or biased images of mental illness). However, correct information does not always helps to reduce stigma. This is likely due to the reality that stigma consists not only of ignorance (Sect. 3.1.7) but also essentially of one-sided, generalising assumptions and emotional reactions. Looking at films and newspaper articles illustrates this problem.

Two studies dealt with the effect of two feature films on attitudes towards people with mental illness. Both films (*Angel Baby*, 1995; *The White Noise*, 2001) describe the psychotic symptoms and crises of people with schizophrenia. The study on *The White Noise* found that the film led to an increase in viewers' desires for social distance (i.e. viewers wanted to have less to do with people with schizophrenia after seeing the film than before) [636]. For *Angel Baby*, a more thorough study evaluated how knowledge and the desire for social distance differed amongst viewers who saw the film—according to whether they saw additional short films with information about schizophrenia or not [637]. Prejudices improved only amongst people who also watched an additional film and worsened amongst those who did not.

Witnessing and experiencing acute psychotic symptoms second-hand, as part of the emotional intensity of a film, seems to worsen attitudes towards the mentally ill. This could be because knowledge about illness alone is not sufficient to reduce stigma, and a presentation focused on symptoms is unhelpful (Sect. 8.1.3). On the other hand, films dealing with depression and using the perspective of those affected often succeed in making the experience and severity of depression vivid and empathetic [638]. The unique perception of time for those with depression is also vividly portrayed by film: the present time flows slowly, the future is locked away and the past with its perceived guilt does not go away [639].

In general news reports, facts alone do not necessarily reduce stigma. Pat Corrigan examined the effect of two newspaper articles that had appeared in the daily papers about 10 years prior [640]. One report described the history and suicide of a mentally ill prisoner as an example of the deadly consequences of the inadequate care system in the US state of Oregon. Another article told the aforementioned story of the mathematician John Nash along with information about the frequent recovery of people with even severe mental illness. Although the report on Nash dispelled prejudice, this effect was not found in readers of the article on suicide and the care system. On the contrary, they were more in favour of coercive psychiatric measures than before. This is a problem for background reporting in the media. Articles that point to inadequate care can help to improve services (as was probably the case in Oregon [640]), but they also carry the risk of encouraging prejudice. Journalists therefore face the challenge of reporting on grievances without adding to the stigma.

7.4.4 IMPACT OF THE MEDIA

Some consequences of the portrayal of mental illness in entertainment, information and social media have been mentioned in the preceding sections. Here we will briefly summarise why the media, besides being omnipresent, is so significant in perpetuating as well as in reducing the stigma of mental illness. In democratic systems, the media is often referred to as the fourth power alongside government (executive), legislation (legislative) and jurisdiction (judicial). It is centrally important to how members of a society absorb and interpret information; in doing so, it can have an enlightening effect or spread disinformation. The media is able to pick up on public attitudes, can reinforce stigmatising representations and can perpetuate negative attitudes in the general public. The media often sets the agenda, focuses public attention on certain areas and also controls what is perceived as relevant [641].

The media thus has a great deal of influence over cultural change as well as on political processes, especially in the area of structural discrimination (Sect. 5.1.8). This is one reason why stigma in the media is sometimes considered a form of structural discrimination [642]. Negative representations also affect self-stigma amongst people with mental illness. In one German study, participants with depression were more likely to agree with negative stereotypes about people with depression after watching a film about the Germanwings crash (Sect. 7.4.2 [643]). Negative media portrayals can increase shame and self-stigma in people with mental disorders, deterring those who are seeking help (Sect. 5.1.7 [644]). A systematic overview of the influence of the media shows the negative consequences of stigmatising reports, both in experimental studies (Sect. 7.4.3) and correlational ones (i.e. the more people recall negative media portrayals, they more likely they are to be prejudiced [645]). The review also found that the impact of both negative and positive media coverage was reinforced by online comments in the newspaper portals that mimicked the tones of the articles.

7.4.5 MEDIA AND SUICIDE

As discussed previously, the stigma of suicide is different from that of mental illness (Sect. 5.2). For the media, suicides and suicide attempts are therefore also a separate issue.

Reporting on Suicides

The media has the capacity to improve knowledge about suicide and counteract prejudice. An Austrian study has shown different media outlets' success with this to varying degrees. Participants who read the tabloid press were more likely to agree with misinformation about suicides (e.g. that people who experience suicidality usually do not communicate this to others) [646]. The media frequently report on suicides by celebrities, for example that of the German national football team goalkeeper, Robert Enke, in 2009, or that of the actor Robin Williams in 2014, as previously mentioned. One risk of such reporting is an uptick in suicides when others attempt to imitate a celebrity's death. This is called the *Werther effect*, after Goethe's epistolary novel from 1774 and is unfortunately an empirically well-documented phenomenon [647]. In the months following Williams' suicide, for example, the number of suicides in Canada increased by 16%, especially among men who were no longer young and used the method he chose. Both of these factors suggest imitation effects [648]. A survey of German newspapers showed that not only did the number of suicides after the death of Robert Enke increase sharply, but those using a similar method to Enke's did as well. Reporting of this death tended not to follow the usual guidelines (Sect. 7.4.7) and thus probably contributed to acts of imitation [649].

Suicide in Films

Suicide is a frequent theme in films and television. In March 2017, Netflix released *13 Reasons Why*, a series that portrays the suicide of a teenager with a plot line centred on her motives for it.

Even before the series' release, warnings were issued against imitation effects on vulnerable young people, especially because the suicide method is discussed in detail. In a longitudinal study, Thomas Niederkrotenthaler investigated suicide rates in the United States before and after the release of the series: a significant increase was observed from April to June 2017 [650]. During this period, about 100 more young people took their own lives than in comparable periods of other years. The effect was stronger for girls than for boys and was limited to this age group. Although this study is not proof that the series caused these additional suicides, it provides a strong indication. Statistically, the effect may not be strong. But due to the widespread distribution of such films and shows online, even small effects can lead to many suicides.

Experimental studies in the form of a survey questionnaire collected after a film can provide clearer evidence of the influence of films on suicidal behaviour. In one RCT, participants watched either a film that ended with the suicide of the main character or a film in which a mental health crisis was overcome. Especially for participants who, before seeing the film, had already considered their lives not worth living, the first film increased suicidality, and the second film about overcoming the crisis reduced it [651]. In contrast to the aforementioned Werther effect, the suicide-preventing effect of such a positive presentation is called the *Papageno effect*, named after the character in Mozart's opera *The Magic Flute* who overcame his suicidality [652].

Suicide Prevention Through the Media

Media campaigns can be used for suicide prevention. There are several possible starting points: they can inform the general public so that people know how to better recognise warning signs and help those affected, they can remove stigma to create an atmosphere in which people can seek help without fear of discrimination, and they can reach out to risk groups to encourage them to seek help. A systematic review of 20 individual studies examined the effectiveness of various media initiatives of this kind [653]. The overall results are encouraging: public knowledge and attitudes improved, as did (in most cases) the willingness to seek help. Some studies showed a decrease in suicides.

Social Media

In April 2018, the Swedish DJ with the artist name Avicii died by suicide. That his death was by suicide was made public nearly a week after his passing was announced. The method of suicide was relayed a while later. In the four weeks after his death, about three million tweets were sent containing his name. An analysis of these Twitter messages showed how many people worldwide exchanged information about his death and in what ways [654]. The news of his suicide led to more sustained attention than that of his death. The suicide method attracted less attention—there were, however, users who occupied themselves intensely with the method. The study showed that social media is a quick method by which to detect risky media reporting and identify vulnerable people.

Self-inflicted injuries can occur without suicidal intent, for example by cutting as a means of emotion regulation. This nonsuicidal self-injury has been commonly shared through images on social media. It is somewhat unclear how worrying the effects of this are. One British study on Twitter, Instagram and Tumblr has given the all-clear, concluding that most of such messages do not glorify self-harm but rather seem to facilitate mutual exchange and support [655]. A German study has confirmed this finding and additionally revealed that such images are not only very common, but that images of severe self-harming are also commented on more often. This form of attention could of course be problematic, and these images (and the self-harm they depict) could become more frequent [656]. There is an extensive evaluation of more than 10,000 contributions (and individual interviews) on the topic of self-harm in the digital age of social media that underscores the role and import of peer support [657].

Web Pages on Suicidality

One topic that can only be touched upon here is websites that advocate suicide and disseminate suicide methods. Research suggests that such sites increase the number of suicides by teaching people how to take their own lives. In Germany, for example, the frequency of internet searches for the keyword phrase 'carbon monoxide poisoning' is clearly correlated with the sharp increase in suicides caused by this method [658]. A survey of US and German-language websites on suicidality showed that positive websites (e.g. that help to deal with suicidal thoughts or prevent suicide in crisis) were more prevalent than negative ones that provided information on suicide methods. However, negative websites tended to have a higher ranking and were therefore easier to find online [659]. Healthcare professionals should therefore discuss (dis)information from the internet with their patients openly, and as part of suicide prevention, the visibility of positive websites could be improved.

7.4.6 REASONS FOR STIGMA IN THE MEDIA

Profit

Whether through the news or movies, most media products are also produced for commercial reasons. This need not be considered inherently bad—it is simply a condition under which media content is produced and understood. Nor is this situation new. The Roman poet Horace wrote some 2000 years ago: 'Aut prodesse volunt aut delectare poetae' (Poets either want to be useful or to entertain; *Ars poetica*, 333). Even then, it was necessary to consider whether a text should be useful as a piece of information or should be offered as entertainment. For media professionals today, this question is fundamentally the same. From a producer's perspective, viewership of news and entertainment shows should be as high as possible, and a lot of clicks on an online platform promises income. The media is therefore often inclined to give information a back seat to provide better entertainment [660]. Bizarre, acute psychological symptoms and crises, especially in the context of violence, seem to be better suited for entertainment and attract more interest from audiences than displays of people who are doing well: 'Being well is dead boring because mostly people are much more interesting when they're ill. They just are' ([660], p. 31). However, this statement expresses a cliché. How people with mental illness find their way back into life after crisis can be a rich and complex theme, and anything but boring. This is obvious from reports of personal experience, such as those of Thomas Melle (Sect. 5.4.2 [314]).

Ignorance

There is no particular reason why media professionals should be more knowledgeable about mental illness than the general public. This is all the more true as economic constraints often leave journalists little time for research of their own. Moreover, many so-called experts, including psychiatrists, often have a biased opinion anyway (Sect. 5.1.2). But a reporter's lack of knowledge, exhibited through their published work, can ultimately contribute to widespread repetition of certain (negative) stereotypes about people with mental illness.

Anna Mueller investigated a local media outlet's reporting on the frequent suicides of young people and public attitudes towards them in a small midwestern US town [661]. Media attention was given, above all, to the suicides of those young people who had been successful and appeared 'perfect' in the time leading up to their deaths, and whose deaths thereby seemed difficult to explain. The media offered as an explanation for the suicides the pressure to perform that is widespread among young people. This argument is not without problems—it could make suicide appear as an understandable solution to a problem (Sect. 7.4.7). Presumably due to the prejudice and taboo surrounding mental illness, the media did not discuss depression as a (concomitant) cause of the suicides; seeking help for depression was thus not presented as a possible solution.

Mueller concluded that while such media coverage can contribute to suicide incidents and make it more difficult to seek help, this coverage is based on the prevailing attitudes which influence the media in turn. This has implications for antistigma interventions in the media sector (Sect. 7.4.7). Since the media are (also) a product of society, it does not suffice to point the finger at media professionals.

Pictorial Stereotypes

In addition, the media have a long tradition of showing depictions of people with mental illness. Sander Gilman described this history in his striking book *Seeing the Insane* [662]. In the 18th century, the idea spread that conspicuous psychological features and personality traits were reflected in the shape of the head and face. The intensive study of these forms and the facial features or expressions of the human being is called physiognomy. The multivolume *Physiognomic Fragments* by Swiss writer Johann Caspar Lavater, published from 1775 onwards, bears witness to this. Physiognomy had a comprehensive influence on the psychiatry of its time. In 1801, for example, French psychiatrist and reformer Philippe Pinel drew the heads of an 'idiot' and a 'madman' to compare their facial proportions with the classical ideal of the Apollo Belvedere. As could be predicted, this comparison did not favour the mortals ([662], p. 73). The drawing of a melancholic woman by Belgian reform psychiatrist Joseph Guislain (1797-1860) showed her with a darkly shaded face. Thus the associated colour of melancholy (black bile; Sect. 2.1.1) was clearly presented to the viewer ([662], p. 226). In this way, images convey ideas of the time about the causes of illness and the way the ill look different.

These illustrations were later followed by photographs of psychiatric patients, which were presumed to show visible signs of various illnesses. Protruding eyes, as can be seen from some thyroid diseases (e.g. Graves' disease), are an old imagerial sign of insanity [663]. As a consequence of this motif, a clinical textbook of the late 19th century shows a woman with Graves' disease and strongly protruding eyes staring upwards in a 'mad' way ([662], fig. 300, p. 234; Fig. 7.3). This way of staring has little to do with the thyroid gland but does show the power of the pictorial tradition that associates protruding eyes and madness. The depiction carries on in Peter Lorre's

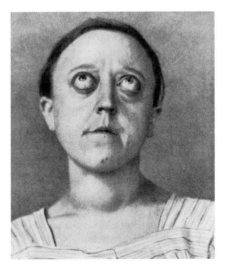

Fig. 7.3 **Woman with Graves' disease from an atlas of clinical medicine, ca. 1895.** (Science History Images, Alamy stock photos.)

cinematic roles (Sect. 7.4.1). Media that emphasise the visible difference of people with mental illness find their inspiration in these depictions.

Cultural Knowledge and Self-Assurance

The media transports cultural knowledge; they are called the storytellers of our time [609]. The presentation of mental illness is often influenced by currently prevailing views and models of illness. In the Western world, for example, the idea that traumatisation caused by war causes mental illness pervaded following the Vietnam War. This led to an abundance of Hollywood films about Vietnam and veterans with posttraumatic stress disorder.

Films explain the world, and worldviews are a human need—they make the confusing, often absurd details and hardships of life easier to understand (Sect. 3.3.3, 'Belief in a Just World'). Therefore depictions of mental illness and violence, such as in the films described, also serve as explanations of why someone becomes violent: he was not one of us, but one of them, which is why he could commit such an act [609]. Sander Gilman described the calming effect of such depictions (Sect. 3.1.4):

> Our shock is always that they are really just like us ... Then we no longer know where lies the line that divides our normal, reliable world, a world that minimises our fears, from that world in which lurks the fearful, the terrifying, the aggressive. We want—no, we need—the 'mad' to be different, so we create out of the stuff of their reality myths that make them different.
>
> ([664], p. 13)

The differentness of the 'madman' explains the world and calms us, because it places the source of our fear in him. It also implies that the cause of violence and other evils, for example, is part of the person himself, this ill person who is so different from us. This relieves the observer of the task of dealing with the social causes of mental illness, such as poverty or deficiencies in the care system [609]. It also serves to justify the system in which 'lunatics' are disadvantaged (Sect. 3.3.3).

7.4.7 ANTISTIGMA INTERVENTIONS IN THE MEDIA SECTOR

Stigmatising media content is common; simultaneously, positive media reports can in fact reduce stigma. The question therefore arises as to whether and how targeted interventions can improve the portrayal of mental illness in the media. This type of antistigma intervention is discussed here. Interventions in general are presented at a later point (Chapter 8 ff.).

Media Guidelines

Guidelines are intended to help journalists provide factual and balanced reporting that does not increase stigma. Various recommendations and guidelines are available. Those of the Carter Center, founded by former US President Jimmy Carter and his wife Rosalynn and committed to the training of journalists in this area, are well known in the United States (https://cartercenter.org). They recommend using appropriate language (Sect. 1.2) when referring to prevention and treatment options and when dealing with topics of recovery. In Germany, there are similar recommendations from the *German Alliance for Mental Health* (Sect. 12.2; https://seelische-gesundheit.net).

With regard to suicide, there are the 2008 WHO reporting guidelines [665] and country-based recommendations, such as the German ones provided by NASPRO (German National Suicide Prevention programme; https://suizidpraevention-deutschland.de; Sect. 5.2.3). The key points of these recommendations are not to write about suicides in a lurid way or on the front page; not to give details about the method and place; to avoid romanticising, glorifying or presenting the suicide as inevitable; and to refrain from giving rash explanations ('She took her own life because …') or remote diagnoses by so-called experts. It is also helpful to point out that a suicide is usually the result of a mental illness or crisis for which help is available (and thereby promote solutions other than suicide).

Courses for Media Professionals

Another approach is the active training of journalists or journalism students to improve reporting on the topic. As a rule, these programmes focus on education (i.e. the provision of information) (Sect. 8.1). Very few studies worldwide have investigated the effectiveness of such training [645, 666]. And the results of the studies that are available are quite sobering: for journalists, hardly any positive effects were observed; some of them were even negative. This may be due to the brevity of the intervention and the fact that none of the lecturers taking part in the programme had lived experience of mental illness (see the next paragraph). For journalism students, the evaluations turned out to be slightly better.

Contact and Involvement of Peers

With regard to antistigma interventions in general, including those outside the media, contact between the target group (here media professionals) and people with personal experience of mental illness is one of the most effective ways of reducing stigma (Sect. 8.4). A thoughtful documentary filmmaker once said something that is applicable to more than just television: 'Television can make the visible invisible' ([660], p. 36). The social reality and personal experience of mental illness can easily get lost in the constant media drumbeat. In contrast, the inclusion of people with mental illness in the form of *citizen journalism* helps. In Canada, people with mental illness who were not already professional journalists were enrolled in a course on citizen journalism and trained in the production of videos on mental illness. Compared with videos by professional journalists on the same topic, theirs were much more positive and dealt with recovery or stigma and less often with violence or crime [667].

7.5 Stigma and the Law

Law permeates all areas of our lives. With regard to the stigma of mental illness, there are numerous areas of law involved, from social law to the prohibition of discrimination on the grounds of disability, including mental disability (in Germany, art. 3 para. 3 of the German Constitution and the UN-CRPD; Sect. 7.5.2). This prohibition is more comprehensively regulated in the German Equality Act of 2010. Since law refers to general procedures, it is particularly relevant to structural discrimination. However, a ban on discrimination on grounds of mental illness is likely to reduce also public stigma and self-stigma. Legal standards contribute to making such discrimination less acceptable. This applies to the general public (reduction of public stigma) as well as to people with mental illness, whose self-esteem can be enhanced by legal protection (reduction of self-stigma). Without trying to be all-inclusive, we focus here on five main aspects of stigma and legal discrimination.

7.5.1 STIGMA AND SOCIAL JUSTICE

The stigma of mental illness is a question of social justice. While legal regulations and protections alone are not sufficient to prevent discrimination, the fight against discrimination is all the more difficult without them. The law holds both practical and symbolic significance: standards influence social attitudes.

What is fair? This question has occupied mankind for thousands of years. In negative terms, justice is not about everyone receiving the same or equal amounts. The conditions for when and where we all start out in life differ greatly, particularly in terms of talent, wealth and health. What can a society do to distribute scarce resources fairly when our individual conditions are so diverse? Followers of utilitarianism, since Jeremy Bentham and John Stuart Mill in the early 19th century, want to distribute goods in such a way that the total sum of benefits for all would be as great as possible. One problem with this is that the interests of minorities are not given enough consideration as long as the majority benefits. This approach suggests that if social and health policy are geared to the approximately 95% of the population without serious mental illness, it is acceptable that the seriously ill 5% fall by the wayside.

American philosopher John Rawls (1921–2002 [668]) formulated his own *Theory of Justice*, which addresses this problem of utilitarianism. To develop rules for a just social order, Rawls designed a fictitious starting situation that he called the 'original position'. Imagine if people knew nothing about their personal starting positions in society (e.g. with regard to talent, money, power or health). With this *veil of ignorance* about their own starting point, they would agree on certain rights to freedom and the stability of society, and they would impartially advocate a fair distribution of resources—for the benefit of those who, due to illness or disability, might have a disadvantaged starting position in life. According to Rawls' veil of ignorance, everyone would want even the worst starting position to be one that is acceptable—it could possibly be their own. Though not the neatest comparison, it would thus be fair for people with severe mental illness to be given the necessary resources and support to make the best of their situation (even if this does not remove their illness or disability).

Despite some important differences, Rawls' position is not too far away from the *capability approach* of Indian Nobel Prize winner for Economics Amartya Sen (b. 1933 [669]). This approach is influential in current debates surrounding social and development policy. A key assumption of his approach is that people, for their own well-being, need the freedom of choice to live and be the way they want to. Sen's starting point is that to be able to assess social justice and the condition of people in a society, it is not sufficient to only take a view on resources or subjective satisfaction. This is because people with disabilities or who have experienced social exclusion are often unable to use resources that are theoretically available. Similarly, people who have become demoralised by their poverty or being excluded may express satisfaction even though they objectively have no option of living a different life (Sect. 5.1.1, 'Experience and Expectation of Stigma').

Sen distinguishes between modes of functioning and capabilities: functionings are states and activities (beings and doings), such as being able to read or learning to read. Capabilities are realisable modes of functioning and the freedom to choose between them and thus determine one's own life. Those who starve out of necessity do not have the capability to eat, but those who fast voluntarily have this capability. The functioning of hunger in both examples is the same, but the capabilities and freedom of choice are completely different. The possibilities of achieving certain modes of functioning depend crucially on the individual person and his or her social environment. People with mental illness suffer from a lack of capabilities if they cannot work because of their illness or because of stigma or lack of support. Sen thus emphasises the role of social factors for a just society as well as the well-being of the people in it. In its focus on self-determination and freedom of choice, the capability approach is highly compatible with the recovery concept (Sect. 5.1.6 [670]).

Solidarity is a term often used in this context. The word comes from the *obligatio in solidum* of ancient Roman law (Lat. solidus: massive, whole) and means accepting total liability for each other: we stand all for one and one for all in the event of fateful danger or loss. Solidarity in this original sense is an intermediate stage between legal obligation and voluntary human kindness [671]. The solidarity concept is particularly important in regards to stigma—solidarity with people with mental illness can be a powerful message for antistigma interventions (Sect. 8.1.4 [672]).

7.5.2 THE UN CONVENTION ON THE RIGHTS OF PERSONS WITH DISABILITIES

In 2006, the UN General Assembly adopted the UN Convention on the Rights of Persons with Disabilities (UN-CRPD), which was drawn up with the active participation of associations of people with disabilities. This Convention on the Rights of Persons with Disabilities is ratified law, including in the EU and the United Kingdom. The UN-CRPD applies to all 'who have long-term physical, mental, intellectual or sensory impairments' (Art. 1) and thus explicitly includes people with serious mental illness. Whereas disability was previously seen as the deficit of the disabled person, the UN-CRPD is based on a social concept of disability. Disability therefore arises out of the interaction of the person's impairment with barriers in his or her environment (Preamble [e]). The phrase 'I'm not disabled, I'm being disabled' puts it more simply. This concept applies to a wheelchair user who is unable to access a building due to the lack of a ramp or lift and to autistic people who cannot work in an open-plan office due to their impairment and are hindered from participation in working life if not given a quiet, individual office (Sect. 5.4.1).

The UN-CRPD is based on the concept of dignity, the principle of nondiscrimination and the principle of self-determination. All of these are outlined as inalienable rights of people with disabilities. And if a person cannot exercise their rights because of a disability, their rights should not be exercised by a representative. Rather, she should be supported in her decision-making (Art. 12(3)). The education system should contribute to the full development of awareness regarding the dignity and self-esteem of persons with disabilities (Art. 24, para. 1[a]). However, this comes up against common prejudices and discrimination in society. In this respect, the UN-CRPD calls for antistigma work. Article 8, Awareness Raising, meant 'to combat stereotypes, prejudices and harmful practices relating to persons with disabilities', explicitly demands this. Another important principle of the UN-CRPD is that people with disabilities are not seen negatively or as deficient human beings but rather as enrichers of a diverse society (Preamble [m]). The right to social inclusion established by the UN-CRPD therefore benefits people with disabilities as well as society as a whole. The protection against discrimination also extends to associated persons (i.e. relatives of people with disabilities) [673].

The implications of the UN-CRPD for people with mental illness are diverse. In addition to the aforementioned basic principles, there are specific regulations. Article 25 formulates the right to 'the enjoyment of the highest attainable standard of health without discrimination on the basis of disability'. This includes rehabilitation (see also Art. 26), early intervention and community-based care (on existing deficits in these areas, see Sects. 7.3.1, 7.3.3). Article 27 deals with 'the right of persons with disabilities to work, on an equal basis with others', including 'assistance in finding, obtaining, maintaining and returning to employment' (Art. 27 [e]). This reads like a brief description of Supported Employment; however, this psychosocial intervention has hardly been implemented in German-speaking countries so far (Sect. 7.1.2). All in all, the UN-CRPD has great potential to improve the situation of people with mental illness. But its implementation is only partial, even in Western countries. Many hope it will be helpful in the gradual elimination of existing deficits affecting people with mental illness.

Article 33 obliges signatories to verify their implementation of and compliance with the UN-CRPD. People with mental illness must be involved in the preparation of these reports (Art. 4(3)). For this purpose, as in other countries, there is a monitoring office in Germany at the German Institute for Human Rights in Berlin (https://institut-fuer-menschenrechte.de/en). The institute prepares regular reports that are also submitted to the United Nations. On the basis of these and other reports, WHO published a 2018 overview of the situation of people with intellectual or mental disabilities living in institutions in Europe (including residential and nursing homes) [674]. This group is particularly threatened by restrictions of their rights due to the severity of their disabilities and the often remote location of the facilities. The study therefore examined compliance with human rights, as defined in the UN-CRPD, in institutions from 31 European countries. The results were sobering. In many cases, fundamental rights such as legal capacity, self-determination, dignity, freedom, security, protection from ill treatment and violence had been violated. Sexual abuse was reported. Provisions were very rarely made for meaningful employment and activities. There were too few opportunities to complain. In most cases, there was no plan to improve recovery and social participation and no possibilities for housing outside the institution. The majority of residents would have liked to leave their respective institutions but had nowhere to go [674].

7.5.3 GERMAN FEDERAL PARTICIPATION ACT

The German Act to Strengthen the Participation and Self-Determination of People with Disabilities, or Bundesteilhabegesetz (BTHG), was passed in 2016. The law was both inspired by the UN-CRPD and driven by a desire to curb further costs for integrated care for people with disabilities. The BTHG amended large parts of the Social Code Book IX (rehabilitation and participation of people with disabilities) and Social Code Book XII (social welfare). The changes came into force gradually from the beginning of 2017 to the beginning of 2020. In 2023, a regulation will follow as to who is entitled to integrated care benefits.

In the BTHG, *individual case support* is extracted from SGB XII and integrated as a new part 2 into SGB IX. This has the advantage for service users that assets and income count for less in relation to benefits. However, support is now only granted by application (§ 108 SGB IX). The consequences of this so-called application requirement on everyday life are unclear. There is a risk that people with serious mental illness or addictions may not apply for benefits or appeal within the time limit. The application requirement thus raises the access threshold to assistance ([675], p. 337 f.). Organisations providing so-called supplementary independent advice on participation therefore need to increase support to eligible applicants. Given the complexity of the German social and healthcare system (Sect. 7.3.3), this is a daunting task.

Participation planning is now regulated by the BTHG. The rehabilitation provider has to agree on the goals, type and scope of benefits in coordination with other providers and the person entitled to benefits (i.e. the disabled person) (§ 19 SGB IX). In the overall planning procedure for the coordination of aid, the beneficiaries are to be involved at every level—in line with the UN-CRPD. Service users have a right of choice here. They can refuse to live in institutions, for example, and instead live independently in supported accommodation (§ 104 SGB IX). This wish should be complied with if and when reasonable and possible. Implementation remains to be seen, and the issue of housing in this respect will remain challenging (Sect. 7.2.6).

In the area of work, the BTHG brings an important innovation: the *budget for work* (§ 61 SGB IX). People with disabilities can take a job in the general labour market, and the employer can receive up to 75% of the costs of the employee's wages for an unlimited period of time. The benefits include, if necessary, a job coach to provide support in the workplace [675] and thus forms an important element of Supported Employment (Sect. 7.1.2). How this budget will prove its worth in practice remains to be seen. But it does offer the opportunity for inclusion through work, unlike current sheltered employment workshops from which it is difficult to enter the general labour market.

Since 2008 there has been a so-called *personal budget* for all people with disabilities (§ 29 SGB IX). It is not an additional service but rather a new way of providing services that enables people with disabilities to buy participation benefits independently. The budget is typically a few hundred euros per month.

Model projects for the implementation of the BTHG were carried out in almost all German federal states until 2021. At present, for example in Baden-Württemberg, there is a dispute between the state and the counties about the distribution of costs. At this stage, it is thus not possible to assess the impact of the BTHG. Opinions on its consequences differ widely.

Proponents hope that the paternalistic care model that incapacitates people with mental illness and keeps them in ghetto-like homes or sheltered employment workshops for years will be done away with [542]. Critics see considerable problems in various areas: the separation of social and integrated care introduced by the BTHG unnecessarily increases fragmentation in this area of the support system. People with severe mental illness may have particular difficulties in coping with the bureaucracy of the social welfare authorities. With the BTHG, the benefit administration no longer addresses the social–psychiatric institution but rather the benefit recipients themselves. If they are unable to open or answer their mail, they may be threatened with benefit cuts or, in extreme cases, homelessness.

Conclusion

The BTHG could have a paradoxical effect: instead of supporting empowerment (as was hoped for), high demands on service users could make legal guardians for the seriously ill unavoidable. There will undoubtedly be pros and cons to this system, and it will be all the more important to prevent discrimination against people with severe mental illness.

7.5.4 RIGHT TO VOTE

The Federal Electoral Act (§ 13, nos. 2 and 3) that was in force until June 2019 did not allow those in Germany with a legal guardian for their affairs, including many people with mental illness, to vote in elections. The same applied to people who had committed a criminal offence but were exempted from criminal responsibility due to mental illness (§ 20 StGB) and were thereby being held in a forensic psychiatry hospital (§ 63 StGB). Eight members from both these groups formally objected to this law. The German parliament, the Bundestag, rejected their complaint. How difficult it was to remove this restriction of fundamental rights, even with recourse to the UN-CRPD, was shown by a subsequent study commissioned by the federal government [676]. In 2016, after weighing up the matter over 300 pages, it advised against complete deletion of voting rights exclusions. The case thus finally ended up before the German Federal Constitutional Court, which in January 2019 declared the Federal Electoral Act unconstitutional (2 BvC 62/14). First, the regulation violated the principle of the universality of elections and deprived the people of their central democratic right to participate in elections. Second, the law violated the prohibition of discrimination on the grounds of disability (Art. 3(3), sentence 2 of the German Constitution). An exclusion from the election is possible in principle, such as when an individual person with a disability cannot form a political opinion. But this has to be justified in concrete terms. Neither the presence of a guardian nor the existence of a previous offence in a mostly temporary state of incompetence justifies the prohibition of one's right to vote. In addition, this exclusion was proven to be applied arbitrarily: in Bavaria, about 200 people were excluded from voting, whereas in Bremen, fewer than 10 were excluded (respectively per 100,000 adult citizens). Those differences are objectively incomprehensible. As a result of the ruling, these exclusion regulations were removed from the Federal Electoral Act in 2019. In the version of the Federal Electoral Act that has been in force since 2019 (§ 13), the voting rights of individuals can only be revoked with a court judgement. Restrictions on voting rights are an important indicator of persistent structural discrimination worldwide: a legal overview of 167 countries showed that only a minority of countries do not have restrictions on voting rights for people with mental illness [677].

From a stigma perspective, the decision of the German Federal Constitutional Court is a clear example of how stubbornly such discrimination persists, and how courts can choose to put an end to cases of structural discrimination that have been around for decades. But this court decision is also a call for decategorisation (Sect. 3.2.2). Previously, people were excluded from elections on the basis that they belonged to a strongly labelled category (e.g. comprehensive legal guardianship, patient in a forensic psychiatry hospital). But the court pointed out that to justify an exclusion from voting, the individual case must be examined. This is therefore a matter of the individual's rights taking precedence over the assumed category or group.

7.5.5 BAVARIAN MENTAL HEALTH CARE ACT

At the beginning of 2018, there was a lively debate about the draft of a new Bavarian PsychKHG ('Glossary'). It would regulate when and how people with mental illness could be admitted to a psychiatric hospital, even against their will. A central point of contention was the planned establishment of a database of people who were involuntarily admitted. It was intended to record data for at least 5 years and would contain information about individuals who had been admitted to a psychiatric hospital against their will as well as their diagnoses. This seemed disproportionate to the issue at hand: if someone with psychosis or an addiction disorder wanders through traffic in a confused state, or if a young mother with postnatal depression becomes depressed and suicidal, it is possible that the police will take the person to a psychiatric ward against his or her will. But to additionally store this person's data for years as a perceived threat to society would be inappropriate, especially because no significant danger emanates from a person like this outside of acute situations. Incidentally, such a file would probably have deterred many from seeking help, further increasing the barrier to service use in crisis situations (Sect. 5.1.7). In addition to this specific provision, the bill often referred to hospital treatment orders of forensic psychiatry (for people who have committed a crime in a state of suspended or reduced culpability). This focus on the supposed general danger posed by people with mental illness would have further reinforced the stigma of mental illness.

There were massive protests from service users (Sect. 6.1), relatives, mental healthcare professionals and social psychiatry associations, hospitals and various professional groups, as well as through a large online petition (on protest as an antistigma strategy, see Sect. 8.3). In the wake of these protests, the drafted law was heavily revised, and the planned database of involuntary admissions was abandoned. The Bavarian PsychKHG was passed in its new form in 2018 and is now similar to the PsychKHGs of other German federal states that have been amended in recent years [606]. On a positive note, the new law will mean that from 2021, crisis services will be set up everywhere in Bavaria for people in mental distress of all kinds. These services can defuse crises by phone and mobile teams. To what extent they will reduce the number of hospital admissions and improve overall care remains to be seen.

CHAPTER 8

Reduction of Public Stigma

This chapter focuses on the reduction of public stigma. Three key questions are discussed:

1. Who is prejudiced and discriminates against individuals with mental illness? These can be people in one's personal life, in positions of power or in the general public.
2. What is public stigma reduction focused on? Is it about knowledge, prejudice or behaviour/discrimination (Sect. 3.1.2)?
3. What strategies are used to reduce public stigma: education, a change in terminology, protest or contact? The chapter is divided into sections exploring these four strategies. As with all strategies, they should not only aim at reducing stigma but also at building positive attitudes: acceptance, recovery orientation and the commitment to equal rights for people with mental illness.

8.1 Education

8.1.1 PRINCIPLE OF EDUCATION

Education is about removing stigma as an expression of ignorance or distorted pseudoknowledge (Sect. 3.1.7) by replacing myths or false stereotypes with facts. Instead of assuming 'People with mental illness are incompetent and cannot do demanding work', the general public should be taught that 'People with mental illness can work. They are represented in all professions and at all career levels, from unskilled workers to corporate executives'.

It is commonly believed in our culture that once a person knows 'enough', they will behave 'properly'. This line of thinking is one of basic optimism: people do not behave badly (i.e. in a discriminatory way) if they know better. Socrates in the fifth century BC seemed to believe this as well, as he would engage other Athenians in long discussions about defining justice and other concepts. As is well known, Socrates not only made friends by doing this but was sentenced to death by his fellow citizens—a warning of the resistance that certain educational approaches can trigger. These days, the transfer of knowledge (or what is meant to be such a process) is omnipresent offline and online. Employees of every company rush from one form of training or educational programme to the next.

8.1.2 SUCCESS CRITERIA FOR EDUCATION

The success of educational approaches can be assessed using two criteria: penetration and impact. *Penetration* refers to the percentage of the target group that is reached through the initiative. This varies greatly depending on the target group: if a mental health education programme is a regular part of a school's curriculum (for an example, see Sect. 5.7), penetration of student cohorts is likely to reach almost 100%. But when it comes to websites or posters, penetration of the general public often approaches zero. Research on large-scale online campaigns in the United States paint a sobering picture: in one study, not even one-thousandth of the general public visited the website—and of those who did, almost all left the site after less than a minute [678]. One problem here is 'preaching to the converted'. These websites, amongst others, mostly reach those who are already receptive to the campaign. In addition, people who have visited a website or seen a poster in passing usually forget about it quickly. Therefore in regard to educating the general public, the question arises as to whether the scarce resources of antistigma work really should be put towards posters, websites, etc.

For education as an antistigma strategy, the decisive *impact* criterion is, as for all other strategies, behavioural change. Do employers hire more people with mental illness (or ensure that they keep their jobs) after an education campaign? Do people with mental illness report fewer experiences of discrimination as a result of nationwide education campaigns targeting the general public?

8.1.3 PROBLEMS OF EDUCATION

Is More Better?

We live in a world bursting with information. This fundamentally challenges our assumption that more information is simply 'good'. In the health sector, this leads to a problem whereby the amount of information available is no longer manageable, and its quality can hardly be assessed (Sect. 1.5). This phenomenon is also called information overload. A filtering problem (i.e. recorded information can no longer be filtered and organised) ensues, and the processing mechanisms of both individuals and societies collapse [679]. Incidentally, impaired filtering is also a model for the development of psychoses. Just as people with psychosis can be swamped by sensory stimuli, so too can we as a society be overwhelmed by the exponentially accelerating production of knowledge.

An overview of psychoeducational programmes (not about stigma but about illness education) for patients with a wide variety of illnesses has shown that these well-intentioned programmes often have an undesirable side effect: the participants suffer afterwards from information overload [680]. Here, too, a social gradient is evident in the sense that people with a low level of education and low social status suffer even more quickly from information overload. In other words, those who need information particularly urgently because of their level of education are often less able to absorb it.

Conclusion

Education as an antistigma strategy must therefore address how the information is to be carefully selected, such that it can be absorbed and effective.

Does Education Lead to Behavioural Change?

One basic assumption is hardly ever questioned: if people know more about health and illness prevention, they will behave more healthily. A large American study has investigated this assumption using the example of the measles, mumps and rubella (MMR) vaccination [681]. There has long been a widespread misconception that this vaccination causes autism. In the study, almost 1800 parents randomly received one of five types of information:

1. explicit correction of the misinformation contained in the misguided belief
2. information on risks of the measles, mumps and rubella illnesses
3. a dramatic story about children suffering from the consequences of MMR
4. option 3, with the addition of pictures of the children
5. information on bird feeding (as a control group).

All of the types of information (1 to 4) were reliable; materials were provided by the US Centers for Disease Control and Prevention. Before and after being provided the information, all of the participants' knowledge about vaccination risks was recorded in addition to their intentions of having their next child vaccinated. Although knowledge did increase, the willingness to vaccinate did not increase on average for participants, nor for any of the intervention types (1 to 4). On the contrary: parents who were vaccination sceptics at the beginning and had received the correction of the misinformation (1) were even less willing to have their child vaccinated afterwards. Both types of stories (3 and 4) also paradoxically led to vaccinations being considered even more dangerous.

The study provides impressive evidence that even factual, good education can achieve the opposite of its goal [2]. There are two explanations for this:

1. People with preexisting, fixed opinions (i.e. vaccination sceptics, but more or less all of us) do not like being told what to think. This leads to increased resistance to the point of view of those trying to advise.
2. Information is often selectively received in such a way that it confirms one's own viewpoint (motivated social cognition [174]).

8.1.4 WHAT MESSAGE SHOULD EDUCATION CONVEY?

What message should educational programmes and initiatives convey to reduce the public stigma of mental illness? Given the overload of available information, this is not a trivial question. Let us take health education about HIV as a comparative example [2]. The message is: condoms! Even in the area of HIV stigma, messages can be simple: HIV is not contagious with protected sex, and there is no reason to maintain social distance! What then would be the analogous message for the stigma of mental illness? That it is noncontagious? Be nice to sick people? Be inclusive? That's hardly likely to work. One problem here is that people being addressed with such messages may think, 'I don't have any prejudices anyway', and therefore they will not feel that they have been (or need to be) addressed. Three educational messages have been used and studied and will be briefly presented below [2]: normality, pity and continuum.

Normality?

'People with mental illness are just like you and me'—this could be a slogan to emphasise the normality of the illness. In view of the prevalence of mental disorders (in around 30% of all people) (Sect. 2.2.1), this approach appears plausible at first glance. However, it has not proven to be particularly helpful.

First, there is a well-known precursor: the campaign for colour-blindness in the fight against racism in the 1960s. People in the United States would learn of their sameness and that they could ignore skin colour. Not only was this well-intentioned approach ineffective, but it had the additional disadvantage of making it more difficult for black people to affirm their group and identity. Black people increasingly rejected this notion of colour-blindness and instead put their efforts towards cultivating pride in their group ('black is beautiful'). As a parallel, people with mental illness are involved in *Mad Pride*.

Second, mental illness is rarely visible from the outside. The normalcy approach puts the onus on people with mental disorders to try even harder to pass as 'normal' (Sect. 4.3.7). Yet this makes it more likely to keep one's illness hidden (which comes with all its known disadvantages, particularly social withdrawal) (Sect. 5.1.4).

Third, programmes to combat the public stigma of mental illness have frequently used normalising messages: mental illness is an *illness like any other* (e.g. like diabetes). But by equating mental illness with physical illness, there is a conceptual proximity to biological models of illness that do not reduce the stigma (Sect. 5.1.2). This illness like any other approach is well understood by the general public but tends to reinforce prejudices [178].

Finally, the message of normalcy has two undesirable side effects. First, it makes it more difficult for people with mental illness to be self-confident and proud of their identities and life stories when they are supposed to be 'normal' (whatever that means). Second, it prevents an important reaction on the part of the general public: solidarity, here understood as standing up for each another in a community (Sect. 7.5.1). If people with mental illness are to be 'normal', there is no spectrum, no horizon, of common experience that the general public can learn to appreciate. More helpful is the attitude that 'it is normal to be different'.

The more the public realises that mental illness is not 'normal' but rather a deeply human experience, the more they can show solidarity. That would not be the worst attitude, especially for those affected by self-stigma and shame. Peer support could also be made more difficult by messages of normalcy, because it consists of mutual support within an in-group that is not 'normal' (for in-group or with Goffman 'the own', see Sect. 4.3.6).

Pity?

Pity can lend itself to a readiness to help. Campaigns to support children with cancer or the victims of a natural disaster, for example, successfully use images and messages that arouse pity. Is pity therefore also suitable as a message against the stigma of mental illness? Service users reject pity. They don't want handouts or condescension, they want equality (*parity, not pity*—in the spirit of the UN Convention on the Rights of Persons with Disabilities; Sect. 7.5.2). Suppose an educational programme against stigma used images of people with severe mental illness who were homeless and lying in rags on the street, or living helplessly in a nursing home. Both could arouse pity. But such messages reinforce two perceptions that are prerequisites for stigma: an imbalance of power and the perception of difference (Sect. 3.1.4). Members of the general public would consider even more that people with mental illness are weak, powerless and very different from themselves [2].

Continuum?

There is a continuum between complete mental health and a state of well-being on one end and severe mental illness and disability on the other (Sect. 1.6). Diagnoses can cause stigma by falsely suggesting that there is a categorical divide between being healthy (without a diagnosis) and ill (with a diagnosis). It is therefore important to emphasise the continuum (rather than the diagnoses) in order to reduce stigma. In an online randomised controlled trial (RCT) conducted with the general public, reinforcing the continuum led to a reduction in stigma [682]. It is not clear whether this approach has an effect on behaviour and how long the effect lasts. In another study, a continuum model resulted in participants from the general public seeing greater similarities between themselves and people with schizophrenia [683]. This can be interpreted as a recategorisation, a decrease in the perceived differences between *them* and *us* (Sect. 3.2.2). Another RCT investigated the effectiveness of a workshop for mental healthcare professionals. The workshop reinforced continuum thinking as hoped but did not reduce stigma [576]. This approach is plausible, but whether it has a sustainable effect for everyday life remains unresolved.

The continuum approach is consistently implemented by the *Hearing Voices Network* (https://hearing-voices.org). It was created in the 1980s in Holland in collaboration with Patsy Hage, a voice hearer; Marius Romme, her psychiatrist; and his colleague Sandra Escher [684]. The network uses the following assumptions: hearing voices in itself is not pathological, but rather a common human experience that can make sense; many voice hearers do not have an illness and do not need treatment; hearing voices can have its origins in traumatic events, and understanding these events can in turn ease the burden of hearing voices. The network emancipates itself from psychiatric approaches, not least because psychiatric drugs often do not silence voices and have many side effects. Hearing voices is also, almost without exception, pathologised in psychiatry and as a symptom (especially of schizophrenia) leads to labelling (for the gentleman from Bayreuth who wanted to keep his voices, see Sect. 6.1). In contrast, the Hearing Voices Network by way of peer support (Sect. 7.3.4) and self-help approaches offers a space where voice hearers can exchange their experiences.

8.1.5 WHAT EDUCATIONAL PROGRAMMES ARE THERE?

Tony Jorm has differentiated between four types of educational programmes [88]: (1) for the general public, (2) in educational institutions and schools, (3) *Mental Health First Aid* and (4) online interventions. Among the first group, Jorm includes Australian *beyondblue*, which aims to improve knowledge about depression, as well as the *Alliance Against Depression* (Sect. 5.2.3). Programmes in schools are plausible, particularly because they achieve high penetration rates in contrast to programmes for the general public (Sect. 8.1.2); they impart students with knowledge about mental illness and available resources for help and treatment (Sect. 5.7). Mental Health First Aid is a programme developed by Jorm to provide first-aid skills for dealing with mental crises and illnesses (similar to first-aid courses for medical emergencies). The course lasts for 2 days and deals in detail with the symptoms of various mental disorders. Participants then should learn five things: assessing the risk of suicide, non-judgemental listening, providing information, encouraging people to seek professional help and peer support/self-help. Finally, as far as the fourth type of education is concerned, online information can be found in incalculable quantities and of highly varying quality.

8.1.6 DOES EDUCATION WORK AGAINST PUBLIC STIGMA?

Doubts about the effectiveness of education in reducing stigma are not new. Gordon W. Allport wrote in 1954:

> It always has been thought that planting right ideas in the mind would engender right behaviour. Many school buildings still display the Socratic motto, Knowledge Is Virtue. But the student's readiness to learn facts ... depends upon the state of his attitudes. Information seldom sticks unless mixed with attitudinal glue. ([76], p. 451])

What is the research evidence? Experimental studies on the effectiveness of education say little about its true effect on the general public. Online or laboratory studies can show a strong reduction in stigma among those taking part in the intervention [685]. But the best intervention does little if it does not reach the general public (i.e. does not achieve a high penetration)—and this is often the case (Sect. 8.1.2). Another problem is the aforementioned information overload. In an artificial study situation, study participants (usually) listen and take in information—but this is different in everyday life when switching between the smartphone, lunch and the gas pedal. Because these issues of applicability in real life are often overlooked, the effectiveness of education is overestimated, at least for the general public. Finally, it is important to note that in real life, the drivers of stigma—from self-esteem enhancement to system justification and social order—are far more influential than they would be in a lab setting (Sect. 3.3).

Some nationwide campaigns have chosen education as a focus and reached large parts of the population, such as beyondblue in Australia or Time to Change in England. An evaluation of beyondblue showed it has good effects on knowledge about depression but no clear effects on stigma [686]. In an RCT, Pat Corrigan examined the effects short videos could have [687]. About 500 participants watched either a beyondblue video with three men talking about depression as a treatable illness, a video in which a man talked about his depression and subsequent recovery, or a video on cleaning teeth as a control group. None of the videos led to an increase in the willingness to seek help when needed. Only the recovery video led to a decrease in prejudice. The study provides an important clue: education that focuses on problems and solutions/treatments is less balanced and effective than an individual's personal account of the ups (recovery) and downs (illness) of his life. This type of narrative should be helpful in replacing stigma with positive attitudes (for contact, see Sect. 8.4; for recovery, see Sect. 5.1.6).

Sara Evans-Lacko, Claire Henderson and Graham Thornicroft found more encouraging evidence for Time to Change in England (Sect. 12.1 [688]): about half of the studied population knew about the campaign, and this group was found to be less prejudiced against people with mental illness. In a more recent evaluation, those who knew about Time to Change were more willing to disclose their own possible illness and seek help if necessary [689]. It is important to note that Time to Change also used contact (Sect. 8.4) as a strategy, which likely helps to explain its effectiveness. This is matched by findings from California in a study of almost 2000 participants with mental health problems: during an antistigma campaign with educational and contact elements, people who had taken note of the campaign were more likely to seek treatment. However, this seemed to be because of an increased individual need for help rather than a decrease in public stigma [690].

The project *psychenet—Hamburger Netz psychische Gesundheit* (Hamburg Mental Health Network, https://psychenet.de) has been active in the Hamburg region since 2011. In cooperation with marketing companies, psychenet conducted a broad-based media education campaign via posters, postcards and short films in cinemas. Content-wise, society's high prevalence of mental illness was emphasised and possibilities for help were identified. The observed results were sobering [691]: compared to a city without the campaign, almost no effect on attitudes or prejudices was found. Not even 10% of the Hamburg population was familiar with psychenet. This is where the problems of such initiatives become apparent: low penetration and lack of effectiveness. Hamburg colleagues concluded that in the future they should focus on programmes aimed at specific target groups (instead of the indiscriminate, general public).

A European study on the Alliance Against Depression (Sect. 5.2.3) has examined its effect on prejudice against people with depression. To this end, members of the general public in the study were assessed right before and towards the end of the Alliance programme [692]. There was a lack of clear evidence on the intervention's ability to reduce prejudice: prejudice decreased in cities whether they had an Alliance programme or not. The lack of impact the Alliance programme had on suicide rates in that same European study has already been mentioned (Sect. 5.2.3). But the Alliance can of course be valuable in other respects: for example, the *Munich Alliance Against Depression* (https://muenchen-depression.de) offers numerous activities from training for general practitioners to advice for teachers. The Munich Alliance also organises the Munich *Mental Health Week* (https://woche-seelische-gesundheit.de), which consists of many individual events. Furthermore, peer support, writing workshops and visits to patients in psychiatric clinics are offered in Munich and at many other Alliance sites.

The effectiveness of *Mental Health First Aid* has been thoroughly investigated. A meta-analysis summarised 18 controlled studies (including 14 RCTs) with a total of almost 6000 participants [693]. Amongst course participants, the programme was found to have a positive impact on illness recognition, knowledge about treatment options and willingness to provide first aid to others in the spirit of the programme. However, the overarching goal of the Mental Health First Aid programme is that people with mental health problems who receive help by trained first aiders are better off than those who do not. Unfortunately, there is no evidence of positive programme effects on those aid recipients. For example, in several RCTs, teachers or parents were trained in Mental Health First Aid and the subsequent well-being of their adolescent students or children was assessed. But no positive programme effects on the adolescents were found [693, 694].

Although Mental Health First Aid appears to have positive effects on course participants, effects on stigma amongst course participants were minimal (and immeasurable 1 year later) [693]. What is the reason for this after an intensive 2-day course? There are several possible explanations:

- First, Mental Health First Aid is a programme with the clear aim of increasing the number of people seeking help in mental crises of all kinds. This is a common goal of antistigma work (Sect. 1.3), and this goal is likely achieved by Mental Health First Aid.

- But as a side effect, the focus on symptoms, risks of untreated illness and treatment needs could emphasise the differentness of people with mental illness—which prevents stigma reduction.
- Information overload is a further problem. At one point when I was already working in psychiatry, I was a guest of Tony Jorm in Melbourne and attended a Mental Health First Aid course. The amount of material on symptoms and psychopathology was extensive. And ultimately, the programme's five recommendations for action (previously mentioned) are more complex than they appear: who can learn to listen nonjudgementally in just a short part of a seminar? Many psychotherapists hardly manage to learn this even after years of training.

The effectiveness of online interventions on mental health knowledge has also been examined. However, the formats of these interventions differ widely, ranging from classic text-based psychoeducation to educational games on social media and fully automated multimedia programmes that facilitate seeking help. A review of 14 experimental studies showed mixed effects [695]. Although the programmes improved participant knowledge, there was no effect found on participants actually seeking help. Effects on stigma varied greatly. One possible explanation for these results is that better knowledge about treatment options does not necessarily lead to more requests for help, especially if stigma (as a known barrier to seeking help [Sect. 5.1.7]) is not simultaneously removed. If this interpretation is correct, it further indicates the limitations of educational approaches.

Using numerous individual RCTs, meta-analyses have examined the effectiveness of education in reducing public stigma [696, 697]. Educational programmes varied greatly in intensity, from short texts to extensive training. Overall, negative attitudes of adults were not only minimally reduced, but this effect also disappeared a few months after each respective programme. The effects of education were weaker than those of contact (Sect. 8.4). However, studies with young people showed a different picture: here education was more effective [696]. According to the results of a large RCT conducted by Bruce Link among 12-year-old students in Texas, the educational intervention had a positive effect on attitudes, the desire for social distance and the willingness to seek help for one's own psychological problems [698]. The effects were maintained over 2 years. A contact intervention in the same RCT showed no effect.

Conclusion

Adults absorb vast amounts of information and pseudoinformation on mental health/illness over the course of many decades. It is therefore unsurprising that educational programmes, with even more information, achieve little as interventions. Since our culture considers knowledge and education to be fundamentally helpful, the benefits of education in reducing stigma (at least among adults) are overestimated [2]. This is all the more true as human and financial resources for anti-stigma work are limited—as is the attention of the general public. Therefore only educational programmes that require minimal resources (e.g. online interventions that require few personnel and are not cost intensive) or reach the entire target group (e.g. school programmes; Sect. 5.7 [471]) should be considered worthwhile. School programmes have the advantage that education among young people is more effective [696] and that attitudes are more malleable in this age group. In addition, in these cases, combining education with contact (directly at school or indirectly in the form of online videos) seems to be more helpful and successful than education alone.

8.2 Changing Words

Terms and labels are not only hollow words. In the field of mental illness, diagnoses can lead to labelling and thus stigma (Sect. 1.6). The term 'schizophrenia' is particularly controversial. According to expert discussions on diagnostic classifications, this is due in part to the fact that the *group of schizophrenias*, as Eugen Bleuler called it [280], comprises very different states and clinical courses. For some, the term thereby loses much of its meaning (Sect. 5.3). And yet schizophrenia is one of the most stigmatised illnesses in the general public. For this reason, attempts have been made, particularly in East Asian countries, to replace schizophrenia with a less negative term in order to reduce the stigma (e.g. 'integration disorder' in Japan in 2002) [699]. As is common in the antistigma field, these term-change initiatives have good intentions. However, there are two simple questions:

1. Are they 'good' at reducing public stigma?
2. Does the approach have side effects?

8.2.1 CRITIQUES OF THE WORD-CHANGE APPROACH

As for unintended consequences, Pat Corrigan has pointed out some problems with the word-change agenda [2].

First, this approach treats the removal of stigma as child's play: 'Let's just change the name, and the stigma is gone!' This is naive and ignores how stubbornly stigma is ingrained in societies through both historical and cultural processes (Sects. 2.1, 3.3). In a sense, this approach plays down stigma as a cosmetic problem and makes a mockery of the suffering and discrimination of those stigmatised. This trivialisation is also a problem for antistigma initiatives that are struggling for resources or are trying to address persistent structural discrimination. Decision-makers will be led to believe that resources are unnecessary, and that a change of the term is easy (and cheap).

Second, the approach runs the risk of being seen as hair-splitting by insiders. The people who propose and discuss integration disorder or *Bleuler syndrome* as alternative terms for schizophrenia are not the main target group of antistigma work. These term-change advocates therefore tend to be preaching to the converted. Effective antistigma work, however, must first and foremost reach members of the general public who do not want to have anything to do with 'lunatics' and have not engaged with the problems associated with the schizophrenia concept.

Third, the effects of a term change on stigma are likely to be short-lived. Suppose we replace the term schizophrenia with the term integration disorder in Western countries tomorrow. We would be able to foresee that, in a survey of the general public soon afterwards, there would be hardly any prejudice against people with integration disorder. But this would be a trivial, unsustainable result. The survey would simply show that people are unfamiliar with the new term and that negative stereotypes (i.e. integration disorder = danger) are not yet pronounced. These results would likely change over the years: once the general public had understood that 'the lunatics who live in the nuthouse have integration problems', the old prejudices would apply to the same people, with or without a new name. What if, instead of spending money on an effort and survey like this one, we donated money directly to peer-support groups?

Fourth, public attention and resources for all types of antistigma work are very limited (Sect. 8.1.3). Members of the general public are concerned about many social issues: climate change, migration, burglaries, diesel engines. Activists against the stigma of mental illness have to fight hard to be heard above the din. And so it is questionable whether it is a good investment to advocate for a name change instead of dealing with real and consequential problems (e.g. equal rights in employment, voting rights).

Fifth, there will never be one name that satisfies everyone. Countless terms have been suggested as an alternative to schizophrenia, and no agreement is in sight. Who should have the power to determine the new term? The voice of the service users should be the decisive one. Yes, schizophrenia is a stigmatised term, but some people with schizophrenia prefer this expression. In the 1980s, a self-help movement called *Schizophrenics Anonymous* was founded in the United States and later became internationally active. Not everyone may like the term, but no one is entitled to tell people which words they can and cannot use (especially for their own illness).

This leads to the sixth problem. Language-choice activists sometimes act as a word police: the word schizophrenia will be forbidden, and only integration disorder (or whichever term) is allowed. This style of proscriptive thinking and speaking can offend and alienate others, which in turn distances them from the original goal (i.e. to reduce discrimination). Not only do people dislike being told what to (not) think but also become even more resistant to change. There is also the risk that the general public will conflate antistigma work with a fixation on political correctness. To me, this kind of word policing seems not only presumptuous but also a distraction from the actual topic (Sect. 1.2): 'I don't care what you call it. We just need to make sure people stop robbing me of my life goals because of my mental health history' ([2], p. 113). Additionally, and especially when it comes to stigma, respect for what people choose to call their own experience is necessary and must be foregrounded.

Finally, consider two final problems with this approach. First, the word-change agenda often allows those who adopt it to feel good and justified: 'I now only say integration disorder, so I'm good and do something against stigma.' This attitude, called *slacktivism*, refers to pseudoengagement primarily aimed at the well-being of those who use these terms. They believe they have done a lot, but in reality making a concrete effort to help people with mental illness would be a much greater service (versus wasting time on online likes or on being the word police). Second, I know of no faster way to derail antistigma work than to argue over words (for an example, see Sect. 1.2). Regardless of whether it is service users talking amongst themselves or a discussion between people with and without experiences of mental illness, the dispute over words prevents concentration on the real issues.

8.2.2 EFFECTIVENESS OF THE WORD-CHANGE APPROACH

What does the research say? There is no convincing evidence from East Asia that a change in terms has reduced the stigma associated with schizophrenia. One study examined millions of Japanese newspaper and television reports between 1985 and 2013 on schizophrenia or, after the change in terminology in 2002, on integration disorder. The proportion of negative reports did not decrease significantly after 2002 [699]. In Taiwan, over a thousand newspaper articles were examined on schizophrenia or, after the change in terminology in 2014, on *dysregulation of thinking and perception*. The proportion of articles associating the illness with crime, violence and suicide remained unchanged after 2014 (33% before, 34% after the terminology change [700]).

Advocates of the word-change approach hope for long-term cultural changes as a result of less stigmatised terms. I am not aware of any data on this, and I predict that this optimistic hypothesis will be difficult to confirm or refute. A term change could be the cause or consequence of a cultural change, or it could take place in parallel without any causal connection.

Conclusion

The approach is likely a waste of resources. It is not conceptually convincing, nor does the data show its effectiveness. Arguing over words will not prove helpful. Change is more difficult and proceeds differently.

8.3 Protest

Protest is an obvious strategy against the harms and consequences of stigma: 'Stop discrimination—it's wrong!' Protest can be directed at the infringement of a discriminated group's rights. There are numerous historical examples of protests that have reduced discrimination. There is of course the classic example of the civil rights movement led by Martin Luther King Jr in the

United States in the 1960s, which inspired significant changes in the structural treatment of black people through its protests. Today, protests are usually initiated by groups that identify discrimination and mobilise against it via organising (in person or online). Protests are often reactive spurred by wrongful depictions in the media or in company advertising, political decisions or drafted legislation. Methods of protest include writing letters, emails or other social media messaging, product boycotts, and demonstrations. Protests can also be an opportunity for antistigma workers to exchange views and collaborate.

Some reports have shown protests to be effective (e.g. in response to advertisements that mock people with suicidality). In England, the sale of a 'mental patient' Halloween costume (which included a hatchet) was stopped after a protest was organised (Sect. 7.4.1). In large numbers on social media, people with mental illness had decided to share completely ordinary pictures of themselves with the tagline: 'This is what a real "mental patient" looks like!'

An example concerning the legal system is the successful protest against the draft of the Bavarian PsychKHG (Sect. 7.5.5). Following protests by many associations and individuals, the law was extensively revised and became less discriminatory in tone and content. The judiciary can also assume a corrective function when protests have failed. One example is the discriminatory exclusion of many people with mental illness from being able to vote in Germany. Protests were of no avail; the exclusion was finally annulled by the highest court in 2019 (Sect. 7.5.4).

There are hardly any studies on the effectiveness of protest. In one RCT, Pat Corrigan examined how members of the general public would react to one of three intervention strategies against public stigma [701]: protest, education or contact. During the trial that applied the protest strategy, participants were shown examples of discrimination in a lecture. They were then encouraged by (simulated) protestors to renounce the discrimination ('Whoever thinks like that should be ashamed!'). In contrast to the other two strategies, protest did not lead to an improvement in attitudes: participants did not think that people with various mental disorders were less to blame for their conditions, nor did they think that recovery was more likely.

A problem of protest is that it does not tend to improve the attitudes of the target group (e.g. a company's advertising department) but can in fact worsen them. This is because it is notoriously difficult *not* to think about something when encouraged ('Don't think about a pink elephant!'). Additionally, the attitude of moral superiority that some people associate with protest leads to the aforementioned objection: 'I will not be told what to think!'

In antistigma work, one therefore has to consider when protest can be applied sensibly and where it can change behaviours (even if broader prejudice persists). For example, antistigma activists could protest a company that discriminates against people with mental illness in its procedures or personnel policy or that uses discriminatory messages in its advertising. Even if the employees of the advertising department do not abandon their personal prejudices as a result, they could still change their company behaviours and policies out of self-interest. Given the sheer number of people affected in the population by mental illness, it is surprising how seldom those affected make use of their economic power (Sect. 2.2.1). Only a small proportion of service users and their allies would have to be mobilised in order to gain influence and protest certain discriminatory practices. To do this, however, one would have to overcome a lot of bickering over words and differing perspectives (Sect. 1.2, end of Sect. 8.2.1).

Conclusion

Public protest can reduce discriminatory behaviour. Little research data is available on the impact and conditions of its effectiveness. The lack of such evidence does not mean that protest does not work. Instead, one should weigh up the chances of success when protesting (e.g. against planned legislation or companies), consider what that success looks like and form alliances. It should be kept in mind, however, that attitudes of individuals can worsen as a result of protest.

8.4 Contact

8.4.1 PRINCIPLES OF CONTACT

In 1954, Gordon Allport formulated the hypothesis that prejudices between members of different social groups can be reduced through group contact [76]. It is important that the contact is positive and that the general conditions are favourable, because confrontation or hostile interactions between groups can reinforce prejudice. Allport identified four conditions under which contact should take place in order to be effective:

1. Equal status established between the members of both groups (i.e. no overt status differences, such as employer/employee or doctor/patient).
2. A common goal (e.g. a shared project).
3. Cooperation (i.e. working together without negative messages about one other during contact).
4. Support from management or other authorities for the contact. For example, a contact intervention for company employees will work better if the boss makes it clear to everyone: 'Today we have an important visitor with valuable experience of their own—listen carefully, we can all learn a lot!' [2].

Studies on the effects of contact have demonstrated two other favourable conditions: the contact should not be superficial, and group membership on both sides should be obvious (group salience [702]). Finally, it is important that the members of the minority are typical representatives of their group. When a contact intervention for antiracism uses contact with Barack Obama, it is easier for (white) addressees to say, 'Yes, Obama is smart, but he's an exception.' Such subtyping (i.e. Obama as a subtype/exception) allows prejudices to persist (Sect. 3.2.8; cf. John Nash, Sect. 8.4.3).

Early studies have shown that contact under these conditions reduces racial prejudice. When white people work in a team alongside black people or live together in housing estates, this leads to better attitudes on both sides (amongst both white and black people) [685]. Prejudice decreases not only against individuals (e.g. the individual black person in a team) but also against the whole group. The effect tends to be stronger among members of the majority (white) population than with members of the minority (black) group. Pettigrew has carried out a meta-analysis of several hundred individual experimental studies with a total of over 250,000 participants and found clear effects: more contact leads to less prejudice. If the conditions do not match Allport's recommendations, the effect is reduced (though it does not disappear altogether) [97].

What does contact change, and how does it work? Contact seems to be effective on many levels, starting with a decrease in the fear of members of the out-group. Pettigrew has called this mechanism *uncertainty reduction*. This is plausible, since there is often uncertainty when dealing with representatives of other groups: what does the other person think of me, and what are his intentions (Sects. 4.1 and 4.2)? This can make social interactions awkward and difficult. Positive contact effectively allows this uncertainty to be reduced. At the same time, empathy and the ability to see the world from others' perspectives increase due to contact. After making contact, members of a group tend to perceive those of the out-group as individuals—the others are no longer all the same (Sect. 3.2.5). The perception of individuals becomes more nuanced, based more on individual characteristics and less on group stereotypes. Interestingly, contact seems to have more of an effect on emotional reactions than on stereotypes: people may continue to think that the others act or are a certain way, but when they meet a member of that group, they are more likely to like them [702]. Contact seems to be effective even without any additional elements (mere exposure [702]), such as when people with mental illness are simply working in a larger team, with equal participant status.

An important form of contact is friendship formed between members of different groups. Friendship meets all the criteria for favourable contact conditions and is one of the best ways to permanently break down prejudice. It also helps if, for example, a person without mental illness knows another person without mental illness who is friends with someone with schizophrenia (this is referred to as 'extended contact'). Just knowing about the relationship between his friend and the person with schizophrenia can reduce his prejudices.

Contact seems to strengthen even more when people talk about themselves (self-disclosure [703]). This makes us more recognisable as individuals and makes it more difficult to pass sweeping judgements on the basis of others' group memberships.

8.4.2 DOES CONTACT REDUCE THE STIGMA OF MENTAL ILLNESS?

In view of these rather robust findings from decades of social–psychological and other research, the question arises as to the effectiveness of contact in reducing the stigma of mental illness. A meta-analysis investigated the effectiveness of education (Sect. 8.1.6) and contact interventions in studies published up to 2010 [696]. In adults, both education and contact showed improvement in attitudes and behavioural intentions, but contact was found to be more effective. Direct contact was more effective than contact via video (i.e. when a participant would watch a person with mental illness talk about himself in a video). The picture was, however, different for young people: here, education and contact had the same effect on behaviour, and education had an even better effect on attitudes.

A more recent meta-analysis has summarised the effectiveness of contact on mental illness stigma using a total of about 100 studies from 24 countries with approximately 26,000 participants [704]. The study examined the influence of different types of contact and conditions. This is critical, otherwise it would be easy for incomparable situations to be compared (Sect. 1.5). However, the following also applies here: if no individual studies have examined and compared certain factors, not even the best meta-analysis can provide information on their link. Seven types of contact were differentiated by the study:

1. personal contact (a face-to-face exchange),
2. contact through a lecture (member of the stigmatised group gives a lecture to participants),
3. video contact (participants see member of the stigmatised group on a screen),
4. vicarious contact (participants observe other people having contact with members of the stigmatised group),
5. e-contact (e.g. in a chatroom online),
6. imagined contact (participants imagine they have contact with a member of the stigmatised group),
7. extended contact.

The study made further distinctions, of which only two are mentioned here: mere contact (i.e. people with mental illness are in contact with majority group members without any other agenda) and contact combined with education (i.e. people with mental illness talk about themselves and their history during contact). The meta-analysis also examined whether the diagnosis of the person with mental illness is consistent with the outcome measure of the contact type: a person with schizophrenia talks about herself (contact and education), and the attitudes of the participants towards people with schizophrenia (or, more generally, towards people with mental illness) are subsequently measured. This is helpful, because the data will show whether increased positive attitudes after a contact intervention regarding one diagnosis will then generalise to people with any psychiatric diagnosis.

What are the results of this meta-analysis? Contact had a moderately strong effect on attitudes, emotional reactions and behavioural intentions; effects on actual behaviour were almost never examined [704]. In terms of the effectiveness of the contact intervention, it did not matter whether prejudice against people with the same disorder as the person in the contact intervention was measured: the contact intervention improved attitudes towards people with mental illnesses in general (i.e. all disorders). Fortunately, this suggests that contact has a positive effect on attitudes towards a broad group, irrespective of diagnosis. This is, incidentally, a further argument for a cross-diagnostic approach to antistigma interventions (Sect. 1.6). Mere contact was also shown to be effective, but only short-term effects were examined and were somewhat weaker than those from contact through education. As far as it could be assessed on the basis of the available studies, the type of contact did not affect the strength of the effect (e.g. video contact had a similar effect to personal contact). The connection between the length and intensity of contact and effect remained unclear [705].

Even imagined contact proved to be effective. It has been suggested for some time that vividly imagining contact with an out-group member can in principle reduce prejudice. For those who find this astonishing (and I confess: I do), the authors of a meta-analysis on the effectiveness of imagined contact offer a quote from Graham Greene: 'When you visualised a man or a woman carefully ... when you saw the lines at the corners of the eyes, the shape of the mouth, how the hair grew, it was impossible to hate. Hate was just a failure of imagination' ([706], p. 3). This points to the fact that successful contact, imagined or not, brings the humanity of one's counterpart to the fore—and thus protects against dehumanisation (which favours extreme discrimination) (Sects. 2.1.2, 3.1.4). Unfortunately, imagined contact can also be harmful. A series of studies found that prejudice against people with schizophrenia only decreases when imagined contact is explicitly positive [707]. In other words, the way imagined contact is enacted matters: when participants influenced by negative stereotypes about schizophrenia imagine the contact to be negative, their prejudices get worse.

The meta-analysis showed that the effects of contact remained just as strong 4 to 12 months after the intervention as they were shortly after [704]. Particularly strong effects were observed in contact interventions amongst healthcare professionals. On one hand, this is encouraging. Prejudices can be reduced if the contact intervention consists of positive contact (according to Allport). On the other hand, this result is sobering. This target group has frequent and intensive contact with people with mental illness (Sect. 7.3.1), but their everyday interactions with people with mental illness seem to be a far cry from Allport's favourable conditions: too rarely on equal terms, not cooperative enough, etc. This suggests how changing practices within the healthcare system towards increased cooperation and genuine, shared decision-making would improve not only care procedures but also the attitudes of professionals.

Another meta-analysis has specifically investigated the question of whether contact in the form of a video breaks down prejudice among schoolchildren [708]. Videos proved to be as effective as personal contact. Long-term effects were not investigated but, for the time being, videos are a promising approach that can be implemented well (at least in schools). This applies to videos in which people with mental illness talk about themselves. (It should be noted that the situation is different when it comes to videos that contain hallucination simulations, which are used time and again by pharmaceutical companies for advertising purposes. The simulated world depicted here is usually one of terror and strangeness. Unsurprisingly, the approach does more harm than good—even if it used for an antistigma strategy with good intentions [697].)

Contact and Self-Stigma

When people with mental illness participate in contact interventions, their own self-stigma can be reduced alongside the public stigma of the target group. They usually take a leading role in the intervention and are shown sincere interest; both counteract self-stigma. A Spanish study supports this assumption [709].

Contact and Social Change

Contact leads to the reduction of prejudice. However, a significant part of stigma involves structural discrimination (Sects. 3.1.5, 5.1.8). Without structural changes, stigma cannot decrease in the long term. Contact interventions have therefore been criticised: they could make everyone be nice and like each other—but for this very reason they could make efforts for social change and for improving the situations of disadvantaged groups more difficult. However, we can imagine a positive structural effect from contact: members of the general public, whose attitudes improve through contact, may be more willing to form coalitions with the discriminated group and take joint action against structural discrimination [702]. Contact may also make members of the minority aware of their relative social disadvantage and thus increase their motivation to work for social change. More recent longitudinal data suggest that contact increases the willingness to fight for social change [710].

8.4.3 WHAT SHOULD CONTACT INTERVENTIONS LOOK LIKE?

Pat Corrigan, in cooperation with researchers and peers, has compiled suggestions for contact-based antistigma programmes [711]. There are five critical components to consider:
1. *Peer leaders:* The programme is led by peers who have undergone training and are remunerated. The peers should fit the target group as closely as possible. If the target group is that of police officers, a police officer should act as peer (i.e. a police officer with lived experience of mental illness).
2. *The target group:* It should be clearly defined (e.g. employers), and the content of the presentation should fit the group's needs. The ideal outcome, which is encouraged, must be tailored to it as well ('Employers hire people with mental illness').
3. *The staff:* Lecturers and programme leaders, as well as the advisory board or equivalent body, should be peers. Otherwise, those being addressed will be given the harmful message that peers can talk about themselves but cannot manage or run a programme.
4. *The message:* The narrative given about one's own mental illness should contain challenges and impairments caused by the illness (hospital stays or similar). The narrative is otherwise not credible. It should also contain successes and recovery despite and with the illness, focusing on the respective addressees and the goal ('People with mental illness can work well').
5. *The follow-up survey of the target group:* Did the programme work? Has it changed attitudes or behaviours? How sustainable are the effects?

In comparison to the aforementioned meta-analysis [704], a few points stand out here. First, Corrigan's approach [711] favours personal contact. Second, the content of the programme is important; in other words, it is about a combination of contact and education. This combination is plausible and widely used. However, in view of the findings of the previous meta-analysis [704], other approaches, such as mere contact (whereby it must be clear during the intervention that the person is a peer, otherwise it is not contact in the sense used here), are also conceivably effective. There are still very few studies on what kind of contact will sustainably reduce discriminatory behaviour [705].

Another point that is important to note: the peer in a contact intervention should only moderately disconfirm the stereotype (cf. Obama at the beginning of Sect. 8.4.1). If John Nash (1928-2015), who had schizophrenia and was awarded the Nobel Prize for Economics, had been part of a contact intervention (e.g. in a video), his contact would not have necessarily been helpful. 'Nash is different, but my neighbour is crazy, I don't want anything to do with him.' Therefore there are online projects like Mutmachleute (https://mutmachleute.de) in which 'completely normal' people with mental illness talk about themselves and their recovery via pictures and text.

8.4.4 *TLC3* AND CONTACT-BASED ANTISTIGMA WORK

Pat Corrigan calls the approach of focused, local contact-based antistigma work *TLC3* (targeted, local, credible, continuous contact [712]):
- *Targeted contact* is aimed at a specific target group, not just anyone. The focus on a target group leads to a reduction in stigma amongst those whose attitudes are particularly important for service users due to their positions of power (e.g. employers, general practitioners, teachers, media professionals, politicians and government officials). The time and place of the programme should also be targeted so that it reaches these participants.

- *Local contact* takes place in a district or county, at a local employers' association or with the police officers of a city. The local focus means that local conditions can be taken into account, and that local stakeholders are known. An antistigma programme that is effective in a big city district may not work as well in a small country town. It is therefore useful to adapt a programme to local conditions—especially if aimed at ethnic or cultural minorities.
- Contact is *credible* if the peers in the contact role come across as convincing to their respective addressees. Employers should ideally be addressed by an employer who has personal experience of mental illness. If this is not possible (e.g. because of the employer's fear of disclosing his own illness), an employer can be accompanied by a peer. They can then speak to employers in tandem: one peer and one employer reporting positive experiences with mentally ill employees. Finally, it increases the credibility of the peer if she has experienced impairments due to the illness but has achieved some of her goals in spite of (and with) it. It is not the high-flyer (John Nash) who is in demand here, but rather someone with experiences of the peaks and troughs.
- Contact should be *continuous*; contact of a one-off nature has a limited effect. Although the effects are measurable, they diminish over time. What helps? Simply repeating the same contact intervention, with the same peer in the role of contact, is probably not ideal. The challenge is to bring the target group into contact in multiple ways, through various channels and with different peers time and again, thus making the contact interventions continuous. This is not easy, and it indicates how far we have to go to achieve real change [2].

8.4.5 IRRSINNIG MENSCHLICH (MADLY HUMAN)

In the year 2000, Manuela Richter-Werling and Matthias Angermeyer founded the association *Irrsinnig Menschlich* (https://irrsinnig-menschlich.de) in Leipzig, Germany. The association started off by visiting schools and doing antistigma work using a combination of contact and education—the school programme is called *Crazy? So What! Mentally Fit at School*. There are now almost 80 regional groups in 11 German federal states plus groups in Austria, the Czech Republic, Slovakia, Poland and the United Kingdom. In 2019, around 36,000 pupils and teachers were accessed on more than 1000 school days. The school programme helps students and teachers talk about the topic of mental health, as well as possibilities for seeking help and prevention when needed. How does the programme work? Peers and professionals (i.e. experts by experience and experts by training) go into school classrooms in tandem. The philosophy is not primarily about psychoeducation—this is where the approach of Irrsinnig Menschlich differs from *Mental Health First Aid* (Sect. 8.1.5). Instead, the life stories of the peers are at the forefront; in this respect, the emphasis is on contact.

A major goal of Irrsinnig Menschlich is secondary prevention (Sect. 7.3.4, 'Prevention'): young people with mental health problems should be empowered by the programme to seek help more easily and earlier, without being hindered by stigma or shame. Choosing young people as the target group makes sense for two reasons: First, various aspects of stigma discourage young people in particular from seeking help (Sect. 5.1.7). Second, mental disorders usually start early and successful prevention can contribute to decades of a happier life. Irrsinnig Menschlich has now expanded its activities from working with schoolchildren to college students and young professionals. Further training for teachers is also offered. The effectiveness of the school projects in particular has been proven several times over [713].

8.4.6 IRRE MENSCHLICH HAMBURG

In the late 1990s, trialogical psychosis seminars in Hamburg gave rise to the association *Irre menschlich Hamburg*, which included Dorothea Buck and Thomas Bock amongst others.

Trialogue means that people with experience of psychosis, relatives and professionals meet and exchange information on equal footing (Sect. 7.3.4, 'Peer Support, Trialogue'). On this basis, the concept of breaking down prejudice through a combination of meetings, contact, information and education was developed. This association has established numerous projects in (secondary) schools and companies. Courses are offered for different professional groups that have unique relationships with and responsibilities towards people with mental illness. In addition to programmes for healthcare professionals, there are programmes for police officers, teachers, journalists and prison officers. Other trialogical events take place in the cultural sector, such as through films and theatre performances.

The effectiveness of this programme has been examined in various ways: one RCT showed positive effects of a trialogical intervention on the attitudes of medical students towards people with mental illness [714]; another course for prison staff reduced their desire for social distance as well as their negative emotional reactions towards prisoners with mental illness [715]. The association cooperates closely with the Hamburg University Hospital. Since the 1990s, a comprehensive network for prevention has formed around a trialogical citizens' initiative, with fixed partners. The work of the association is characterised by its regional focus (TLC3, see Sect. 8.4.4) and the trialogue. A key piece of literature is the trialogical brochure: *It Is Normal to Be Different* (available at https://irremenschlich.de).

8.4.7 BASTA

BASTA (the alliance for mentally ill people [*Basta!* is 'Enough!' in Italian]) is a Munich-based antistigma campaign. It was founded in 2001 and, in cooperation with Werner Kissling and colleagues at the Department for Psychiatry of the Technical University of Munich, carries out contact-based interventions with peers and relatives (https://bastagegenstigma.de). The projects focus on the areas of school, police and culture, primarily in Bavaria (though there are also nationwide projects in schools). The programme resembles the approach of Irrsinnig Menschlich (Sect. 8.4.5), whereby peers and professionals visit school classrooms in tandem. The police project takes place on an ongoing basis within Bavarian universities' police training programmes. In seminars run jointly by peers, family members and professionals, they learn about mental illness and what police officers can do to ensure that crises are well-managed. Cultural projects range from poetry slams, to public art displays, to film days on the subject of mental illness.

Conclusion

Contact is currently the most promising strategy for reducing stigma amongst members of the general public, at least for adults. The effects are stronger than with education and last for a while. So far, however, the effect of contact on behaviour (discrimination) has hardly been investigated. Contact not only helps to reduce stigma amongst those who receive the contact intervention but could also benefit the peers leading the interventions (i.e. empowerment, self-stigma reduction) and promote social change.

One problem with the contact strategy, however, is that personal contact in small groups requires considerable time and financial resources. Newer approaches (videos, imagined contact) could be helpful in this regard and should be evaluated.

CHAPTER 9

Strategies Against Self-Stigma

Like public stigma, self-stigma has different components: thinking (stereotypes), emotional reaction (prejudice) and behaviour (discrimination). But with self-stigma, all of these aspects are directed at oneself. For instance, if a man suffers from self-stigma, he may think: 'Because I have a mental illness, I must be stupid'. He may disrespect himself, be ashamed of his illness or even despise himself [271]. This is damaging to his self-esteem and will ultimately alter his behaviours when he no longer believes he can set or achieve his life goals. This state of demoralisation due to self-stigma is also called *Why try* (Sect. 5.1.3).

Programmes that aim to reduce self-stigma must take on these negative consequences and challenges. Self-stigma should not be seen as an individual fault, defect or personal problem. On the contrary, self-stigma is the internalisation of social attitudes; the problem is thereby a social one and people who suffer from self-stigma or shame deserve every type of support. As long as public stigma persists, there will be self-stigma. It is therefore worthwhile to take a look at programmes in this area. Programmes that focus on and strengthen empowerment are also important; self-stigma and empowerment can be imagined as opposite poles of a continuum [79].

In this chapter, various approaches are briefly presented with regard to their content, effectiveness and limitations (Sect. 9.1). One example we focus on is the HOP programme, which supports participants in their decisions for or against disclosure of their own illnesses (Sect. 9.2).

9.1 Approaches to Reduce Self-Stigma

9.1.1 PSYCHOEDUCATION

As with initiatives against public stigma (Sect. 8.1), psychoeducation is also a popular strategy to fight self-stigma. The premise is that people with mental illness will agree less with negative stereotypes about themselves and their group if they know more about their mental illness and related stigma. Psychoeducational antistigma programmes typically provide information on the forms, causes, course and treatment of the mental illness; on public and self-stigma and its consequences; and on ways of coping with stigma.

The programmes usually consist of groups led by professionals and are typically delivered via several lessons over a few weeks. The approach of psychoeducation is plausible insofar as we agree on self-stigma as the one-sided, negative and distorted stereotyping of oneself. However, this educational approach is optimistic (as to public stigma, see Sect. 8.1.3); it assumes that the correction of such distortions or errors directly and fundamentally influences self-stigma (including its emotional and behavioural components).

Is there data on psychoeducation's effectiveness? Wolfgang Gaebel and his German colleagues have presented an important randomised study on this question [716]. A total of 462 people with schizophrenic or depressive disorders participated in psychoeducation led by professionals. These study participants were divided, with one-half receiving standard psychoeducation without a focus on stigma and the other half participating in an additional three sessions focused on experiences of discrimination, self-stigma and coping. The success of the antistigma psychoeducation was assessed by measuring self-stigma, empowerment and quality of life. One of the strengths of this study was its lengthy observation period: participants were interviewed one year after the end of the programme. The results were sobering: in none of the outcome measures did participants from the antistigma psychoeducation score even slightly better than those in standard psychoeducation. Even before this study, the approach of reducing self-stigma through professional psychoeducation seemed optimistic; this study provided definitive evidence that this is in fact a dead end.

In the United States, Alicia Lucksted and Amy Drapalski developed *Ending Self-Stigma* as a professional-led, psychoeducational self-stigma reduction programme consisting of nine sessions. A large randomised controlled trial (RCT) found that it did not have clear effects on self-stigma at the end of the programme; all effects had disappeared after six months [717]. In one meta-analysis on the effectiveness of interventions against self-stigma, evidence of psychoeducation having positive effects was found [718]. However, the studies were often of poor quality, the effects were weak and the programmes were very different from one another in content and length (and thus incomparable). Additionally, many of the programmes used psychoeducation as one strategy amongst many. There is therefore little to be said for giving priority to psychoeducation as a strategy against self-stigma (which corresponds to findings in the area of public stigma, Sect. 8.1.6).

9.1.2 COGNITIVE THERAPY

Cognitive therapy (CT) is rooted in the thinking of psychotherapist Aaron Beck and uses thought patterns and event evaluation in order to alter feelings and behaviours. Here, self-stigma is seen as distorted and harmful thinking ('Yes, I am mentally ill, and therefore I cannot achieve anything'). The thought can then be questioned and corrected ('Actually, I do take care of my family, I meet with friends, and soon I will work again—I have a mental illness, but I can achieve many goals'). Cognitive therapy uses other strategies to combat self-stigma as well: normalising psychological symptoms on a continuum to feel less *different*, building social skills to cope with stigma and dealing with stressful emotions (including shame) or behaviours (including social withdrawal). However, meta-analyses show a lack of strong studies regarding this approach, and thus there is no clear indication of its effectiveness [718].

9.1.3 NARRATIVE-COGNITIVE THERAPY

For many years, American-Israeli researchers Phil Yanos, David Roe and Paul Lysaker have presented important work on the topics of self-concept and self-stigma. They have developed a comprehensive programme for reducing self-stigma: *Narrative Enhancement and Cognitive Therapy* (NECT; narrative refers to telling one's own life story). The inclusion of narrative in this approach is based on an old insight: we all tell our life stories over and over again, and by doing so continuously construct our present self-image.

NECT is an extensive programme that involves 20 group sessions led by professionals and contains three elements: psychoeducation about stigma, cognitive therapy (Sect. 9.1.2), and work on one's own narrative. Through the latter, participants are supported in developing their life story anew; away from the typical focus on deficits, illness and shame; and towards strengths, empowerment, meaning and much more. Studies have suggested that NECT is effective [718]. A recent RCT involving people with schizophrenia found positive effects, especially among outpatients and in terms of social withdrawal [719]. In some cases, the effect was maintained over several months. Therefore, NECT is a promising approach. However, the programme is quite lengthy and intensive, which is a challenge in terms of implementation and funding.

9.1.4 PHOTOVOICE

Photovoice is an initiative that helps people regain their voices by making their perspectives clear through photography. Since the 1990s, photovoice has been an increasingly popular method of participatory social research for and by people with mental illness [720]. 'Participatory' means that researchers do not simply observe a social group; group members (e.g. people with mental illness) actively participate as co-researchers by taking their own pictures with a camera (or by drawing or other artistic expression). The pictures can show participants' social environments, their character, or things they feel are symbolic representations of their situations. In photovoice projects by people with mental illness, images have been created that illustrate stigma: stigma as a cage in which they are perceived as only *ill* or as nonhumans that live on the fringes of society [721]. By taking the pictures themselves, members of discriminated groups (who are often treated as background objects) become the subject. The method itself contributes to empowerment, to correcting the powerlessness of marginalised groups, and thus to social justice [722]. Photovoice is more than photography. The photos are discussed jointly, often in a group [720]: what can be seen on them? What really happens 'behind the surface'? How does the picture relate to the lives of the participants? What can be changed about the issues the picture is pointing to?

After all this, it seems plausible to use photovoice successfully amongst people with mental illness for their empowerment and against self-stigma. Zlatka Russinova has examined the effectiveness of photovoice in the context of an RCT [723] and found an improvement in the areas of self-stigma, stigma management and recovery among participants who jointly addressed the topic over the course of 10 photovoice sessions. Photovoice is a creative approach to self-stigma. One of its strengths is the active role of the participants (compared to psychoeducation, for example). However, its effectiveness cannot be reliably assessed after only one study.

9.1.5 SELF-HELP AND PEER SUPPORT

One of the many strengths of peer support is that the approach itself leads to empowerment and reduces self-stigma: a peer helps other peers. Peers have a lot to say and give because of their own experiences, especially regarding recovery (often more than professionals). By helping others, a peer is also a role model for others: there is life after the crisis, and one's own experience is valuable. Peer support is therefore likely the best way to replace self-stigma with empowerment. As with public stigma, this is not just a matter of removing something negative (self-stigma) but also replacing it with something positive (empowerment, recovery). Fortunately, many such self-help groups and networks exist across Europe, such as EX-IN in Germany (EX-IN is an abbreviation for 'experienced involvement': https://ex-in.de/ex-in.europa).

Self-help and peer support are the best ways to fight self-stigma. This applies both to self-help groups and peers who work as experts by experience (Sect. 7.3.4) and to specific antistigma programmes run by peers (for HOP, see Sect. 9.2). This assessment is increasingly supported by data: evidence from a systematic review has found that peer support has positive effects on self-stigma, especially among people with depression [724].

Conclusion

Interventions can reduce self-stigma, though available studies on the topic are limited (in quality and number). This makes a clear assessment difficult.

- Psychoeducation's effectiveness is overestimated and is likely to be helpful only as one component among several in a complex intervention.
- Both Narrative Enhancement and Cognitive Therapy (NECT) and creative-participatory approaches such as photovoice seem promising.

- Regardless of the content, group programmes have a better effect than programmes for individuals. This makes sense: sharing mutual experiences of self-stigma and stigma management with others helps.
- It remains to be seen whether future approaches to reducing self-stigma will be able to cater specifically to the needs of individuals (e.g. photovoice in the case of low empowerment, NECT to address a person's deficit-oriented view of his or her own life history, and HOP in the case of stigma stress) [718].

9.2 Honest, Open, Proud (HOP)

Another approach to supporting people with mental illness is the peer-led group programme *Honest, Open, Proud* (HOP), presented in this section (for more information, see [215]). The HOP programme supports participants in their disclosure decisions (i.e. in deciding whether and how to tell others about their mental illness).

9.2.1 IDENTITY AS *MENTALLY ILL* AND DISCLOSURE

Similar to how diagnoses are received differently—from helpful to stigmatising (Sect. 1.6 [7])—peers vary in their approaches to having the identity of a person with mental illness. People with mild or temporary mental illness may refuse to identify themselves as *mentally ill* and thus avoid the consequences of stigmatisation altogether [725]. As mentioned in Section 5.1.3 (insight and self-stigma), identity or self-concept as a person with mental illness is not bad or good per se—it rather depends on what the person associates with that identity. Socially, too, identity as a mentally ill person and identification with the in-group can lead to discrimination by others on one hand and to social support from said in-group (e.g. in the area of mutual-help groups or peer support) on the other [192]. Finally, studies have shown that recovery (Sect. 5.1.6) promotes the development of a positive identity that is not limited to the illness: 'I *am* not the illness, I *have* the illness'.

People with mental illness, like members of sexual minorities, often face the difficult decision whether to disclose this aspect of their identity amidst widespread prejudice. Disclosure of one's illness, or keeping it hidden, is not simply 'good' or 'bad'—its consequences depend strongly on the environment and on the person (Sect. 5.1.4 [726]). In a hostile environment, the disadvantages of disclosure are likely to outweigh the benefits. Conversely, disclosure often makes social support possible. The decision for the individual therefore remains complex and situation dependent. The personal impact is also important to consider: for many, but not all, secrecy can lead to ruminations, a stressful division between public and private roles, and a feeling of diminished authenticity [726]. In contrast, acknowledgement of one's own achievements (in spite of and with mental illness–related impairments) can produce a sense of pride in a person. Moreover, regardless of the goals one has achieved, awareness of one's own identity and the authenticity that comes with that is enough to deeply alter and improve a person's self-image [727].

9.2.2 THE HOP APPROACH

The HOP programme was developed by Pat Corrigan and colleagues in Chicago as a peer-led programme that supports participants with mental illness in making disclosure decisions. This evolved in light of the complexity of aforementioned identity and disclosure challenges. The HOP participants are empowered to make self-determined and confident decisions for or against disclosure of their illness in different environments. Persuading participants to disclose is not the aim. On the contrary, secrecy, such as in a stigmatising work environment, can be a good solution.

In cases like this one, HOP would support well-considered nondisclosure as long as it is driven by neither shame nor self-stigma ('empowered nondisclosure', as service user and HOP group facilitator Chris White has put it).

9.2.3 HOP FORMAT AND CONTENT

HOP consists of three sessions of about two hours each. The sessions are typically offered once a week over the course of three weeks. In newer versions of HOP, a booster session is scheduled after one month. Structured workbooks for group facilitators and participants that include case vignettes, tables, illustrations, worksheets, and individual and group exercises are available for all HOP programmes. In the following paragraphs, an overview of the content in Lessons 1 through 3 and the subsequent booster session (Lesson 4) is provided.

In Lesson 1, participants first discuss to what extent they see themselves as people with a mental illness—in other words, how central the illness is to their identity. As explained previously, this has implications for disclosure decisions and consequences and is therefore an important starting point. Possible motives for disclosure are then worked out (e.g. the desire for social support or the need to be authentic). The main part of the first lesson deals with the advantages and disadvantages of disclosure depending on different environments. (Disclosure in the workplace, for example, involves different opportunities and risks than with family members.) Advantages and disadvantages are then further differentiated by distinguishing between long-term and short-term consequences and weighing them up according to participants' personal significance. Finally, Lesson 1 covers the goals participants would like to achieve with a possible disclosure and what they expect after disclosure—clarifying these goals and expectations in turn influences disclosure decisions. At the end of the first lesson, and after weighing up the pros and cons, participants should be able to make a preliminary decision for or against disclosure. They may also choose to postpone their decision if they need more time to deliberate.

Lesson 2 deals with the five levels of disclosure. The underlying idea is that secrecy and disclosure are located on a continuum that ranges from avoiding social contacts at one end ('I avoid everyone, so that nobody can find out about my illness') to broadcasting one's own experience at the other end ('I talk about my illness on YouTube to inform others and reduce the stigma'). In between (from the second to the fourth level), there is secrecy (without social withdrawal), selective disclosure to some individuals and indiscriminate disclosure without actively sharing one's own experience. The advantages and disadvantages of these five levels are discussed for different contexts. An important and often helpful learning experience for HOP participants is that disclosure decisions are not all-or-nothing choices. Instead, participants can learn to move flexibly on the continuum of disclosure depending on the context.

Lesson 2 also deals with two other important topics for preparing disclosure decisions. First, participants learn how they can test the waters before a possible disclosure and thus find suitable addressees. For example, a woman with mental illness could refer to a TV series about people with mental illness that she has seen in order to start a conversation with a work colleague. If the colleague reacts with prejudice, the participant knows that caution is required and that the colleague may not be suitable as a disclosure addressee. Second, participants role-play with one another to find out how others' negative reactions to their own disclosure may affect them. If they feel hurt, this is an indication to be careful with disclosure.

Lesson 3 develops ways and means for participants to tell their stories if they so choose. Examples of stories from other people with mental illness are the starting point in the HOP workbook. This is followed by a guide to crafting the participant's own story, which lists in biographical order life stages and experiences with illness and recovery as well as stigma experiences and how to cope with them. Depending on the addressee and the target for disclosure, the contents are revised. The aim is to be able to tell a story that conveys only that which is appropriate and helpful for the narrator and addressee. As a group exercise, participants can tell each other their stories—often a very important and moving moment in the HOP programme. Lesson 3 is concluded by reflecting on the experience of telling one's own story, collecting information on peer support for disclosure decisions and recapitulating what has been learned.

About one month after Lesson 3, decisions and experiences with disclosure or nondisclosure are dealt with in Lesson 4. Participants discuss whether and why they decided for or against disclosure after Lesson 3 and how a possible disclosure took place. Previous experiences with self-help programmes and peer support are also discussed. Finally, HOP participants work out the possible new points of view for or against disclosure as well as potential changes in their stories based on new experiences.

9.2.4 GROUP FACILITATORS AND PARTICIPANTS

HOP is a peer-led programme. The group facilitators have their own experience in coping with mental illness and disclosure decisions. This makes them credible to participants and competent as group facilitators. In addition, it is helpful if group facilitators share a specific background or experience with the participants that is relevant to disclosure decisions. For example, HOP groups for soldiers with mental illness in the German military are led by soldiers who have dealt with a mental illness. This corresponds to the principle of credibility in interventions against public stigma (Sect. 8.4.4). What constitutes leadership also has some flexibility: in our study with HOP for adolescents who were predominantly being treated as inpatients, HOP groups were led jointly by a young adult peer and a young healthcare professional. As far as the number of group facilitators is concerned, two peers per group have proven to be a good solution.

Although they typically do, it is not required that participants have a psychiatric diagnosis. It is also not important whether they are currently undergoing treatment. Their own experiences with mental illness and disclosure decisions are key. The groups should have about six to eight participants. If the number of participants is much smaller or larger, a lively group exchange can become difficult to focus. The HOP groups are closed in the sense that no new participants should join after the first session.

9.2.5 HOP FOR DIFFERENT TARGET GROUPS

The original HOP programme was designed for adults with mental illness; since then, HOP has been adapted for different cultural contexts and target groups (developers of these versions are shown in parentheses in the list below [215]). These programmes have been formed in the spirit of participatory research and in cooperation with the target group [728]. Stigma is socially and culturally determined—an intervention that works in one country may not be effective in another. Stereotypes also differ with regard to different groups (e.g. different mental illnesses compared to suicidality) (Sect. 5.2).

These are some of different HOP versions currently available:

■ for young people and students with mental illness (McKenzie, Urbashich & Corrigan, United States)
■ for parents of mentally ill children (Ohan, Australia)
■ for people with experience of suicidality (Sheehan, United States)
■ for soldiers (Rüsch and colleagues of the German military) and veterans (Andra, United States)
■ for people in early stages of dementia (Bhatt, United Kingdom)
■ for mental healthcare professionals with mental illness (Scior, United Kingdom)

Information about different HOP versions and workbooks is available in English (http://hopprogram.org) and German (http://uni-ulm.de/med/iws) [215].

9.2.6 THE NAME

HOP was originally called *Coming Out Proud*. Due to the ongoing misunderstanding that it could be about the disclosure of homosexuality, it was renamed Honest, Open, Proud (HOP) without a change in content. The German name *In Würde zu sich stehen (Stand up for yourself With Dignity)* was created in cooperation between peers, professionals and researchers in Kilchberg and Zurich, Switzerland [729]. As far as the terminology is concerned, the workbook refers to mental illness, but participants are free to choose other descriptors (e.g. mental crisis)—in both their HOP groups and daily lives. The terms they choose for this are part of their personal identity and disclosure decisions (Sect. 1.2).

9.2.7 DOES HOP WORK?

HOP supports people with mental illness in their disclosure decisions. As mentioned above, (non)disclosure is a key response to experienced or anticipated stigmatisation by others and to self-stigma. It is therefore expected that HOP will reduce the distress associated with disclosure decisions and with stigma (i.e. stigma stress, self-stigma). It could also bring about improvements in other areas, such as self-esteem, quality of life and depression.

Four RCTs regarding HOP have been made available so far [215]. The first RCT, conducted amongst Swiss adults, showed a decrease in stigma stress, decisional conflict regarding disclosure and secrecy [729]. A RCT in California with adults confirmed the reduction of stigma stress and found positive effects on self-stigma and depressive symptoms (in women) [730]. In another US RCT, HOP was found to reduce self-stigma and stigma stress in college students [731]. For young people with mental illness, HOP was evaluated in a southern German RCT and showed positive effects not only on stigma variables (including stigma stress and self-stigma) but also on quality of life, depression, recovery and attitudes towards treatment [472]. In this study, HOP showed good cost-effectiveness in terms of improving quality of life. The HOP programme may work particularly well in young people because their social networks and ways of dealing with a (usually quite new) illness are still in flux. A meta-analysis of these four RCTs, and a still unpublished RCT of a HOP version for suicide attempt survivors, found positive effects on stigma stress by the end of the programme and on self-stigma about one month later [215].

Conclusion

Although the data so far is encouraging, the long-term effects of HOP have not yet been investigated. It also remains unclear whether HOP participants who decide to disclose are better off or whether empowered nondisclosure is equally helpful. The HOP programme may also help to reduce public stigma by promoting strategic and successful disclosure. If disclosure goes well, more positive contact between members of the general public and people with mental illness can be established. Contact is the best strategy against public stigma (Sect. 8.4). However, this hypothesis has not yet been tested.

HOP is a compact, three-session programme that can be offered flexibly to different target groups in different settings. Through HOP, participants can learn to deal strategically with disclosure decisions and stigma. From a public health perspective, and in order to achieve robust change, HOP should be combined with programmes that reduce public stigma. Two reasons for this should be considered: First, people with mental health problems must not be left to cope with a stigma for which they are not responsible. Second, only by improving public attitudes can we create a society free of prejudice in which disclosure, positive contact, and social inclusion can thrive.

CHAPTER 10

Reduction of Stigma as a Barrier to Help-Seeking

One goal amongst the many in antistigma work is to facilitate seeking help and service use (services agenda, Sect. 1.3). This means reducing the various forms of stigma that act as barriers to seeking help (Sect. 5.1.7): the fear of labelling and public stigma, self-stigma and shame, and structural discrimination that contributes to a lack of accessible and high-quality mental healthcare (which is why avoiding help can be a reasonable choice).

10.1 General Public and Healthcare System

Because many aspects of stigma make it difficult to seek help (Sect. 5.1.7), a number of antistigma programmes aim to facilitate seeking help directly or indirectly. First, programmes that combat public stigma can encourage requests for help: as public attitudes improve, the fear of being labelled due to seeking help diminishes. This is supported by the fact that antistigma programmes aimed at the general public increase, at least to a small extent, the tendency to seek help for oneself when needed (Sect. 8.1.6 [689]).

More specific are antistigma programmes geared towards healthcare professionals (Sect. 7.3.2) and initiatives to reduce structural discrimination in the healthcare system (Sect. 7.3.4). These programmes aim for better quality and availability of support. There are also educational programmes for the general public or risk groups that want to improve knowledge about mental health, prevention, treatment and early help-seeking options (e.g. *Mental Health First Aid*, Sects. 8.1.5, 8.1.6).

10.2 Self-Stigma, Shame and Relatives

Insofar as self-stigma, shame and *Why try* (Sect. 5.1.3) prevent people with mental illness from participating in treatment, approaches to reducing self-stigma can facilitate seeking help. The Honest, Open, Proud (HOP, Sect. 9.2) programme, for example, has been shown to increase the willingness of young people to seek professional help in a possible future crisis [472]. This result makes sense: disclosure to at least one healthcare professional is a prerequisite for service use—and HOP aims to increase self-confidence when deciding whether to do just that. Any intervention that strengthens the sense of empowerment within and amongst people with mental illness can facilitate autonomous decisions to seek help. As has been discussed, this is not about driving people into the arms of psychiatry. Rather, people should be able to decide freely, without shame or fear of stigma, for or against any kind of professional or non-professional help (Sect. 1.3). Shared decision-making can help here by providing service users with good information and enabling them to decide for or against treatment on an equal footing with professionals (Sect. 7.3.1, 'Interactions Between Patients and Professionals'). Janine Berg-Peer (Sect. 6.2) points out that prejudice against relatives can also be a barrier to seeking help (i.e. if relatives do not want to listen to accusations from professionals during treatment and as a consequence may not encourage their ill family member to seek help). Therefore interventions against this form of family stigma are another way to facilitate service use.

10.3 Evidence

My colleague Ziyan Xu has systematically investigated which interventions (with or without a focus on stigma) facilitate seeking help for mental illness or mental health problems [732]. In her meta-analysis, Xu summarised 98 individual studies, including 91 randomised controlled trials, with a total of almost 70,000 participants. Most of the studies came from the United States, Australia or Europe (in that order). The respective interventions were directed at various target groups: the general public, people with mental illness, people with symptoms and thus an increased risk of mental illness, family doctors, relatives and so forth. For all of these groups, the interventions aimed to facilitate seeking help in the event of one's own mental illness or that of a patient (e.g. family doctor intervention) or relative.

What were the results? First, programmes facilitated the search not only for professional help but also for self-help (e.g. peer support). Clear effects were found only for interventions aimed at people with mental illness, people with increased risk/symptoms and family doctors. Interventions for relatives were not studied as much; no significant effect was found, although the trend was positive. Interventions for the general public had no effect.

What kinds of intervention help? Three main types came to the fore:

■ programmes that improve knowledge on mental health, prevention and treatment (mental health literacy, Sect. 3.1.7)
■ programmes with a clear antistigma focus
■ programmes that clarify the help-seeking motivation of participants (such as motivational interviewing, which is often used in substance use services to clarify personal goals and drives—not too different from the shared decision-making process mentioned previously)

Programmes aimed at more knowledge and programmes against stigma were both effective in the short term; after a few months, their effects were still noticeable but no longer statistically significant. Programmes to clarify help-seeking motivations had long-term rather than short-term effects. As far as procedure was concerned, programmes worked best when using personal contact rather than informational materials or online resources. Here, too, there is a parallel with interventions against public stigma (Sect. 8.4).

CHAPTER 11

Reducing Structural Discrimination

Structural discrimination takes place in certain social contexts and systems (Sect. 5.1.8). To be effective, interventions against structural discrimination must start with the structure itself. They have therefore been addressed in the respective areas of work (Sect. 7.1), housing (Sect. 7.2), healthcare (Sect. 7.3.4), media (Sect. 7.4.7) and law (Sect. 7.5).

Structural discrimination refers to all social processes in institutions and social subsystems that disadvantage people with mental illness. Public stigma and structural discrimination are processes that reinforce each other and, in a vicious cycle, affect both attitudes and the distribution of resources in society. One intervention cannot achieve fundamental improvements. And changes will not be seen quickly—these efforts are part of a marathon. But as my brother tells me, long-distance running can be fun.

That structural discrimination is persistent should not discourage anyone. Change is possible and not limited to, say, the successes of sexual minorities in their fight against stigma and discrimination. Considerable changes over the course of a few decades are also possible for those affected by illnesses: as late as the 1970s, women with breast cancer often encountered stigma and reacted with secrecy and shame. The healthcare system was perceived as a burden, unhelpful and paternalistic (almost as psychiatry is perceived by some people today)—a *disease regime* of professionals prevailed [733]. This fortunately went through a fundamental change in the following decades.

Which approaches reduce structural discrimination? It is worth taking a look at widespread racism against black people and its often fatal consequences (see the film *Queen & Slim*, 2019; Sect. 4.2.6 [145]). Programmes against structural discrimination of black people tend to target central issues where discrimination is institutionalised: interventions in predominantly black and low-income neighbourhoods to improve living conditions, interventions in the criminal justice and judicial system to reduce the incarceration rate of black men, and interventions in the health system, where black people are disadvantaged [734].

Similarly, there are two things that can be done to reduce structural discrimination against people with mental illness:

- It must be made clear to all those involved that self-determination and recovery of people with mental illness is a task for all policy areas (mental health in all policies, Sect. 2.3.3). This ranges from the Ministry of Defence for matters relating to soldiers with mental illness (end of Sect. 5.1.7) to the Ministries of Justice and the Interior (not to mention the Ministry of Health and Social Affairs).
- Service users and their allies will have to select and focus on core areas where change is urgent. Possible choices include initiatives to enforce the rights laid down in the UN Convention on the Rights of Persons with Disabilities (Sect. 7.5.2), measures to facilitate employment (Sect. 7.1) and the expansion of peer support within and outside the healthcare system (Sects. 7.3.4, 9.1.5).

Finally, a reduction in discrimination will not be enough. The active and equal participation of people with mental illness in decision-making processes must be simultaneously enforced. This also applies to science: less research should be done 'on' or about users or survivor researchers—more must be done through and with them [26, 27]. This shift is ultimately about power over resources and interpretation, and thus for many professionals it may take some getting used to [735]. Professional researchers are not superfluous: they can contribute their expertise, particularly in the systematic evaluation of the effectiveness of antistigma programmes. They can also be valuable partners for structural improvements in the social and healthcare systems.

CHAPTER 12

Nationwide Antistigma Campaigns

Initiatives against public stigma are most promising when they take place locally (Sect. 8.4.4). The same applies to programmes against self-stigma (e.g. through peer support or peer-led groups, Sects. 9.1, 9.2). The situation is different for efforts that fight structural discrimination and thus require political and legal mobilisation (Ch. 11). The question therefore arises as to what role cross-regional and nationwide antistigma programmes can play. This will be discussed briefly in this chapter (without claiming to be exhaustive).

12.1 Antistigma Campaigns From English-Speaking Countries

In the English-speaking world, nationwide antistigma programmes are quite common. In England, the *Time to Change* campaign (https://time-to-change.org.uk [736]) was very active between 2007 and 2021 (when it officially ended). The campaign and its evaluations were supported by millions of pounds from the National Lottery Community Fund, Comic Relief and the British Department of Health and Social Care. Its aims were to educate the general public, establish contact programmes and reduce the experience of discrimination reported by people with mental illness. Time to Change used a variety of strategies, including mass media such as television, newspapers and online public service announcements; contact interventions of all kinds; and art projects. Besides the general public, Time to Change engaged various target groups: employers, teachers and students, and media professionals. In the final phase of the campaign (2016–2021), the public relations work was aimed particularly at younger men with lower incomes—a group particularly affected by stigma [737]. The effectiveness of Time to Change was continuously and thoroughly evaluated by Claire Henderson, Sara Evans-Lacko, Graham Thornicroft and their colleagues. Repeated population surveys showed that during the Time to Change campaign, attitudes of the general public slowly but surely improved [737, 738]. Newspaper coverage of mental illness also became more positive and less dominated by negative stereotypes [620].

The Scottish *See Me* programme (https://seemescotland.org [739]) is funded by the Scottish government and managed by the Scottish Association for Mental Health and the Mental Health Foundation. Its approach is more grassroots than Time to Change and relies less on mass media. Instead, See Me advocates for a social movement that would bring stigma and discrimination based on mental illness to an end. The main target areas are young people and the employment and social and healthcare systems. Particular attention is paid to human rights that are violated by discrimination (Sect. 7.5.2); co-production (i.e. joint development and communication of the content by peers, professionals, relatives and citizens); and intersectionality (i.e. the particular stigmatisation of social groups with multiple marginalised identities; Sect. 5.5). Finally, See Me places a strong emphasis on cultural initiatives, particularly in the context of the Mental Health Arts and Film Festival in Glasgow [740].

The Canadian programme *Opening Minds* [741] has a clear profile as well: the aim is to reduce discrimination amongst four target groups (young people, healthcare professionals, journalists and employees); the strategy for all target groups is contact-based (Sect. 8.4) and involves the creation of a network for local initiatives to exchange their best practices and useful methods.

Opening Minds refrains from using mass media, which is considered inefficient in view of limited resources [742]. A strength of this Canadian approach is the clear focus and concentration on contact programmes as the most sustainable strategy.

12.2 The Situation in German-Speaking Countries

An external perspective can be instructive. The *Global Anti-Stigma Alliance* has been in existence since 2012 as a platform for national antistigma programmes from around the world. Included in the alliance are programmes that take place in English-speaking countries and in numerous continental European countries (e.g. Denmark, Holland, the Czech Republic and Spain). German-speaking countries are completely absent (for an overview, see https://time-to-change. org.uk). This is regrettable and speaks to the lack of political prioritisation of the issue in the German-speaking world.

There are, however, more clearly-defined antistigma coordination projects operating within Germany. This includes the *German Mental Health Alliance* (https://seelischegesundheit.net). It is derived from the *Open the Doors* campaign of the World Psychiatric Association in the 1990s, which focused on schizophrenia. The Alliance is supported by the German Federal Ministry of Health, as well as by the German Association for Psychiatry, Psychotherapy and Psychosomatics (DGPPN), and its chairman is the psychiatrist and former DGPPN president Wolfgang Gaebel. The Alliance provides a platform for the exchange of information between over 100 individual organisations, from self-help groups to professional and political associations. The approach is primarily psychoeducative (i.e. the population should learn more about prevention of mental illness, including its prevalence and treatments). Another focus is working with media professionals. In their annual autumn mental health action week, various themes and affected groups are promoted, such as the children of mentally ill parents. Especially in view of scarce resources, the work of the Alliance is commendable and provides a good overview of activities in Germany. However, the effectiveness of this work cannot be assessed, as no systematic evaluations have been published [743].

12.3 Who Pays?

In times of scarce resources, the question arises as to who should pay for nationwide antistigma campaigns. This brings us back to the topic of health economics (Sect. 2.2.4). The social costs of mental illness each year in Germany alone are in the hundred-billion-euro range. If antistigma programmes can reduce these costs, they are economically well-justified.

There is much to suggest that antistigma programmes are cost-effective. Studies show that the experience of discrimination in healthcare is associated with greatly increased health costs, regardless of the extent of psychological symptoms [744]. One possible explanation is that people do not seek the help that is available, or seek it too late, due to fear of labelling, self-stigma or past negative experiences with treatment or practitioners. This leads to acute crises and higher costs, particularly in the form of inpatient treatment. Paul McCrone has developed a detailed model of the economic effects of antistigma campaigns [745]. It is based on the assumption that a decrease in public stigma and self-stigma would result in more people seeking help of any kind, psychological symptoms improving, employment and tax-payment rates increasing and dependency on welfare benefits decreasing. Model calculations on this basis indicate that antistigma campaigns are a very good investment—even if only short-term consequences are taken into account and major cost drivers such as early retirement are not included.

The fact that there are no adequately financed nationwide programmes in the German-speaking countries is absurd. The costs would be a pittance compared to the social consequences of mental illness—not to mention the human consequences, which cannot be estimated in monetary terms, for the stigmatised and those closest to them. Both should be reason enough to launch such long-term programmes. This is not a matter of installing an elaborate programme from the top down, under the chairmanship of some psychiatrists (Sect. 12.4). Rather, this would require supporting and evaluating peer-led, local contact initiatives for selected target groups and establishing a practice network, such as in Canada (Sect. 8.4.4).

12.4 Who Sits in the Driver's Seat?

Stigma and discrimination take place because of a power imbalance that disadvantages the stigmatised group. This means that stigma can only be changed effectively and credibly *by* people with mental illness, not for them or over their heads. Imagine if I, as a man, were chairman of a programme to reduce discrimination against women in workplace settings; or that I, as a white man, led a campaign against racism in Germany. Not only would that not be credible; it would be absurd. To avoid any misunderstanding: every stigmatised group needs allies within the general public and within target groups (e.g. employers). I should of course participate as a white professional in an initiative against racism—but by taking a back seat, not the driver's seat.

All of this sounds more obvious than it is. Psychiatrists and other professionals have tendencies to paternalise—an expression of (benevolent) stigma. This could explain why psychiatrists sometimes chair antistigma programmes. But this is the wrong approach. They can undoubtedly participate and cooperate but, contrary to their habits, should do so by taking on an assistive role [746]. Putting peers with first-hand experience in charge effectively communicates that these peers, and the initiative they are running, are competent. Professionals can make their contribution as allies in reducing stigma in the healthcare system (Sect. 7.3). They can also help to reduce the taboo by speaking out about their own experiences of mental illness, which are by no means uncommon amongst professionals (as they are everywhere in society, Sect. 7.3.1).

Switching from being in control to taking a back seat is not always easy for professionals, as it is a question of relinquishing power. But this is precisely why doing so is so important. The key decisions must be made by peers. In this space, I advocate for a power differential in favour of those with experiences of mental illness.

CHAPTER 13

Stigma and Discrimination Related to Mental Illness in Low- and Middle-Income Countries*

Gurucharan Bhaskar Mendon ▪ Yukti Ballani ▪ Anish V. Cherian

▪ Petra C. Gronholm ▪ Graham Thornicroft ▪ Santosh Loganathan

I am not attentive as before and have become quite forgetful. People at home tell me I should not work, but I am a graduate and I feel I should be working. Due to my illness my interest in getting married has also decreased. I at times feel different, and dependent on tablets. Educating people about mental illness through books and TV can decrease the stigma and hopefully improve attitudes of people towards the mentally ill. Education should also begin with children who should be educated according to their capacities.

Earlier I used to earn around Rs 30,000 in the Gulf, where I was away from my family. People's attitudes towards the mentally ill can be improved, especially in the rural areas by giving examples of cured people, i.e. promoting contact with patients doing well.
—Both quotes are from service users with schizophrenia, in India

Low- and middle-income countries (LMICs) constitute approximately 80% of the global population, and approximately the same proportion of individuals with mental illness reside in these countries [747–750]. And yet, on average 76% to 85% of these individuals with mental health problems do not receive any form of treatment, while those who do receive care are most likely not receiving evidence-based treatment [751].

This discrepancy between the mental health needs of persons with mental illness and the availability and delivery of appropriate and accessible healthcare services is referred to as the 'treatment gap' [752] (Sect. 5.1.7). On average 75% of people with severe and common mental disorder in LMICs do not have access to specialised mental health services, leading to a higher disease burden within the community [753–759]. As an example, the National Mental Health Survey of India found an overall treatment gap of 70% to 92% across conditions [760], and 79.1% for depression in particular [761], which is one of the commonly diagnosed conditions in the primary healthcare setting. Generally, treatment costs and low quality of available mental healthcare services are known to add to the treatment gap.

A number of different barriers have also been reported to give rise to this situation, often categorised as demand-side barriers (including decreased perceived need as a result of limited mental health awareness, sociocultural beliefs, values, norms and stigma) and supply-side barriers

*The authors were supported by the UK Medical Research Council in relation to the INDIGO Partnership (MR/R023697/1) award.

(including limited or inequitable distribution and access to resources). Prevalent sociocultural beliefs may particularly affect the ways in which individuals seek help and support for their concerns, with additional distress experienced due to not knowing where to go for help, cost, transportation, confidentiality, individuals feeling that they can handle the problem on their own, beliefs that treatment will not help, thinking the problem will resolve itself or fear of being hospitalised [762] (Sect. 7.3.3).

Appropriate help-seeking behaviours can facilitate effective treatment, when people with mental illness are informed and choose amongst different pathways to reach out to mental healthcare service providers. This decision is then commonly influenced by standard referral pathways, accessibility of mental health services and other resources, and is often associated with a treatment delay. Individuals may reach out to general health and primary care practitioners, doctors, religious healers, nurses, social workers, police or voluntary agencies. Faith healers or spiritual practitioners form a significant pathway as the primary contact in the mental healthcare systems of LMICs [763–767] (Sect. 5.8).

Health systems in low-resource settings may encounter common obstacles to help-seeking behaviours, which include a lack of infrastructure that might reduce mental illness stigma, such as proper screening and detection of psychosocial problems, legislation and policy implementation, training programmes for health professionals and so on [754, 764, 766, 768–771]. Scarcity of financial resources may also prove to be a hindrance for service delivery, since only about 2% or less of the national health budget is allotted to mental health in developing countries [772].

It is within this wider context of global mental health that we shall discuss, first, the cultural aspects and explanatory models of mental illness across LMICs, followed by examples of such beliefs from various settings. We will then cover societal and structural aspects of mental illness stigma, related mental health legislation and policies in LMICs, and provide an overview of antistigma interventions conducted in these settings. We will also talk about stigma in relation to integrating mental health treatment within the primary healthcare sector and provide proposals for stigma reduction strategies in LMICs.

Stigma has been defined as an 'attribute that is deeply discrediting' [8] that describes the situation of an individual as being 'disqualified from full social acceptance' [8]. Thornicroft and colleagues [773] defined stigma in terms of three core components: problems related to knowledge (ignorance or misinformation), attitudes (prejudice) and behaviour (discrimination) (Ch. 3). Stigma is not only confined to the persons with mental illness but also results in affiliate stigma (also called courtesy stigma or stigma by association against family members, professional caregivers and even mental healthcare facilities [774–776]) (Sects. 5.6, 6.2).

As a construct, stigma within any culture is multifaceted, including the cognitive, affective and behavioural responses of perceivers, self-stigma and stigma by association along with processes maintained by structural and ideological systems [777]. Considering all these levels at which stigma may impact the mental healthcare status of a country, the development of antistigma interventions in LMICs seems to be an important step towards bridging the treatment gap [732]. However, efforts towards this goal have not been as fruitful compared to those seen in high-income countries. It may be that a lack of consistent evidence, cultural differences and high costs of interventions makes it challenging for similar programmes to be extrapolated from the latter to the former [778]. Semrau and colleagues [779] also state that effectiveness and coverage of interventions are determined by the factors associated with existing healthcare systems, and difficulty in knowledge exchange and application of the research findings is a barrier in implementing mental health literacy programmes in LMICs.

A systematic review of antistigma interventions was conducted by Mehta and colleagues [780] and Thornicroft and colleagues [781], and it was reported that of the 11 studies that were conducted in LMICs, 8 had a less than 4-week follow-up and only 3 had longer follow-ups. It was also observed that most of the interventions adopted education, entertainment and psychoeducation strategies for stigma-reduction, but none of the studies assessed any behavioural outcomes. It was reported that interventions in India, Turkey and China resulted in slight improvements in attitude, whereas knowledge in various target groups remained the same after postintervention assessment. In a similar vein, Heim and colleagues [782] found that most anti-stigma programmes in LMICs use theoretical information and lecture-based methods to achieve a range of goals, but the effects of these particular methods have been mixed. It was also noted that the studies had a range of values for associated risk of bias and no study was reported on adequate cultural adaptation of measures and scales employed.

These findings reflect on the need to better understand the nature of existing stigma in LMICs, such that effective interventions can be developed to reduce the same while keeping the specific contexts in mind.

13.1 Cultural Aspects and Explanatory Models of Mental Illness Across LMICs

This problem started since many years ago at first we went to [small town] and visited an astrologer. After that we went to [another small town]. There they told us somebody had given her something to eat, that is why her mind has got damaged, we paid him a thousand rupees. In another temple we have paid 1000 rupees and 500 rupees for a hen's sacrifice, total 1500 we have spent but there was no improvement. Then, the priest told us that what we had spent for that hen was small and not sufficient. Again, we have given 1000 rupees for hen, even then there was no improvement. Totally we have spent around three and half lakh (Indian Rupees) for hospitals and temples. There was no improvement with all this. Only now, she has improved with this medication.

(A MOTHER OF A SERVICE USER WITH OBSESSIVE-COMPULSIVE DISORDER IN INDIA)

Cultural, social, moral and religious teachings often influence beliefs about the origins and nature of mental illness and can shape attitudes towards the mentally ill, thus directly affecting clinical realities and experiences [783]. These present an idea of what 'normal' should look like, and anything perceived as different is strange and likely to be disqualified from full social acceptance [8]. Thus the specific sociocultural beliefs held by and within a culture, along with certain structural inequalities in power, add to the social exclusion and stigmatisation of certain populations at individual, interpersonal and societal levels [784]. As the body of beliefs and values varies across cultures, these differences can accordingly model stigma related to mental illness, which in turn would affect the specific and sometimes uniquely attached feelings, attitudes and behaviours. These are often targeted in antistigma interventions, and hence the understanding of individual and cultural beliefs about mental illness is essential for the valid measurement of stigma and implementation of these approaches to existing mental healthcare systems in LMICs. Generally, the implementation of such interventions might be more fruitful if they are based on traditionally available and culturally congruent healing treatments and approaches accompanied by reintegration of persons living with mental illness into the community [785].

Prior research on effective interventions for stigma reduction in LMICs has established conflicting outcomes across communities, which suggests inadequate cultural adaptation and lack of availability of culturally validated scales and methodologies used to measure variables related to the stigma construct. Several factors have been identified as having an adverse social impact of the illness on the person diagnosed and their caregivers, such as concerns about marriage (ability to get married, problems caused by the illness in the existing marriage), autonomy, social devaluation, fear of avoidance/rejection by others, uneasiness about disclosure, feelings of shame and embarrassment about their or their relative's condition [786–789].

Other studies have also observed how specific cultural and sociodemographic variables, such as place of residence and gender, can produce differences in participant responses. As an example from India, two separate studies conducted by Loganathan and Murthy [790, 791] found that individuals with schizophrenia, living in urban areas and men in general felt the need to hide their illness and avoided illness histories in job applications, and those in rural areas experienced more ridiculing, shame and discrimination. Women with schizophrenia were particularly likely to experience problems related to their marriage or household, and their families experienced distress and uncertainty about their long-term security and future due to the added stigmatisation of divorce and separation [791, 792]. It was further reported that women diagnosed with depression experienced higher degrees of stigma, which was also linked with domestic and structural violence [793]. These manifestations of stigma could represent culturally specific impacts of stigma, where the specific nature of the negative consequences of stigma associated with mental illness varies between settings, depending on values and 'what matters most' (e.g. marital prospects) in a given context [794].

Among other beliefs, culture exerts its most fundamental influence through the categories we employ to define a concern as a problem, how the problem is then understood and which solutions to the problems are acceptable to the culture [795]. For instance, nonmedical and external causal beliefs (such as karma [Sanskrit for 'act', see 'Glossary'] and evil spirits) may be found as the basis of a person's own explanatory model of their condition and could thus influence help-seeking behaviours and pathways [788]. These beliefs would then likely have discrepancies with a mental health professional's explanatory model, especially if their expertise is derived from a disease-centric understanding of the patient's condition. After receiving even such evidence-based care, the patient might not comply with the expert's instructions, creating a barrier to seeking the appropriate healthcare services [783].

Now, for a better understanding of how stigma can vary across cultures, we shall outline examples in LMICs across the world.

13.2 Southeast and East Asia: India, Nepal, Pakistan, Bangladesh, China, Thailand

Although this continental area covers diverse and differing cultures, the values and beliefs held by these countries are often found to be along common lines [796]. For instance, the prevalent values of conformity to norms, emotional self-control, collectivism, family recognition through achievement and filial piety may contribute to the stigma related to mental illness in this region. The perspective of viewing mind and body as one entity might reflect on the way people experience, explain and seek help for psychological distress and symptoms (which are often attributed to the body rather than the mind) and hence, on our understanding of stigma within these contexts [797].

In *India*, cultural beliefs around 'karma', 'dosha' (Sanskrit for 'that which is at fault', see 'Glossary'), 'supernatural powers', punishment by God, alignment of astrological stars through time, disturbed relational factors, psychosocial factors (like stress and trauma) and environment sanitation (infection and contamination) as major causes for mental illness are prevalent [798–800]. Existing evidence supports that cultural systems can shape the experience of mental illnesses such as depression, where the patient might express somatic complaints for culturally salient symbols, like the belief in karma and associated difficulty in perceiving symptoms as health-related concerns [801]. In other instances, like a particular healing temple in south India [802], explanatory models were in alignment with these cultural systems, and the resulting treatment of mental illness was found to be nonstigmatizing and contextually appropriate to the individual's personality [784, 803]. As a culturally valued space, this temple provides a potentially supportive environment for treatment wherein short stays were effective in managing illness in the absence of other treatments.

In *Nepal*, mental health concerns are associated with the term 'kalanka', a blemish or a spot, that can lead to harmful misrepresentation or slandering of individuals [804]. Gender roles are considered an important component of culture-bound rules, norms, behaviours and practices, and these may influence the experience and explanatory models of those associated with mental health concerns in specific ways. For instance, psychological distress observed with Nepali mothers is often attributed to family- and gender-related factors, and the patient's responses to this distress is likely to be based on a fatalistic worldview [805–807].

In *Pakistan*, individuals are likely to misattribute symptoms of various mental illnesses due to conventional and religious beliefs around entities such as 'jinn' and 'jaadu-tona'. Support was then likely sought from traditional healing practices rather than getting professional help, particularly during their initial presentation [808]. A number of sociodemographic variables also tend to influence perceptions of mental health and illness in this community; for instance, beliefs in the jinn are more common in individuals within the lower socio-economic strata [809].

In *Bangladesh*, stigma around mental illness is widespread with supernatural causes commonly being placed within the explanatory models of many individuals. Inadequately disseminated information about available pathways for seeking help and aforementioned stigmatisation has been seen to lead to delay or lack of appropriate care [810]. High levels of social stigma and associated feelings of denial may also give rise to similar consequences of social isolation, rejection and discrimination [811, 812].

In *China*, traditional beliefs (such as those associated with Confucianism) hinder the understanding of mental illness by depicting it as punishment for sins in past lives [813]. Mental illness stigma directly affects the supportive ties that link a person to the community ('quanxi wang'), and a moral 'defect' is further assigned to patients and their families as a threat to the existing way of life [814, 815]. In another study, early discharge (i.e. before completion of treatment) was noticed among men because of the cultural emphasis on reporting back to work as early as possible [816].

In *Thailand*, the cultural belief system often includes animist and supernatural concepts, which state that ghost, God and spirit possession can cause mental illness for an individual's past deeds and bad actions, which leads to stigma. Aside from these Buddhist concepts, the animist concept of 'kwan', or life force, is also prevalent and is said to leave the body when a person has a mental illness. Social stigma seems to be a major concern within this culture, to the extent that medical students might steer clear of choosing to specialise in psychiatry because of the stigma involved [785, 817].

13.3 The Middle East and North Africa: Saudi Arabia, Jordan, Iran, Lebanon, Libya, Tunisia

The culture within this region tends to value concealing emotions and keeping one's family honour intact at all times, which might present barriers to seeking professional mental healthcare and add to the stigmatisation of those individuals who seek help, along with bringing shame upon their family [797]. People living with mental illness may also be perceived as dangerous, pessimistic or immature [818]. Because there is a deeply ingrained sense of patriarchy within this culture, men with mental illnesses may be branded as weak or incapable of carrying out their social roles and responsibilities, whereas women may be shamed into not reporting their concerns, which often present somatically before being recognised as mental health concerns [797, 819].

In *Saudi Arabia*, religious beliefs seem to emphasise shaming of specific conditions such as substance abuse, as consumption in general counts as socially inappropriate behaviour, thus making way for stigma around related disorders [820]. Poor knowledge and understanding about psychiatric problems has also led to the belief that supernatural causes such as 'jinn' (demons), 'seher' (magic), 'hasad' (evil eye), sorcery, God's punishment, weak faith, weakness of character, and social and financial stress cause psychiatric conditions. Visiting 'sheiks' for the Holy Quran, usage of blessed water, offering prayers and seeking help from faith healers/traditional therapists where they get the head bandaged, with the bony prominences as anchors, were considered the predominant treatment methods for mental illness (sheikh/sheik is Arabic for 'elder': in Islam, this is an honorific title given to the leader of a tribe, a spiritual master or a religious scholar [821–823]). Acceptance of God's will in the form of 'destiny' and belief in the healing power of traditional methods forms another part of the predominant, often stigmatizing attitude towards treatment of mental illness [822–830]. It should also be noted that most of the available literature on mental health–related stigma is based on samples that might not be adequately representative of the society [831].

In *Jordan*, culture is communalistic to which changes come slowly—this emphasises a family- and community-based approach in resolving mental health concerns. This also indicates that stigma around mental illnesses hinders recovery and quality of life of the family members along with the patient [832, 833]. Sociocultural factors were found to play an important role in the way healthcare professionals, patients and their families view mental illness and related conditions [834, 835].

In *Iran*, a qualitative study conducted by Taghva and colleagues [836] found that a culture of 'perfectionism' might contribute to stigma around mental illness and may also act as a barrier to self-disclosure and seeking help. Mental health concerns are also associated with themes such as negative judgement, shame and social isolation [836, 837], which translate into low social sup- port, high social stigma and low quality of life for caregivers of persons living with mental illness [838].

In *Lebanon*, most individuals living with mental illness are first examined by a religious or spiritual healer, whose task is to free the patient from the believed causes such as the evil eye, jinn (the devil), sehr (black magic) or punishment from God for a committed sin [839, 840]. Indi- viduals who adhere to these beliefs and explanatory models are likely to receive emotional support from family and friends and tend to experience less public stigma when compared with their counterparts. In a study of beliefs regarding mental health held by religious leaders in the country, most participants had a well-informed and even educated view about mental illness, but a stig- matising and discriminatory attitude was also noted [841].

In *Libya*, high levels of social stigma are reported around mental illness, where psychiat- ric facilities might be perceived as 'frightening' places meant to serve 'crazy' individuals. Formal mental healthcare services are often only sought as a last resort, when traditional approaches (healers and 'sheiks') have been unhelpful and the concerns are urgent, acute or severe [842].

In *Tunisia*, individuals are likely to experience stigma for seeking help for mental health con- cerns in both institutional and noninstitutional settings (often employing nonspecialists and/or traditional healing methods). Stigmatization may also result in attribution of mental health con- cerns to moral faults or weaknesses by mental healthcare professionals [843].

13.4 Sub-Saharan Africa: Uganda, Ghana, South Africa, Ethiopia

Cultures within this region tend to share beliefs of communalism, social role flexibility and spiritualism, which attach a positive value to the connectedness of individuals within the group; each person contributes to the culture through their assigned role. The general understanding and explanations of mental illness are often based on stereotypes and supernatural occurrences (e.g. spirit possession, punishment from God due to one's sins, the evil eye, bewitchment, ancestral curses). Traditional healers commonly provide primary mental healthcare services in this region, particularly in low-income and/or rural settings. It might thus be advantageous to take steps for the integration of their services with formal approaches such that the community benefits from a more holistic healthcare system and reduced stigma levels [785, 844].

In *Uganda,* specific mental illnesses may not be accepted culturally (e.g. depression is rather expressed as 'alluhire', an idiom for distress) or may not be recognised as an illness in the first place (as is the case with dissociative disorders) [845–847].

In *Ghana,* the community is likely to view mental illness as dangerous and unpredictable so that persons living with such conditions are often disliked and shunned and may experience violence and harassment [848, 849]. The acceptable route to seek help involves visiting traditional and faith healers who might hold inaccurate and even harmful beliefs around mental health. For instance, 'aggressive' and 'disruptive' behaviours are often considered as direct evidence of a mental illness and lead to inhumane treatment like chaining of the individual. It is also likely that persons with mental illness would be thought to have intellectual deficits [848, 850, 851].

In *South Africa,* Sorsdahl and Klein [852] reported that certain illnesses (e.g. schizophrenia and substance abuse disorders) are more likely to be stigmatised than other conditions (e.g. posttraumatic stress disorder [PTSD]). This may be indicative of what the community perceives as mental illnesses, given that schizophrenia and PTSD were considered as the most and least representative of a psychiatric disorder within this sample.

In *Ethiopia,* it was found that individuals are inclined to hold the belief it is possible for a person to be fully cured from mental illness in some manner. This further correlated with higher stigma levels against individuals living with mental illness, possibly due to the respondents' expectation that these conditions necessarily have fast cures, thus disregarding their sometimes chronic nature. A link was found between occurrence of mental health problems and poverty, stress, and rumination; also, it was reported that the place of residence might be a strong predictor for stigma in the respective community, with higher levels being reported from rural areas in comparison to urban areas [853].

13.5 Societal/Structural Aspects of Mental Illness Stigma in LMICs

The stigma construct has expanded to include structural stigma, that is, 'societal-level conditions, cultural norms and institutional policies that constrain the opportunities, resources and well-being of the stigmatized' [854] (Sects. 3.1.5, 5.1.8; Ch. 7). Essentially, structural stigma can be viewed as an indicator of poor mental health outcomes [854]. Inadequate legislation and policies related to mental health concerns, and lack of political will to make appropriate changes, contribute largely to the existing stigma (Sect. 7.5). The legal framework would also impact the implementation, organisation and planning of mental healthcare systems and provide for limited financial and resource allocation by the government [766, 768, 855] (Sect. 7.3.3). The behavioural consequences of this type of stigma (structural discrimination) hinder adequate access and equitable provision of mental healthcare services across LMICs [766].

13.6 Mental Health Legislation and Policies in LMICs

Saxena and colleagues [753] observed that discrimination against people with mental disorders is not just widespread but also often codified in law (Sect. 7.5). Persons with mental illness may often be denied the right to vote, from entering into contracts and in some countries, even from entering into a marriage [677, 856]. In 2014, the UN Committee on the Rights of Persons with Disabilities expressed a general comment stating that 'perceived or actual deficits in mental capacity must not be used as justification for denying legal capacity'; words such as 'mad man', 'demented' and 'deranged' included in legislature are considered to increase the stigma towards mental illness, as they may not be well defined [856]. In some countries, existing legislature was reformed in accordance with these comments. For instance, the Mental Healthcare Act 2017 in India now includes a more exact definition of mental illness and related terms, along with specifying that a person may only be classified as living with such an illness with respect to their treatment and not within any societal or cultural terms that may be stigmatizing ([857], pp. 4 f.). However, lack of mental healthcare, social structures, and poor academic and economic empowerment policies for particular populations, such as women living with mental illness, may attribute to their social exclusion, which could be a violation of various human rights [677, 856, 858]. It is further reported that 41 (22%) of countries, including 26 (45%) of low-income countries, particularly exclude mentally ill people from benefits of the general healthcare systems [753]. The resulting gaps and inadequacies need to be dealt with in the strengthening and development of appropriate mental health legislation, policy plans and systems specific to the needs of a country. The primary functions of the mental health legislation include provision of legal protection of fundamental human rights and wellbeing of affected and stigmatised individuals while reinforcing the framework and timeline stipulated in related mental health policies [859, 860].

Poor governance, often due to inadequate funding of integrated mental healthcare systems, may be the biggest challenge in strengthening policy, legislation and healthcare systems in LMICs [860]. For a needs-based, comprehensive assessment of mental health systems in LMICs, the World Health Organization (WHO) has developed the WHO Assessment Instrument for Mental Health Systems (WHO-AIMS) [753]. It recommends deinstitutionalisation of mental healthcare, integration of mental health into general healthcare systems and the development of community mental health services as the most important steps in the process of drafting improved legal frameworks and plans. Others have suggested participation of a range of stakeholder groups to initiate evidence-based efforts [860, 861].

In Southeast Asia, several countries do not have distinct national level policies or legislations for mental health. The existing legislation may be decades old and hence not in keeping with current needs; there are also reports of only partial implementation of these legislations [862]. Within the Middle East and North African regions, 6 out of 20 countries do not have a mental health legislation and 2 do not have a mental health policy. There is no information for Mauritania and Comoros [863]. In Africa, 46% of countries either do not have separate policies for mental health or have not yet implemented them [864]. A total of 58 LMICs across the world have completed the WHO-AIMS assessment, including Nigeria, South Africa, Jordan, Sudan, Bangladesh and China; the results of these could be used to build on the aforementioned structural and legislative inequalities. For instance, Bruckner and colleagues [865] used data from these assessments to report on the mental health workforce gap, with the aim of helping policy makers scale up existing human resources to meet their country's specific needs.

13.7 Antistigma Interventions in LMICs

LMICs have carried out a number of antistigma programmes using different methodologies, as seen with the Time to Change campaign (Sect. 12.1) in India, which relied on the theory of social contact and media campaigns to raise mental health awareness; The Real Test (an antistigma campaign) and *Khoutweh Khoutweh* (an e-mental health initiative) in Lebanon; and the #TalkAboutIt campaign, which encouraged persons with mental illness to freely talk about their conditions in Pakistan.

These programmes often rely on social contact to raise public awareness by the way of media campaigns, peer programmes, and so forth. In these programmes, persons recovered from mental illness share their experiences with the community and hence clear misconceptions about mental health. However, such disclosure of one's experience with mental disorders (which is central to strategies other than social contact as well) presents certain risks, like the possibility of being labelled and experiencing discrimination by the community [866] (Sect. 5.1.4). Furthermore, although there is general evidence that social contact can play a major role in the reduction of prejudice, stigma and discrimination, there is no strong evidence about the efficacy of such anti-stigma interventions, especially across longer-term contexts in LMICs [678, 702, 776, 781, 867].

In comparison to high-income countries, the development of stigma-reduction strategies at both regional and national levels has been inadequate in LMICs [778]. This could be because the latter often face scarcity of financial resources for large-scale antistigma campaigns, in which case utilizing local facilitators and adding cultural perspectives in said interventions might be helpful [815, 868].

The studies that have been carried out in various LMICs targeted different groups of people, including persons with lived experience of mental illness, their family members, service providers, healthcare students/trainees, researchers, policymakers and organisations, students and teachers/youth leaders, and the general community (see Table 13.1 for further details). Short-term, one-off or cross-sectional intervention studies have been associated with positive outcomes and changes in knowledge and attitude [781], but it was noted in some studies that the positive effect of these interventions was not retained in posttest evaluations [869–871]. One notable exception is a study by Maulik and colleagues [872], which utilised a longitudinal approach for the assessment of an antistigma campaign conducted for two general rural communities in Andhra Pradesh, India. The design included a three-month antistigma intervention accompanied with provision of primary healthcare based services for 12 months and follow-ups at three points across a two-year span. The study found positive intervention effects, but it lacked a control group. For mental health literacy interventions in LMICs, audience segmentation strategies are recommended for desegregating a heterogenous population to homogenous target groups. The interventions are more effective when targeted on specific audiences; segmentation strategies are also cost-effective and useful when based on sociocultural variables [873].

Some examples of antistigma interventions conducted in LMICs (with the respective methods, outcome measures and results) are provided in Table 13.2.

TABLE 13.1 ■ Target Groups of Antistigma Interventions in Low- and Middle-Income Settings

Stakeholder Group	Examples
Persons with lived experience and their family members	Individuals with schizophrenia [869, 874] Family members/caregivers [875–878]
Service providers	Lay health workers [879] Care assistant workers [880] Community health workers [881, 882] Primary healthcare workers [883] Primary care nurses [884] Psychiatry residents/specialists [885]
Healthcare students/trainees	Medical students [886–889] Nursing students [890] Preclinical medical students [871]
Researchers, policymakers and organisations	Policymakers [891] Public sector managers [891] Nongovernmental organisations [891] Professional organizations [892]
Students and teachers/youth leaders	High school students [893] Secondary school students [894] College students [870] Primary and secondary school teachers [895] Youth club leaders [895]
General community	Community members [896–898]

TABLE 13.2 ■ Examples of Antistigma Interventions in Low- and Middle-Income Countries

Study	Country	Target Group	Intervention	Method and Scales	Results
[890]	Brazil	Nursing students, experimental ($n = 56$) and control group ($n = 144$)	Experimental group received six weeks' clinical training for specialised treatment for alcohol abuse/addiction; control group received six weeks' training in mental health	Quasiexperimental controlled pre/post design Attitude Scale Towards Alcohol, Alcoholism and Alcoholics (EAFAAA). The instrument was developed by Vargas for this study	Participants in the experimental group reported significant improvements in attitudes, perceptions, opinions and feelings towards persons with alcohol addiction
[875]	Chile	Family members/ caregivers of persons diagnosed with schizophrenia ($n = 45$)	Psychoeducational programme that consisted of 18 weekly group sessions for caregivers Sessions covered family members' experience with schizophrenia, psychoeducation, communication skills, self-care of caregivers	Randomised controlled trial (RCT) Family Attitude Scale (FAS) General health questionnaire	Psychoeducation improved attitudes towards persons with schizophrenia in postassessment among experimental group; no effect on health perceptions of family members
[894]	China	Secondary school students ($n = 255$): education ($n = 88$), education-video ($n = 94$), video-education ($n = 73$)	Stigma reduction programmes: (1) education (30 minutes demythologizing lecture); (2) education-video based contact (lecture followed by video on mental health experiences); (3) video-education (video followed by lecture)	Three group pretest/ posttest design, one-month follow-up The Public Stigma Scale The Social Distance Scale used in this study was a modified version of a scale developed for secondary school students	Knowledge test and level of contact report Education-video programme improved attitudes at postintervention and at follow-up; knowledge also improved at follow-up
[869]	China	Individuals with schizophrenia with high self-stigma ($n = 66$)	Self-stigma reduction programme (12 group and 4 individual sessions: psychoeducation, cognitive behavioural therapy, motivational interviewing, social skills training and goal attainment programme) and control condition (newspaper reading group)	RCT with six-month follow-up Chinese Self-Stigma of Mental Illness Scale (CSSMIS)	Intervention reduced self-stigma at postintervention but not at follow-up; positive effects also on self-esteem
[880]	China	Care assistant workers ($n = 293$): intervention group ($n = 139$) and control group ($n = 154$)	Both groups received training in financial assistance policy of care assistant workers and mental health knowledge. Only the intervention group received antistigma psychoeducation (control group received traditional mental health training). Both trainings lasted for three hours.	RCT with pretest/ posttest. Perceived Devaluation and Discrimination Scale (PDD) Mental Illness Clinicians' Attitudes (MICA) Mental Health Knowledge Schedule (MAKS)	Intervention reduced perceived discrimination and improved clinician attitudes

Study	Country	Target Group	Intervention	Method and Scales	Results
[886]	China	Medical students (*n* = 205)	Educational intervention to improve understanding about depression Two-arm controlled trial of two different didactic methods (lecture vs. lecture and self-study) Both groups received four classes for total of 1.5 hours	Self-report questionnaire International Depression Literacy Survey (IDLS) Mental Illness Clinicians' Attitudes (MICA)	Lecture + self-study was superior to lecture only with respect to depression knowledge. Only lecture + self-study improved attitudes at follow-up
[896]	Egypt	Community members (*n* = 2274)	National antistigma campaign on mental illness with media/ television (two TV education clips lasting two minutes each on daily basis)	Recall and offer opinion about programme, negative attitudes and behaviour towards person with mental illness In-depth interviews	Improved attitudes among people exposed to the TV campaign
[897]	India	Community members (42 villages; *n* = 1576 at preassessment and *n* = 2100 at postassessment)	Intervention based on education and recovery messages, including personal contact and video-contact tailored to the target population with culturally sensitive resources, such as Indian drama theatre group	Mixed method approach with pretest/posttest design Barriers to Access to Care Evaluation (BACE) Mental Health Knowledge, Attitude and Behaviour Focus group discussion and in-depth interviews	Improvements of attitudes, behaviour and treatment-related stigma, no effect on knowledge Qualitative interviews showed social contact and drama as most effective strategies
[872]	India	Community members (two villages, *n* = 1417)	Intervention based on printed information, education and communication (IEC) materials: brochures, pamphlets and posters. Two videos were made: one of an individual sharing their experience with mental illness and the other for mental health promotion. A local theatre group performed drama on mental illness and seeking help.	Mixed method approach with pretest/posttest design, with a follow-up at 24 months Barriers to Access to Care Evaluation (BACE) Mental Health Knowledge, Attitude and Behaviour (KAB)—16-item questionnaire	Improvements observed in knowledge, attitude and behaviour towards mental health, which were sustained till the scheduled follow-up Reduced perception of stigma towards seeking help
[870]	India	College students (*n* = 50)	One-time education and contact-based two-hour intervention (dance and drama on myths about mental illness plus PowerPoint presentation and direct contact with person recovered from mental illness)	Pretest/posttest design with single group and follow-up after one week Open-ended questions on perceptions of people with mental illness Community Attitudes Towards Mental Illness Scale (CAMI)	Positive effects on feelings and ideas about community mental health, reduced authoritarianism Increased positive description of mental illness, decreased discrimination and labelling

Continued

TABLE 13.2 ■ Examples of Antistigma Interventions in Low- and Middle-Income Countries *(cont'd)*

Study	Country	Target Group	Intervention	Method and Scales	Results
[881]	India	Community health workers (n = 70)	Four days' training to increase mental health literacy (general psycho-education, Mental Health First Aid, practical skills, mental health promotion and providing support)	Pretest/posttest design with follow-up at three months Mental health literacy survey to measure knowledge of mental health (open-ended questions and structured interviews)	Positive effects on understanding about mental illness, illness recognition and knowledge about helpful interventions, and stigmatizing attitudes No effect on beliefs about recovery
[879]	India	Trained lay health workers delivered intervention to persons with schizophrenia and care givers (n = 30)	Community intervention with five components: psychoeducation, rehabilitation, management of treatment adherence, referrals, health promotion	Qualitative interviews to evaluate intervention components	Intervention was acceptable and feasible, but experiences of stigma and discrimination were inadequately addressed
[874]	India	People with schizophrenia and their caregivers (n = 282)	Intervention components: needs assessment, clinical reviews, psychoeducation, adherence management, health promotion, individualised rehabilitation, strategies for dealing with stigma and discrimination, link to self-help groups, and network building	Multicentre parallel group RCT design with 12-month follow-up Stigma-related outcomes for people with schizophrenia: Discrimination and Stigma Scale (DISC); alienation subscale of Internalised Stigma of Mental Illness Scale (ISMI), willingness to disclose illness Stigma-related outcomes for caregivers: knowledge and attitudes about the illness, burden of caring, experiences of stigma and discrimination	People with schizophrenia: no change in stigma between intervention and control group Participants in intervention group were more likely to be unwilling to disclose their illness at 12 months Both groups reported significant reductions in stigma and discrimination from baseline to 12 months Caregivers: no changes in knowledge, burden, reported stigma or willingness to disclose their family members' illness
[883]	India	Primary healthcare workers (n = 150)	One-week mental health training programme facilitated by a manual: lectures, case demonstrations and role play	Pretest/posttest design Attitudinal questionnaire	Positive effect on attitudes of health workers
[876]	India	Case management with four members of one family diagnosed with mental illness; and unknown number of community members	Home visits, individual sessions, collaboration with local government, street play, experience sharing by a person recovered from mental illness, distribution of IEC material and oath taking	Case management Family Burden Schedule (Pai and Kapur) WHO Family Interview Schedule stigma items	Positive effect on burden among family members, significant reduction in stigma perceived by the participating family members, and improved community acceptance and social support

Study	Country	Target Group	Intervention	Method and Scales	Results
[898]	India	Community members (n = 901), caregivers (n = 213), persons with mental illness (n = 223)	Ten psychoeducational group sessions with approximately 100 people in each group, 10 poster exhibitions and street plays Question and answer sessions, distribution of printed materials	Pre- and postexperimental design with random sample Case history forms and semistructured interviews	Improved views about stigma among caregivers and community members Less stigmatizing attitudes among caregivers than community members Attitude change was sustained at three-month follow-up
[877]	Iran	Family caregivers of persons with mental illness (n = 43)	Training programme with in-person communication and small group interaction (information about mental illness, family members role in care, skills to cope with stigma and discrimination); four education sessions of approx. one hour each	Quasiexperimental pre/post study with single group Author has prepared the stigma evaluation questionnaire which was designed for the family caregivers of patients with chronic mental disorders	Reduced prejudice towards ill family member after the intervention
[895]	Malawi	Primary and secondary school teachers and youth club leaders (n = 218)	Three-day curriculum culturally adapted from a Canadian programme (stigma, understanding about mental health and wellness, experiences of mental illness, seeking help)	Pretest/posttest study design Questionnaire designed to measure knowledge and attitudes towards mental health and mental disorders	Positive effects on knowledge and attitudes
[884]	Malaysia	Primary care nurses (n = 206)	Video-based contact intervention (VBCI) for five minutes with psychoeducation and interviews of person with mental illness (experience of mental illness and recovery)	A pre/post, quasiexperimental cross-sectional study Attitude of Nurses to People Presenting with Mental Illness-Questionnaire (ANPMI) Opening Minds Scale for Health Care providers Scale (OMS-HC)	Positive effects on attitudes
[871]	Malaysia	Preclinical medical students (n = 102)	Intervention: (1) educational lecture (90 minutes); (2) face-to-face contact with person recovered from mental illness (45 minutes); (3) video-based contact (40 minutes)	RCT with pre/post assessment and follow-up at one month Scale: Opening Minds Stigma Scale for Health Care Providers (OMS-HC) is a 15-item self-report measure of attitudes and behavioural intentions towards people with mental illness	All three interventions improved attitudes to a similar degree

Continued

TABLE 13.2 ■ Examples of Antistigma Interventions in Low- and Middle-Income Countries *(cont'd)*

Study	Country	Target Group	Intervention	Method and Scales	Results
[887]	Malaysia	Medical students ($n = 122$)	Mandatory eight-week psychiatry training with exposure to person with mental illness	Longitudinal study with pretest/post-test design Attitude to Mental Illness (AMI) Questionnaire has 20 items that examines attitudes towards the causes, treatment and consequences of mental illness and its impact on individuals and society. The AMI was constructed by SP Singh using feedback received from students Attitudes Towards Psychiatry (ATP 30) is a 30-item, Likert-type scale that examines attitudes. The questionnaire was constructed and validated by Burra	Positive effect on attitudes towards people with mental illness and psychiatry only among female, not male students
[882]	Nigeria	Community health workers ($n = 24$)	One-week workshop with theory, discussion and role plays (five modules on concepts of mental health and disorder, skills including communication, assessment, mental status examination [MSE], illness management, common neurological disorders, WHO primary care guidelines for mental health, policy, legislation and integration of mental health in other services)	Pretest/posttest design Participants completed a modified version of the questionnaire originally designed for use in the Kenyan training to assess the knowledge of and attitude to mental health issues before and at the completion of the training.	Positive effects on knowledge and attitudes about mental health problems
[893]	Serbia	High school students ($n = 63$)	Six-week workshop that covered mental health and illness, feeling of stigma and discrimination among persons with mental illness, myths about illness, labelling and stereotypes	Pilot programme: Pretest/posttest design Opinion about Mental Illness Questionnaire (OMI)	Positive effects on social stigma and discrimination and social awareness towards mental illness six months after programme implementation

Study	Country	Target Group	Intervention	Method and Scales	Results
[891]	South Africa	Departments of Health, mental health societies, boards and councils (quant. data requested from n = 31 sources) Policymakers, NGOs, faith-based and public sector managers, organisers, mental health service users (n = 64 qual. interviews)	Survey of antistigma campaigns that used consumer/user involvement, education, public awareness and media, correctional services and social integration programmes	WHO Assessment Instrument for Mental Health Systems Version 2.2 (quant.) and semi-structured interviews (qual.)	Numerous ongoing antistigma campaigns across the country arranged by government and NGOs, targeting different groups (youth, ethnic groups, healthcare professionals, teachers, politicians). School-based antistigma activities are being set up. Service users actively involved in media campaigns, but limited systematic evaluation/peer-reviewed reporting of the effectiveness of these strategies.
[892]	South Africa, Uganda	South Africa: focus groups (n = 15), stakeholders (n = 22). Uganda: focus groups (n = 5), stake holders (n = 12) Self-help groups promoted social inclusion of users	Reorientation of district management, establishment of community collaborative forums, task-shifting, promotion of self-help groups	Qualitative study focuses group discussions and individual qualitative interviews	A common implementation framework increased mental health service accessibility and led to improved attitudes among health professionals
[878]	Thailand	Family members/care givers (n = 91)	One-day psychoeducation: didactic session, group discussion and communication building	Pretest/posttest design knowledge assessment questionnaire was composed of 10 items including definition, etiology, symptoms, and management. The attitude assessment questionnaire had 12 items about attitudes towards people with schizophrenia	Knowledge and attitudes improved
[888]	Turkey	Medical students (n = 135)	Three-week psychiatric training to increase mental health literacy (lectures and clinical work with direct contact), control group with three-week ophthalmology training	Two groups with pretest and posttest design Questionnaire with case vignettes Social distance scale	No intervention effect

Continued

TABLE 13.2 ■ Examples of Antistigma Interventions in Low- and Middle-Income Countries *(cont'd)*

Study	Country	Target Group	Intervention	Method and Scales	Results
[889]	Turkey	First-year medical students (*n* = 60)	Experimental group received education, contact and film about person with schizophrenia; control group without any intervention	Controlled design with pre/posttest and one-month follow-up In this study, a 32-item questionnaire designed for rating the attitudes towards schizophrenia by the Psychiatric, Research and Education Center was used	Positive intervention effects on attitudes with regard to beliefs on etiology of schizophrenia, social distance and care of person with illness at postassessment and follow-up
[885]	Turkey	Psychiatry residents and specialists (*n* = 205)	Online stigma education programme delivered by email; control group did not receive email	Two-group RCT Nine-item questionnaire on stigmatising opinions about mental illness	Positive intervention effect on attitudes towards people with mental illness

The different interventions conducted in LMICs till date have addressed various types of stigma, such as healthcare provider stigma, public stigma, family stigma and consumer stigma/self-stigma. These are discussed in further detail in the following sections.

13.8 Provider Stigma

Stigma and discrimination among healthcare providers is likely to be observed when professionals 'see the illness ahead of the person', which can lead to engagement with the patient in a dismissive or demeaning manner [899] (Sect. 7.3.1). The majority of studies on stigma have focused on provider stigma, and education-based interventions were used to reduce stigma among health and allied professionals [871, 875, 884, 886, 900, 901] (Sect. 7.3.2). The interventions ranged from five minutes to eight weeks of structured conversation and training to the integration of a mental health team into the existing primary healthcare system in a particular country [759, 884, 887].

13.9 Public Stigma

Public stigma relates directly to the community's general reaction towards people with mental illness, which includes negative beliefs about a person or group (e.g. as dangerous or incompetent), negative emotional responses (e.g. anger and fear) and discriminatory behaviour (e.g. avoidance) [902] (Sect. 3.1.5). Interventions have helped reduce public stigma related to mental illness through different means, including lecture/video-based education, media campaigns, collaborative work with local governing bodies, workshops, exhibitions and so on [876, 893, 896, 898] (Ch. 8). Nationwide campaigns and other antistigma activities have been conducted in African countries, but the effectiveness of these programmes has not yet been evaluated [891]. Various creative methods have been conceived to reduce stigma, such as developing and using culturally appropriate street plays in an attempt to increase mental health literacy of a community in India [903]. This study employed formative research to create a needs-based intervention and implicated that details related to this intervention outcome (which are yet to be published) should provide an accurate and relevant picture of the current status and potential improvements with respect to the stigma construct within that community.

13.10 Family Stigma

There is no specific definition for family stigma in the context of LMICs; however, this construct is related to community's negative perceptions, attitudes and behaviours towards a family unit due to the latter's close contact with an individual living with mental illness (Sects. 5.6, 6.2). Resulting responses could be related to culturally pervasive beliefs about mental illness, with labels of being 'unusual', 'dangerous' or otherwise harmful associated with all family members due to potential contamination with these perceivably undesirable and threatening traits [904]. This is reminiscent of the concept of 'courtesy stigma', as defined by Goffman [8]. One study reported that caregivers' attitudes towards mental illness might be less stigmatizing in comparison to those held generally within the community [898]. Interventions for families aimed to support them in coping with public stigma and to reduce prejudice among (healthy) family members towards their ill relatives by adopting methods involving close interaction and psychoeducation sessions through different modalities, which resulted in significant reduction in associated stigma [875, 877, 878].

13.11 Self-Stigma

Self-stigma is the prejudice or stereotype that has been internalised by persons with mental illness (e.g. 'I am dangerous'), which can lead to decreased self-esteem and confidence [902] (Sect. 3.1.5). A cross-cultural meta-analysis found that the more collectivistic a culture is, the stronger the link between perceived public stigma and self-stigma [905]. Interventions focused on reducing self-stigma use techniques such as psychoeducation, cognitive behavioural therapy, motivational interviewing and social skills training (Ch. 9). The effect of these techniques was positive immediately after the intervention, but the effect was not sustained at follow-up [869]. Mittal and colleagues [906] found two major approaches to antistigma interventions developed specifically to combat this type of stigma: either targeting certain stigmatising beliefs directly or leading to empowerment of affected individuals to help them achieve their treatment and life goals (without challenging existing stereotypes about mental illness). There is initial evidence for the efficacy of the former in LMIC settings (in terms of using techniques such as cognitive behavioural therapy and psychoeducation), but interventions for a wider range of mental health conditions need to be implemented and evaluated [907].

13.12 Cross-Country Antistigma Research Efforts in LMICs: The INDIGO Partnership Research Programme

In contrast to the individual studies described above, it is also important to consider how strategies to reduce stigma and discrimination can be implemented across LMICs settings. One such effort is the INDIGO Partnership, an ongoing research programme to develop and test new methods to reduce mental health–related stigma in LMICs [908]. This work is conducted within a broad global antistigma research programme [909] and involves (1) conducting formative cross-cultural research to identify stigmatising language, behaviours, and institutional practices and their underlying mechanisms of action across diverse cultural contexts; (2) establishing a harmonised online evaluation toolkit of culturally adapted research instruments specifically designed for use in stigma-reduction intervention studies; and (3) developing and pilot testing evidence-based, contextually adapted antistigma interventions to target stigma reduction in community, primary care and specialist care settings.

This work is conducted in India, China, Nepal, Ethiopia and Tunisia; these settings represent diverse context in terms of healthcare provision and country-level economic indicators. This variability of the field sites is of importance, as cultural, economic, political and health contexts influence what is stigmatised in a given setting. By developing intervention manuals and adaption strategies that are effective across these contexts, the programme intends to generate findings and materials that can be generalisable to other LMICs settings.

13.13 Integration of Mental Health to Primary Healthcare in LMICs

Globally, individuals with mental illness have reported that service providers in the primary healthcare sector may be a major source of stigma and discrimination due to the impact of negative attitudes related to mental illness commonly held within their community [163, 781, 886, 910] (Sect. 7.3.1). In fact, it is reported that mental health professionals can be stigmatisers, recipients of stigma and agents of destigmatisation all at once [911]. This might result in consequences such as 'diagnostic overshadowing', where health professionals wrongly attribute observable physical symptoms to the patient's mental illness [162], which results in poor diagnosis and treatment along with comparatively lower life expectancy of persons with mental illness [912, 913]. The WHO-conducted mental health Gap Action Programme (mhGAP) intervention gave importance to the integration of mental health services and the primary healthcare sector in an effort to increase scalability of services, especially in LMICs [914]. However, provider's stigma related to mental illness was one of the barriers for the success of implementing mhGAP and other such programmes [915].

Presently, observations related to health inequity, limited progress towards Millennium Development Goals, inadequate human resources and the fragmented and weakened state of healthcare systems in LMICs has resulted in piqued interest in similar efforts aimed at integration [916, 917]. It is hoped that a well-integrated model might help reconcile the long-standing opposition between horizontal and vertical approaches (relating to general healthcare services and specific health conditions, respectively). This approach would still need to be adapted to a particular context. It is important to note here that the tendency to fund selective interventions rather than more comprehensive and systems-wide projects, along with fragmented healthcare governance, are two main barriers for establishing such models in LMICs [917]. Efforts of integration could be facilitated by adapting a 'what matters most' framework, which proposes that antistigma interventions must be informed by local values, moral principles and experiences and integrated with the specific mental health user–provider context of the community [794]. In fact, acknowledging and addressing threats to adaptations of such a framework at local levels helped to achieve attitudinal change and improve behaviour in clinical settings [915]. Overall, regular involvement of service users with healthcare staff helped in strengthening the positive feedback cycle of stigma reduction and thus gaining reassurance in clinical self-efficacy and quality care [915].

Not many interventions with the goal of reducing stigma among healthcare professionals have been conducted globally, and the few existing interventions primarily deal with enhancing mental health education and literacy levels (i.e. they are based on the cognitive 'knowledge' aspect of stigma). These efforts have resulted in relatively short-term behavioural change and medium-term effects at follow-up in about half the studies [781]. Some programmes in LMICs have focused on training primary healthcare workers to identify and treat mental health problems, thus increasing the availability of mental health services at the community level and indirectly resulting in stigma reduction towards mental illness. In Nepal, interventions such as PRogramme for Improving Mental health carE (PRIME) focused on training prescribers for 10 days and nonprescribers for five days to improve communication skills, provision of psychosocial support, psychoeducation and mhGAP training materials, along with appropriate management of cases [918, 919]. Another intervention, the REducing Stigma among HealthcAre ProvidErs (RESHAPE) programme, covered three domains of threats around the framework of 'what matters most' to primary health-care providers to understand barriers to stigma reduction within this population—the survival (related to perceptions of violence related to mental illness), the social (related to the possibility of being shunned by the community because of the provider's association with mental illness) and the professional (related to one's ability to be able to engage and treat a condition well) [915]—due to which changes in perception of mentally ill people as violent were seen as changing; an improved ability to treat mental illness and improved willingness for communication with patients was also reported. Similarly, in India, the District Mental Health Programme (DMHP) was launched under the National Mental Health Programme (NMHP) to focus on ensuring availability of basic mental health services, improving understanding of mental health among primary healthcare (PHC) staff and increasing community participation around mental health. In this programme, understanding about mental illness improved among the targeted population; however, the confidence for treating mental illness still seemed to be lacking. Service users were also unsure about taking help from nonprofessionals at PHCs [920].

DISCUSSION

The components, focus and implementation processes of different antistigma interventions in LMICs vary based on their feasibility and acceptability in the respective social and cultural environments [765]. Other than the barriers to conducting effective antistigma interventions already mentioned, in some instances religious and sociopolitical reasons may act as additional challenges [766, 921]. Insufficient evidence-based information and improper methods of carrying out such campaigns may actually add to existing stigma levels in the community instead of delivering the right content and message.

Most of the antistigma interventions in LMICs have been of relatively short-term duration, although nationwide programmes are currently few and/or ineffective in producing and maintaining structured outcome and behavioural evaluations. These efforts also may not have adequately addressed the self-stigma among people with mental illness [780]. The resulting limited evidence has made it difficult to conclude which interventions would be more appropriate and adaptable across contexts [779]. These observations are indicative of a need for extensive research in this field; specifically, culture-based and context-focused interventions that place importance on gender and family roles and utilise existing resources could be promoted. Policy-level attention for stigma reduction towards people with mental illness is furthermore very essential in LMICs.

Stigma reduction models in these countries are not standardised as of now and often fail to take into account the existing healthcare system. It can be surmised that the inclusion of mental health in the primary healthcare system may aid in promotion of human rights, development of a more holistic approach to stigma reduction and encouragement of help-seeking behaviours [765, 922]. However, training existing primary healthcare staff to provide basic mental health counselling may lead to a heavier workload, as professionals are already managing multiple tasks in the primary healthcare setup. Although a better course of action would be to recruit personnel trained in mental health, this alternative would involve effective planning and funding [923].

Conclusion

The healthcare systems of many LMICs are not yet directed by properly planned policies, legislative and related frameworks that also take into account the construct of stigma, which may present as a barrier affecting the efficacy of said systems across different aspects and levels of the community (i.e. at the interpersonal, intrapersonal, institutional and structural levels).

Research suggests that the construct of stigma is multifaceted and may be derived and maintained by the prevalent and unique cultural beliefs of a country. In contrast to high-income countries, there is a limited evidence base from LMICs regarding the relationship between stigma and culture, which might contribute to the development of culturally appropriate theoretical models of stigma and stigma reduction. Such a model might be particularly helpful in highlighting 'what matters most' for a specific community, as limited or inadequate resource availability is still a major challenge to the development and implementation of antistigma interventions in these countries. The magnitude of this issue can commonly be observed as gaps in financing, governance or workforce, resulting in short-term, relatively unstructured and unsustainable efforts towards stigma reduction.

Most programmes that have been conducted (predominantly in high-income countries) relied on an increase in social contact with stigmatised populations as a basis for stigma reduction (Ch. 8, Sect. 12.1). Although the follow-up testing for some interventions did show associated attitudinal/behavioural changes in favourable directions, longitudinal follow-ups show that these effects might need further maintenance across time. Application of a more continuous evaluation system before, during and after conducting an intervention might provide feedback of context-specific factors affecting penetration of desired effects that help ameliorate, diminish or maintain stigma within the group. The potential scalability of these interventions is also of concern, as hardly any nationwide antistigma interventions have been conducted in LMICs. These settings might benefit from additional support and participation from different national and international stakeholders such that the necessary planning, execution and learning can occur, with the aim of building well-integrated, people-centred healthcare systems.

CHAPTER 14

Looking Back and Ahead

Until now, this book has been a hike through the rugged landscape of mental illness stigma consisting of various peaks and valleys. In some places, productive antistigma work is flourishing (e.g. through peer support), whereas in others, the field remains untilled. I set out at the beginning of this book with two goals (Sect. 1.1): to make stigma recognisable in its various forms and consequences and to show ways of reducing it. I hope that the first goal has been achieved to some extent. How often do I hear from so-called experts and authorities in health services: 'Oh, stigma, that used to be a problem, but today it's no longer an issue!' This remark is itself a barrier to change—where no problem is seen, nothing is done.

As for the second goal, I tried to cut a few paths and cover a multitude of approaches in order not to lose sight of the forest for the trees. Across individual initiatives and their target groups, the question arises as to how fundamental social change can be achieved. In particular, structural discrimination shows that one-off measures will not be enough—stigma resembles, as we have discussed (Sect. 1.1), the ancient sea-god Proteus. Even if we try to stand in his way, he will often achieve his goal of discrimination in some other form.

CONCLUSION

What we need are approaches at different systemic levels, as well as a cultural change. We need a solidarity movement working towards full equality of rights for people with mental illness in all areas of life.

14.1 What Promotes Social Change?

How does social change that improves the situation of disadvantaged groups come about? This is the subject of complex sociological research [924]. A broad cultural movement—such as the LGBTQIA+ rights movement—seems to be necessary for successful, fundamental change. Movements may be more successful if that which is stigmatised is not considered self-inflicted [924]. This will be a serious challenge in the fight against mental illness stigma, especially because biological models that may reduce guilt are not actually helpful as an overall long-term strategy (Sect. 5.1.2). Research on cultural change and societal views of illnesses has found that there are three necessary conditions for a reduction in public and structural stigma, all rooted in the introduction of a new social concept (in our case, of mental illness) [925]:

1. The new concept must be credible and credibly represented by experts.
2. The concept should be compatible with and based on existing opinions and ideologies.
3. Destigmatisation is more likely to occur when members of the general public come to the conclusion that their own fate is linked to that of the stigmatised group.

How might we understand these three factors in the case of mental illness destigmatisation? First, a credible conceptual model of mental illness would underline the importance of its social aspects (Sect. 2.3). The one-sided biological model that currently dominates discourse is unhelpful for antistigma initiatives. Experts of all kinds can help to reduce stigma by integrating social understandings of mental illness (and its consequences) more strongly into science and therapy via a biopsychosocial model. In regard to the second factor, consider how antistigma work can be based on the United Nations Convention on the Rights of Persons with Disabilities (UN-CRPD) (Sect. 7.5.2). The UN-CRPD is internationally known and valid law. It protects people with mental illness from discrimination and can therefore be a powerful reference point for stigma reduction. Finally, mental disorders are so common that almost every family is affected—and individuals themselves can be affected overnight (Sect. 2.2.1). This alone should make it clear that we are all in the same boat, as it were, and must promote solidarity (end of Sect. 7.5.1). From these suggestions, it is clear that enacting the aforementioned conditions to reduce mental illness stigma is plausible and could help create a cultural shift.

CONCLUSION

It is not enough to simply reduce stigma. Positive attitudes centred on empowerment and recovery must be built up to actively support people with mental illness. If our society and all those who form it could inherently value recovery, people with mental illness would be able to better take control of their lives (and, if they wish, engage in antistigma work). They are the agents of change.

None of this will happen without conflict: in order for peers to gain influence and self-determination, other groups must relinquish some of their power. Problems can arise when peers get ready to, for example, work in the psychiatric ward: 'What are *they* doing here? That's *our* job!' The same applies to the management of antistigma programmes (Sect. 12.4).

14.2 Science Fiction?

Some might say that it is difficult to give a prognosis as far as the future is concerned. But let us dare to predict that the stigma of mental illness will stay with us in many different forms for quite some time. Some themes are emerging: Machine learning algorithms will help to measure and understand stigma [926]. Biogenetic research in psychiatry will continue to advance—with or without consideration of social factors. And in regards to biomarkers of mental illness, unanswered questions about labelling (through biomarking), as well as legal protection against discrimination, will arise [927].

The issues surrounding mental illness and its media echo chamber (an important contributor to stigma) will increasingly be negotiated online in real time, and in particular on social media (on Twitter and Avicii, see Sect. 7.4.5). This opens up new spaces for spreading prejudice and for antistigma work. Billions of people enjoy playing online games (Sect. 7.4.2)—use of this medium may also contribute to stigma reduction in the form of 'serious games' and challenges, particularly through simulated contact and confrontation with famous quotations, like this one from Spanish artist Salvador Dali: 'There is only one difference between a madman and me. The madman thinks he's sane. I know I'm mad' ([928], p. 206). Finally, our understanding of the impact of social networks on health (online and offline), as well as social network interventions, will increase [929].

14.3 What Can Be Done

The stigma of mental illness concerns us all. It is not only the problem of those who have a mental illness. It is social injustice. People with mental illness have a right to live without stigma and its consequences. To make progress, we need coalitions (which are not made any easier with ideological squabbling over who may speak for whom). All kinds of ruptures within and between various groups stand in our way. For example, for some service users, psychiatry is (only) part of the problem, and for others it is (also) part of the solution. Professionals don't make it any easier: some consider recovery and empowerment to be newfangled and flowery words, whereas for others, these words are inspiring—to say nothing of the disputes between professionals at care sector boundaries and between schools of therapy.

Every attitude carries with it an argument. However, instead of getting stuck and feeling paralysed, common goals could be sought. Disputes over words and ideological dogmatism change nothing (Sect. 1.2). So while some colleagues think very differently from me, their opinions do not need to stop me from taking an initiative. The German poet Friedrich Hölderlin (1770–1843), who was considered insane in the last four decades of his life and lived with a carpenter's family in Tübingen, wrote in 1812: 'The lines of life are different, like travelling paths and mountain borders.' In this sense, a relaxed and pragmatic approach to dealing with differences of opinion would be helpful. If we cannot agree on some common goals and speak for them as one (i.e. in our dealings with politicians), we will at best achieve a shake of the head.

As far as the options for antistigma work are concerned, it is necessary to examine which approach leads to real change with regard to various legitimate objectives (Sect. 1.3). There is no *single* remedy, or *one* intervention for every type of stigma, in every target group, in every situation. Therefore, interventions must always be adapted to suit local conditions, and their effectiveness and side effects must be evaluated. This is only possible in dialogue with the target group and with the peers who drive the programme (e.g. in contact interventions). Finding a balance between confidence and enthusiasm for antistigma work on one hand and scepticism on the other is undoubtedly challenging. The task to substantially reduce stigma is huge. But without confidence, we will not succeed, and there is reason for optimism. Just as important is healthy scepticism: not every antistigma intervention helps, and some even cause harm. But data show what works and what does not. Even stronger research will be needed to test the feasibility and effectiveness of future adapted interventions in local contexts.

The question remains as to what kind of society we want to live in and what we consider to be fair. With recourse to Rawls (Sect. 7.5.1), social justice is what enables people with disabilities to live their best possible lives. For this to occur, we should not only tolerate our differences and the otherness of others, but also welcome them as part of the diversity of human life. This is best taught by people who have learned to live with being different. A member of the editorial staff of *Ohrenkuss*, a magazine for and by people with Down's syndrome, once wrote unwittingly about diversity: 'Everybody has an opinion from everybody else.' She probably meant to include the word 'different'. But does that really matter? Our thoughts and experiences are inextricably tied to one another; embracing that is what this work is truly about.

antistigma strategies: Three main strategies for reducing public stigma are protest, education and contact (see *contact, education* and *protest* and Sects. 8.1, 8.3, 8.4).

BZgA: Federal Centre for Health Education in Bonn, Germany (https://bzga.de/home/bzga/), with the goals of health education and health promotion, including risk prevention.

contact: Strategy to reduce public stigma by bringing members of the general public (e.g. employers) into contact with peers. This means that people with lived experience of mental illness (peers) interact with the target group (e.g. employers) in a cooperative atmosphere (e.g. in a workshop or joint project). For more information, see *peers*.

DALY: The disability-adjusted life year is a measure for the healthy life years lost through illness and disability. The DALYs cover the years lost through an early death and the years spent living with disability or illness-related impairment. The DALYs therefore allow comparisons of the burden of disease across different types of disease and disability.

DGPPN: Deutsche Gesellschaft für Psychiatrie, Psychotherapie, Psychosomatik und Nervenheilkunde (German Association for Psychiatry, Psychotherapy and Psychosomatics).

discrimination: Behaviour as a result of prejudice ('As an employer I will not hire people with mental illness'); see *structural discrimination*.

dosha: Sanskrit for 'that which is at fault'; types of bodily humours in Ayurvedic medicine (three in total); the relative proportions of these 'tri-dosha' or three doshas is thought of as cause for different illnesses or 'imbalances' in one's body.

education: Reduction of public stigma by replacing false stereotypes about people with mental illness with facts and realistic narratives (Sect. 8.1).

empowerment: Feeling of personal strength, self-determination and control over one's own life. Thus despite having a mental illness, one can have positive self-esteem and not be significantly restricted by prejudice. Empowerment is an important prerequisite for recovery.

FAZ: *Frankfurter Allgemeine Zeitung* (a leading German daily newspaper).

general public: In this book, this generic term refers to the non-stigmatised, 'healthy' or 'normal' public. It includes, amongst others, people in a position of power who may practice discrimination (e.g. an employer or a landlord). It also includes the public that is targeted by the media or those who participate in population surveys.

HOP: Honest, Open, Proud (formerly known as Coming Out Proud) is a peer-led group programme on the topic of disclosure of one's own mental illness (Sect. 9.2).

ICD: International Classification of Diseases and related health problems of the World Health Organization (WHO). Currently the eleventh version (ICD-11) is in use.

IPS: Individual Placement and Support is the best defined and most effective type of Supported Employment (Sect. 7.1.2, 'Supported Employment'). Using the IPS model, people with mental illness are placed directly into general employment without prior training or rehabilitation (hence 'first place, then train'). Participants are supported by job coaches both in their job search and in their new workplace.

karma: Sanskrit for 'act'; in Indian religion and philosophy, 'karma' is the universal connection between cause and effect of one's actions along with the morality behind them; one's bad karma in the past or present is what could be known to result in mental illness.

LMICs: Low- and middle-income countries. According to the World Bank, countries can be classified into high–, upper-middle–, lower-middle– and low–income countries based on the gross national income per capita.

NECT: Narrative Enhancement and Cognitive Therapy is a group programme to reduce self-stigma (Sect. 9.1.3).

OECD: Organisation for Economic Co-operation and Development. The OECD has 36 member states, including the USA, UK, Australia, Canada, Germany, Austria and Switzerland, and regularly presents detailed reports and data, including on health systems.

peer: A person who is similar, has had similar experiences or belongs to your group. In this book, peers refers to people who have lived experience of mental illness or with psychiatric treatment. They can offer *peer support* (i.e. support for others as peers) (Sect. 7.3.4).

prejudice: Agreement with negative stereotype and emotional reaction ('Yes, people with mental illness are lazy, therefore I find them annoying').

professional: In this book, a professional is someone working in the field of psychiatry or psychotherapy with some form of professional training, including nursing, psychology, medicine, social work, occupational therapy, etc. (for *peers*, i.e. experts by experience and not by training, see above).

protest: Strategy to reduce public stigma (Sect. 8.3). Protest can be communicated, for instance, via email, letters or social media against a company advertisement that may mock people with mental illness, against proposed legislation, etc.

PsychKHG: Psychisch-Kranken-Hilfe-Gesetze of the German federal states (also called Psychisch-Kranken-Gesetz or, in Saarland, Unterbringungsgesetz; the names differ slightly between the states). These laws regulate issues such as the involuntary admission and placement of people with mental disorders in psychiatric hospitals in the event of acute danger to themselves or others (Sect. 7.5.5).

RCT: Randomised controlled trial (Sect. 1.5), in which the efficacy of a therapy or an antistigma intervention is tested. Study participants are randomly allocated either to the intervention group or to a comparison group (without intervention). The change in the intervention participants is then compared to those without intervention. This comparison makes it possible to better assess the effectiveness of interventions than, say, pre–post studies (which do not have a without-intervention comparison group).

recovery: Recovery is not only about a reduction in symptoms; above all, it is about claiming the confidence and positive attitude to be able to lead a good, self-determined life even with a mental illness and possible limitations (Sect. 5.1.6). Recovery describes an individual recovery process.

service user: A person with lived experience of mental illness who has used or uses mental health services.

SGB: Sozialgesetzbuch (i.e. German social law) in 13 books, from SGB I to SGB XIV; for example, SGB V covers health insurance, and SGB IX covers rehabilitation and participation of people with disabilities (Sect. 7.5.3).

stereotype: Views about a social group; the association of this group with particular attributes (qualities) (e.g. 'Germans are punctual' or 'people with mental illnesses are incompetent') (Sect. 3.2.3).

StGB: German Criminal Code (Strafgesetzbuch).

stigma/self-stigma: Stigma is a generic term for stereotypes, prejudices and discrimination (for more on these terms, see above). Stigma in this book refers not only to the stigmatised label ('mentally ill') but also to the negative views caused by it that lead to discrimination (Sect. 3.1.4). People with mental illness are exposed to prejudice and discrimination because the illness is perceived by others as a stain or sign of disgrace (Sect. 5.1.1). Members of the general public (see *general public*, including employers or landlords) can discriminate against people with mental illness, which is known as public stigma. People with mental illness can agree with prejudices and apply them to themselves, which is called self-stigma ('I am mentally ill, therefore I must be lazy and incompetent'; Sect. 5.1.3).

structural discrimination: Discrimination of members of a group through the use of rules and procedures, including in institutions, companies, political processes or the legal system (Sect. 5.1.8). This discrimination can be intentional or unintentional. Related terms are organisational, institutional or systemic stigma (see *discrimination* above).

UN-CRPD: Convention on the Rights of Persons with Disabilities, adopted in 2006 at the United Nations (UN). The UN-CRPD has now been ratified and is applicable in law, including in the EU, UK and Switzerland (Sect. 7.5.2).

WHO: World Health Organization of the United Nations (UN).

[1] Finzen A. Stigma and stigmatization within and beyond psychiatry. In: Gaebel W, Rössler W, Sartorius N, eds. The Stigma of Mental Illness - End of The Story? Cham: Springer; 2017. pp. 29–42.

[2] Corrigan PW. The Stigma Effect: Unintended Consequences of Mental Health Campaigns. New York: Columbia Univ. Press; 2018.

[3] Corrigan PW, Al-Khouja MA. Three agendas for changing the public stigma of mental illness. *Psychiatr. Rehabil. J.* 2018;41:1–7.

[4] Oexle N, et al. Self-stigma and suicidality: A longitudinal study. *Eur. Arch. Psychiatry Clin. Neurosci.* 2017;267:359–361.

[5] Smith GCS, Pell JP. Parachute use to prevent death and major trauma related to gravitational challenge: Systematic review of randomised controlled trials. *BMJ* 2003;327:1459–1461.

[6] Patel V, et al. The Lancet Commission on global mental health and sustainable development. *Lancet* 2018;392:1553–1598.

[7] Perkins A, et al. Experiencing mental health diagnosis: A systematic review of service user, clinician, and carer perspectives across clinical settings. *Lancet Psychiatry* 2018;5:747–764.

[8] Goffman E. Stigma: Notes on the Management of Spoiled Identity. New York: Simon & Schuster; 1963.

[9] Birbeck GL, et al. Advancing health equity through cross-cutting approaches to health-related stigma. *BMC Med.* 2019;17:40.

[10] Bolton D. What Is Mental Disorder? An Essay in Philosophy, Science, and Values. Oxford: Oxford University Press; 2008.

[11] Winterling A. Caligula: A Biography. Berkeley: University of California Press; 2011.

[12] Fuchs T. Ecology of the Brain: The Phenomenology and Biology of the Embodied Mind. Oxford: Oxford University Press; 2018.

[13] Leonhard K, Beckmann H. Classification of Endogenous Psychoses and Their Differentiated Etiology. 2nd ed. Wien: Springer; 1999.

[14] Tikkinen KAO, et al. Public, health professional and legislator perspectives on the concept of psychiatric disease: A population-based survey. *BMJ Open* 2019;9:e024265.

[15] Rüsch N, et al. What is a mental illness? Public views and their effects on attitudes and disclosure. *Aust. N. Z. J. Psychiatry* 2012;46:641–650.

[16] Beck U. The Metamorphosis of the World: How Climate Change Is Transforming Our Concept of the World. Cambridge: Polity Press; 2016.

[17] Swinburn BA, et al. The global syndemic of obesity, undernutrition, and climate change: The Lancet Commission report. *Lancet* 2019;393:791–846.

[18] Evans GW. Projected behavioral impacts of global climate change. *Annu. Rev. Psychol.* 2019;70:449–474.

[19] Palinkas LA, Wong M. Global climate change and mental health. *Curr. Opin. Psychol.* 2020;32:12–16.

[20] Marmot M. The Health Gap: The Challenge of an Unequal World. London: Bloomsbury Press; 2015.

[21] Ribeiro WS, et al. Income inequality and mental illness-related morbidity and resilience: A systematic review and meta-analysis. *Lancet Psychiatry* 2017;4:554–562.

[22] Goschler C. Rudolf Virchow: Mediziner, Anthropologe, Politiker. Köln: Böhlau; 2002.

[23] West ML, et al. Forensic psychiatric experiences, stigma, and self-concept: A mixed-methods study. *J. Forens. Psychiatry Psychol.* 2018;29:574–596.

[24] Fazel S, et al. Mental health of prisoners: Prevalence, adverse outcomes, and interventions. *Lancet Psychiatry* 2016;3:871–881.

[25] Zehnder M, et al. Stigma as a barrier to mental health service use among female sex workers in Switzerland. *Front. Psychiatry* 2019;10:32.

[26] Sweeney A, Beresford P, Faulkner A, Nettle M, Rose D, eds. This Is Survivor Research. Ross-on-Wye: PCCS Books; 2009.

[27] Russo J. In dialogue with conventional narrative research in psychiatry and mental health. *Philos. Psychiatr. Psychol.* 2016;23:215–228.

[28] Scull A. Madness in Civilization: A Cultural History of Insanity, From the Bible to Freud, From the Madhouse to Modern Medicine. London: Thames & Hudson; 2015.

[29] Klibansky R, Panofsky E, Saxl F. Saturn and Melancholy: Studies in the History of Natural Philosophy, Religion, and Art. Montreal: McGill; 2019.

[30] Klee E. "Euthanasie" im Dritten Reich: Die "Vernichtung Lebensunwerten Lebens". 3rd ed. Frankfurt: Fischer; 2018.

[31] Roelcke V. Psychiatry during National Socialism: Historical knowledge and some implications. *Neurol. Psychiatry Brain Res.* 2016;22:34–39.

[32] Armbruster J, Dieterich A, Hahn D, Ratzke K, eds. 40 Jahre Psychiatrie-Enquete: Blick Zurück Nach Vorn. Köln: Psychiatrie-Verlag; 2015.

[33] Goffman E. Asylums: Essays on the Social Situation of Mental Patients and Other Inmates. New York: Anchor Books; 1961.

[34] Söhner F, Becker T, Fangerau H. Psychiatrie-Enquete mit ZeitZeugen Verstehen: Eine Oral History der Psychiatriereform in der BRD. Köln: Psychiatrie-Verlag; 2020.

[35] Engstrom EJ. Clinical Psychiatry in Imperial Germany: A History of Psychiatric Practice. Ithaca: Cornell University Press; 2003.

[36] Szasz TS. The Myth of Mental Illness: Foundations of a Theory of Personal Conduct. New York: Harper; 1974.

[37] Foucault M. Psychiatric Power: Lectures at the Collège de France, 1973-1974. New York: Picador; 2008.

[38] Zedlick D. Psychiatriereform in der DDR. In: Armbruster J, Dieterich A, Hahn D, Ratzke K, eds. 40 Jahre Psychiatrie-Enquete: Blick Zurück Nach Vorn. Köln: Psychiatrie-Verlag; 2015. pp. 102–121.

[39] Weil F. Ärzte als inoffizielle Mitarbeiter des Ministeriums für Staatssicherheit der DDR: Das Beispiel der Psychiater. In: Kumbier E, Steinberg H, eds. Psychiatrie in der DDR: Beiträge zur Geschichte. Berlin: Be.bra wissenschaft verlag; 2018. pp. 127–142.

[40] Finzen A. Gutachten zum Abbau von Vorurteilen gegenüber psychisch Kranken und Behinderten. In: Deutscher Bundestag, ed. Bericht über die Lage der Psychiatrie in der Bundesrepublik Deutschland: Zur psychiatrischen und psychotherapeutisch/psychosomatischen Versorgung der Bevölkerung. Bonn: Heger; 1975. pp. 1130–1139.

[41] Wittchen HU, et al. The size and burden of mental disorders and other disorders of the brain in Europe 2010. *Eur. Neuropsychopharmacol.* 2011;21:655–679.

[42] Thom J, et al. Versorgungsepidemiologie psychischer Störungen: Warum sinken die Prävalenzen trotz vermehrter Versorgungsangebote nicht ab? *Bundesgesundheitsbl* 2019;62:128–139.

[43] Mulder R, et al. Why has increased provision of psychiatric treatment not reduced the prevalence of mental disorder? *Aust. N. Z. J. Psychiatry* 2017;51:1176–1177.

[44] Ehrenberg A. The Weariness of the Self: Diagnosing the History of Depression in the Contemporary Age. Montreal: McGill; 2010.

[45] Baxter AJ, et al. Challenging the myth of an "epidemic" of common mental disorders: Trends in the global prevalence of anxiety and depression between 1990 and 2010. *Depress. Anxiety* 2014;31:506–516.

[46] Goldney RD, et al. Changes in the prevalence of major depression in an Australian community sample between 1998 and 2008. *Aust. N. Z. J. Psychiatry* 2010;44:901–910.

[47] Whiteford HA, et al. Global burden of disease attributable to mental and substance use disorders: Findings from the Global Burden of Disease Study 2010. *Lancet* 2013;382:1575–1586.

[48] Vigo D, et al. Estimating the true global burden of mental illness. *Lancet Psychiatry* 2016;3:171–178.

[49] Knapp M, Wong G. Economics and mental health: The current scenario. *World Psychiatry* 2020;19:3–14.

[50] OECD/EU. Health at a Glance: Europe 2018: State of Health in the EU Cycle. Paris: OECD; 2018.

[51] Trautmann S, et al. The economic costs of mental disorders: Do our societies react appropriately to the burden of mental disorders? *EMBO Rep.* 2016;17:1245–1249.

[52] Chisholm D, et al. Scaling-up treatment of depression and anxiety: A global return on investment analysis. *Lancet Psychiatry* 2016;3:415–424.

[53] McDaid D, et al. The economic case for the prevention of mental illness. *Annu. Rev. Public Health* 2019;40:373–389.

[54] Earnshaw VA, et al. Stigma-based bullying interventions: A systematic review. *Dev. Rev.* 2018;48:178–200.

[55] Evans-Lacko S, et al. Childhood bullying victimization is associated with use of mental health services over five decades: A longitudinal nationally representative cohort study. *Psychol. Med.* 2017;47:127–135.

[56] Aceituno D, et al. Cost-effectiveness of early intervention in psychosis: Systematic review. *Br. J. Psychiatry* 2019;215:388–394.

[57] Knapp M, et al. Recovery and economics. *Psychiatrie* 2015;12:162–166.

[58] WHO, Calouste Gulbenkian Foundation. Social Determinants of Mental Health. Geneva: WHO; 2014.

[59] Case A, Deaton A. Mortality and morbidity in the 21st century. *Brookings Pap. Econ. Act.* 2017;2017: 397–476.

[60] Durkheim É. On Suicide. London: Penguin; 2006.

[61] Braveman P, et al. The social determinants of health: Coming of age. *Annu. Rev. Public Health* 2011; 32:381–398.

[62] Priebe S. A social paradigm in psychiatry - themes and perspectives. *Epidemiol. Psychiatr. Sci.* 2016; 25:521–527.

[63] Dean CE. Social inequality, scientific inequality, and the future of mental illness. *Philos. Ethics Humanit. Med.* 2017;12:10.

[64] Bundeszentrale für Politische Bildung, Statisches Bundesamt, et al. Datenreport 2018: Ein Sozialbericht für die Bundesrepublik Deutschland. Bonn: Bundeszentrale für Politische Bildung; 2018.

[65] Jaspers K. General Psychopathology (published in German 1959). 7th ed. Baltimore: Johns Hopkins University Press; 1997.

[66] Gühne U, Weinmann S, et al. (DGPPN) S3-Leitlinie Psychosoziale Therapien bei Schweren Psychischen Erkrankungen. 2nd ed. Berlin, Heidelberg: Springer; 2019.

[67] Mueser KT, et al. Psychosocial treatments for schizophrenia. *Annu. Rev. Clin. Psychol.* 2013;9:465–497.

[68] Evans K. Treating financial difficulty - the missing link in mental health care? *J. Ment. Health* 2018; 27:487–489.

[69] Ma R, et al. The effectiveness of interventions for reducing subjective and objective social isolation among people with mental health problems: A systematic review. *Soc. Psychiatry Psychiatr. Epidemiol.* 2020;55:839–876.

[70] Pescheny JV, et al. The impact of social prescribing services on service users: A systematic review of the evidence. *Eur. J. Public Health* 2020;30:664–673.

[71] Schöck G, Schöck I. Bürgerhelfer in der Psychiatrie: Mehr als "Grüne Damen" im Krankenhaus! In: Zinkler M, Laupichler K, Osterfeld M, eds. Prävention von Zwangsmaßnahmen: Menschenrechte und therapeutische Kulturen in der Psychiatrie. Köln: Psychiatrie Verlag; 2016. pp. 209–217.

[72] Oesterle S, et al. Long-term effects of the Communities That Care trial on substance use, antisocial behavior, and violence through age 21 years. *Am. J. Public Health* 2018;108:659–665.

[73] Wahlbeck K, et al. Interventions to mitigate the effects of poverty and inequality on mental health. *Soc. Psychiatry Psychiatr. Epidemiol.* 2017;52:505–514.

[74] Sayce L. Stigma, discrimination and social exclusion: What's in a word? *J. Ment. Health* 1998;7:331–343.

[75] Nelson TD. The Psychology of Prejudice. 2nd ed. Boston: Pearson Education; 2006.

[76] Allport GW. The Nature of Prejudice. Oxford: Addison-Wesley; 1954.

[77] Link BG, Phelan JC. Conceptualizing stigma. *Annu. Rev. Sociol.* 2001;27:363–385.

[78] Driskell JE, Mullen B. Status, expectations, and behavior: A meta-analytic review and test of the theory. *Pers. Soc. Psychol. Bull.* 1990;16:541–553.

[79] Corrigan PW, et al. Self-stigma and the "why try" effect: Impact on life goals and evidence-based practices. *World Psychiatry* 2009;8:75–81.

[80] Hatzenbuehler ML. Structural stigma: Research evidence and implications for psychological science. *Am. Psychol.* 2016;71:742–751.

[81] Gawronski B, Creighton LA. Dual process theories. In: Carlston DE, ed. Oxford Handbook of Social Cognition. Oxford: Oxford University Press; 2013. pp. 282–312.

[82] Rüsch N, et al. Implicit self-stigma in people with mental illness. *J. Nerv. Ment. Dis.* 2010;198:150–153.

[83] Hehman E, et al. Disproportionate use of lethal force in policing is associated with regional racial biases of residents. *Soc. Psychol. Personal Sci.* 2018;9:393–401.

[84] Hebl MR, et al. Formal and interpersonal discrimination: A field study of bias toward homosexual applicants. *Pers. Soc. Psychol. Bull.* 2002;28:815–825.

[85] Sue DW, et al. Racial microaggressions in everyday life: Implications for clinical practice. *Am. Psychol.* 2007;62:271–286.

[86] Lilienfeld SO. Microaggressions: Strong claims, inadequate evidence. *Perspect. Psychol. Sci.* 2017;12: 138–169.

[87] Barber S, et al. Microaggressions towards people affected by mental health problems: A scoping review. *Epidemiol. Psychiatr. Sci.* 2020;29:e82.

[88] Jorm AF. Mental health literacy: Empowering the community to take action for better mental health. *Am. Psychol.* 2012;67:231–243.

[89] Waldmann T, et al. Mental health literacy and help-seeking among unemployed people with mental health problems. *J. Ment. Health* 2020;29:270–276.

[90] Thornicroft G. Shunned: Discrimination Against People With Mental Illness. Oxford: Oxford University Press; 2006.

[91] Al-Faham H, et al. Intersectionality: From theory to practice. *Annu. Rev. Law Soc. Sci.* 2019;15:247–265.

[92] Crenshaw K. Demarginalizing the intersection of race and sex: A Black feminist critique of antidiscrimination doctrine, feminist theory, and antiracist politics. *Univ. Chic. Leg. Forum* 1989;140:139–167.

[93] Hurtado A. Intersectional understandings of inequality. In: Hammack PL, ed. The Oxford Handbook of Social Psychology and Social Justice. Oxford: Oxford University Press; 2018. pp. 157–172.

[94] Dovidio JF, Gaertner SL. Intergroup bias. In: Fiske ST, Gilbert DT, Lindzey G, eds. Handbook of Social Psychology. 5th ed. Hoboken: Wiley; 2010. pp. 1084–1121.

[95] Rhodes M, Baron A. The development of social categorization. *Annu. Rev. Dev. Psychol.* 2019;1:359–386.

[96] Turner JC. Rediscovering the Social Group: A Self-Categorization Theory. Oxford: Basil Blackwell; 1987.

[97] Pettigrew TF, Tropp LR. A meta-analytic test of intergroup contact theory. *J. Pers. Soc. Psychol.* 2006;90:751–783.

[98] Nier JA, et al. Changing interracial evaluations and behavior: The effects of a common group identity. *Group Process Intergroup Relat.* 2001;4:299–316.

[99] Fiske ST. Stereotype content: Warmth and competence endure. *Curr. Dir. Psychol. Sci.* 2018;27:67–73.

[100] Khalifeh H, et al. Recent physical and sexual violence against adults with severe mental illness: A systematic review and meta-analysis. *Int. Rev. Psychiatry* 2016;28:433–451.

[101] Yee N, et al. A meta-analysis of the relationship between psychosis and any type of criminal offending, in both men and women. *Schizophr. Res.* 2020;220:16–24.

[102] Scheff TJ. Being Mentally Ill: A Sociological Theory. Chicago: Aldine; 1966.

[103] Link BG, et al. A modified labeling theory approach in the area of mental disorders: An empirical assessment. *Am. Sociol. Rev.* 1989;54:400–423.

[104] DeLuca JS. Conceptualizing adolescent mental illness stigma: Youth stigma development and stigma reduction programs. *Adolescent Res. Rev.* 2020;5:153–171.

[105] Link BG, et al. The social rejection of former mental patients: Understanding why labels matter. *Am. J. Sociol.* 1987;92:1461–1500.

[106] Angermeyer MC, Matschinger H. The stigma of mental illness: Effects of labelling on public attitudes towards people with mental disorder. *Acta Psychiatr. Scand.* 2003;108:304–309.

[107] Duckitt J. Differential effects of right wing authoritarianism and social dominance orientation on outgroup attitudes and their mediation by threat from and competitiveness to outgroups. *Pers. Soc. Psychol. Bull.* 2006;32:684–696.

[108] Hill T, et al. The role of learned inferential encoding rules in the perception of faces: Effects of nonconscious self-perpetuation of a bias. *J. Exp. Soc. Psychol.* 1990;26:350–371.

[109] Yzerbyt V, Demoulin S. Intergroup relations. In: Fiske ST, Gilbert DT, Lindzey G, eds. Handbook of Social Psychology. 5th ed. Hoboken: Wiley; 2010. pp. 1024–1083.

[110] Hamilton DL, Gifford RK. Illusory correlation in interpersonal perception: A cognitive basis of stereotypic judgments. *J. Exp. Soc. Psychol.* 1976;12:392–407.

[111] Sherman JW, et al. Attentional processes in stereotype formation: A common model for category accentuation and illusory correlation. *J. Pers. Soc. Psychol.* 2009;96:305–323.

[112] Craft JT, et al. Language and discrimination: Generating meaning, perceiving identities, and discriminating outcomes. *Annu. Rev. Linguist.* 2020;6:389–407.

[113] Macrae CN, et al. Out of mind but back in sight: Stereotypes on the rebound. *J. Pers. Soc. Psychol.* 1994;67:808–817.

[114] Snyder ML, et al. Avoidance of the handicapped: An attributional ambiguity analysis. *J. Pers. Soc. Psychol.* 1979;37:2297–2306.

[115] Crocker J, et al. Social stigma. In: Gilbert DT, Fiske ST, Lindzey G, eds. Handbook of Social Psychology. 4th ed. Boston: McGraw-Hill; 1998. pp. 504–553.

[116] Gerber JP, et al. A social comparison theory meta-analysis 601 years on. *Psychol. Bull.* 2018;144:177–197.

[117] Wills TA. Downward comparison principles in social psychology. *Psychol. Bull.* 1981;90:245–271.

[118] Rosenblatt A, et al. Evidence for terror management theory: I. The effects of mortality salience on reactions to those who violate or uphold cultural values. *J. Pers. Soc. Psychol.* 1989;57:681–690.

[119] Jones EE, Farina A, et al. Social Stigma: The Psychology of Marked Relationships. New York: Freeman; 1984.

[120] Corrigan PW, et al. From whence comes mental illness stigma? *Int. J. Soc. Psychiatry* 2003;49:142–157.

[121] Sidanius J, Pratto F. Social Dominance: An Intergroup Theory of Social Hierarchy and Oppression. Cambridge: Cambridge Univ. Press; 1999.

[122] Furnham A. Belief in a just world: Research progress over the past decade. *Pers. Indiv. Diff.* 2003; 34:795–817.

[123] Rüsch N, et al. Do people with mental illness deserve what they get? Links between meritocratic worldviews and implicit versus explicit stigma. *Eur. Arch. Psychiatry Clin. Neurosci.* 2010;260:617–625.

[124] Madeira AF, et al. Primes and consequences: A systematic review of meritocracy in intergroup relations. *Front. Psychol.* 2019;10:2007.

[125] Jost JT. A quarter century of system justification theory: Questions, answers, criticisms, and societal applications. *Br. J. Soc. Psychol.* 2019;58:263–314.

[126] Lewin K. Resolving Social Conflicts: Selected Papers on Group Dynamics. New York: Harper & Row; 1948.

[127] Ross LD, et al. Social roles, social control, and biases in social-perception processes. *J. Pers. Soc. Psychol.* 1977;35:485–494.

[128] Chow WS, Priebe S. How has the extent of institutional mental healthcare changed in Western Europe? Analysis of data since 1990. *BMJ Open* 2016;6:e010188.

[129] Phelan JC, et al. Stigma and prejudice: One animal or two? *Soc. Sci. Med.* 2008;67:358–367.

[130] Neuberg SL, et al. Evolutionary social psychology. In: Fiske ST, Gilbert DT, Lindzey G, eds. Handbook of Social Psychology. 5th ed. Hoboken: Wiley; 2010. pp. 761–796.

[131] Nesse RM. The smoke detector principle: Signal detection and optimal defense regulation. *Evol. Med. Public Health* 2019;2019:1.

[132] Kurzban R, Leary MR. Evolutionary origins of stigmatization: The functions of social exclusion. *Psychol. Bull.* 2001;127:187–208.

[133] Walsh D, Foster J. A contagious other? Exploring the public's appraisals of contact with 'mental illness'. *Int. J. Environ. Res. Public Health* 2020;17:2005.

[134] Pescosolido BA, et al. The "backbone" of stigma: Identifying the global core of public prejudice associated with mental illness. *Am. J. Public Health* 2013;103:853–860.

[135] Pacilli MG, et al. When affective (but not cognitive) ambivalence predicts discrimination toward a minority group. *J. Soc. Psychol.* 2013;153:10–24.

[136] Stephan WG. Intergroup anxiety: Theory, research, and practice. *Pers. Soc. Psychol. Rev.* 2014;18:239–255.

[137] Steele CM. A threat in the air. How stereotypes shape intellectual identity and performance. *Am. Psychol.* 1997;52:613–629.

[138] Spencer SJ, et al. Stereotype threat. *Annu. Rev. Psychol.* 2016;67:415–437.

[139] Quinn DM, et al. Discreditable: Stigma effects of revealing a mental illness history on test performance. *Pers. Soc. Psychol. Bull.* 2004;30:803–815.

[140] Lazarus RS. Stress and Emotion: A New Synthesis. New York: Springer; 1999.

[141] Major B, O'Brien LT. The social psychology of stigma. *Annu. Rev. Psychol.* 2005;56:393–421.

[142] Ruggiero KM, Taylor DM. Coping with discrimination: How disadvantaged group members perceive the discrimination that confronts them. *J. Pers. Soc. Psychol.* 1995;68:826–838.

[143] Pascoe EA, Richman LS. Perceived discrimination and health: A meta-analytic review. *Psychol. Bull.* 2009;135:531–554.

[144] Beatty Moody DL, et al. Interpersonal-level discrimination indices, sociodemographic factors, and telomere length in African-Americans and Whites. *Biol. Psychol.* 2019;141:1–9.

[145] Orchard J, Price J. County-level racial prejudice and the black-white gap in infant health outcomes. *Soc. Sci. Med.* 2017;181:191–198.

[146] Nystedt TA, et al. The association of self-reported discrimination to all-cause mortality: A population-based prospective cohort study. *SSM Popul. Health* 2019;7:100360.

[147] Testa M, Major B. The impact of social comparisons after failure: The moderating effects of perceived control. *Basic Appl. Soc. Psych.* 1990;11:205–218.

[148] Roth P. The Human Stain. London: Cape; 2000.

[149] Pachankis JE. The psychological implications of concealing a stigma: A cognitive-affective-behavioral model. *Psychol. Bull.* 2007;133:328–345.

[150] Major B, Gramzow RH. Abortion as stigma: Cognitive and emotional implications of concealment. *J. Pers. Soc. Psychol.* 1999;77:735–745.

[151] Cole SW, et al. Accelerated course of human immunodeficiency virus infection in gay men who conceal their homosexual identity. *Psychosom. Med.* 1996;58:219–231.

[152] Rüsch N, et al. Attitudes toward disclosing a mental health problem and reemployment: A longitudinal study. *J. Nerv. Ment. Dis.* 2018;206:383–385.

[153] Pachankis JE, Bränström R. Hidden from happiness: Structural stigma, sexual orientation concealment, and life satisfaction across 28 countries. *J. Consult. Clin. Psychol.* 2018;86:403–415.

[154] Link BG, et al. The effectiveness of stigma coping orientations: Can negative consequences of mental illness labeling be avoided? *J. Health Soc. Behav.* 1991;32:302–320.

[155] Rüsch N, et al. Mental illness stigma: Concepts, consequences, and initiatives to reduce stigma. *Eur. Psychiatry* 2005;20:529–539.

[156] Angermeyer MC, Dietrich S. Public beliefs about and attitudes towards people with mental illness: A review of population studies. *Acta Psychiatr. Scand.* 2006;113:163–179.

[157] Boysen GA, et al. Evidence for blatant dehumanization of mental illness and its relation to stigma. *J. Soc. Psychol.* 2020;160:346–356.

[158] Corrigan PW, Nieweglowski K. How does familiarity impact the stigma of mental illness? *Clin. Psychol. Rev.* 2019;70:40–50.

[159] Angermeyer MC, et al. Changes in the perception of mental illness stigma in Germany over the last two decades. *Eur. Psychiatry* 2014;29:390–395.

[160] Schomerus G, et al. Evolution of public attitudes about mental illness: A systematic review and meta-analysis. *Acta Psychiatr. Scand.* 2012;125:440–452.

[161] Phelan JC, et al. Public conceptions of mental illness in 1950 and 1996: What is mental illness and is it to be feared? *J. Health Soc. Behav.* 2000;41:188–207.

[162] Thornicroft G, et al. Global pattern of experienced and anticipated discrimination against people with schizophrenia: A cross-sectional survey. *Lancet* 2009;373:408–415.

[163] Lasalvia A, et al. Global pattern of experienced and anticipated discrimination reported by people with major depressive disorder: A cross-sectional survey. *Lancet* 2013;381:55–62.

[164] Mestdagh A, Hansen B. Stigma in patients with schizophrenia receiving community mental health care: A review of qualitative studies. *Soc. Psychiatry Psychiatr. Epidemiol.* 2014;49:79–87.

[165] Rose D, et al. Reported stigma and discrimination by people with a diagnosis of schizophrenia. *Epidemiol. Psychiatr. Sci.* 2011;20:193–204.

[166] Evans-Lacko S, et al. Association between public views of mental illness and self-stigma among individuals with mental illness in 14 European countries. *Psychol. Med.* 2012;42:1741–1752.

[167] Freeman W, Watts JW. Psychosurgery: Intelligence, Emotion and Social Behavior Following Prefrontal Lobotomy for Mental Disorders. 2nd ed. Springfield: Thomas; 1949.

[168] OECD. Health at a Glance 2017: OECD Indicators. Paris: OECD Publishing; 2017.

[169] Hyman SE. Psychiatric drug development: Diagnosing a crisis. *Cerebrum* 2013;2013:5.

[170] Weiner B, et al. An attributional analysis of reactions to stigmas. *J. Pers. Soc. Psychol.* 1988;55:738–748.

[171] Dar-Nimrod I, Heine SJ. Genetic essentialism: On the deceptive determinism of DNA. *Psychol. Bull.* 2011;137:800–818.

[172] Johnson EC, et al. No evidence that schizophrenia candidate genes are more associated with schizophrenia than noncandidate genes. *Biol. Psychiatry* 2017;82:702–708.

[173] Border R, et al. No support for historical candidate gene or candidate gene-by-interaction hypotheses for major depression across multiple large samples. *Am. J. Psychiatry* 2019;176:376–387.

[174] Keller J. In genes we trust: The biological component of psychological essentialism and its relationship to mechanisms of motivated social cognition. *J. Pers. Soc. Psychol.* 2005;88:686–702.

[175] Lebowitz MS, Appelbaum PS. Biomedical explanations of psychopathology and their implications for attitudes and beliefs about mental disorders. *Annu. Rev. Clin. Psychol.* 2019;15:555–577.

[176] Angermeyer MC, et al. Biogenetic explanations and public acceptance of mental illness: Systematic review of population studies. *Br. J. Psychiatry* 2011;199:367–372.

[177] Schomerus G, et al. Causal beliefs of the public and social acceptance of persons with mental illness: A comparative analysis of schizophrenia, depression and alcohol dependence. *Psychol. Med.* 2014; 44:303–314.

[178] Pescosolido BA, et al. "A disease like any other"? A decade of change in public reactions to schizophrenia, depression, and alcohol dependence. *Am. J. Psychiatry* 2010;167:1321–1330.

[179] Lebowitz MS, Ahn WK. Effects of biological explanations for mental disorders on clinicians' empathy. *Proc. Natl. Acad. Sci. USA.* 2014;111:17786–17790.

[180] Rüsch N, et al. Biogenetic models of psychopathology, implicit guilt, and mental illness stigma. *Psychiatry Res.* 2010;179:328–332.

[181] Wigand ME, et al. Causal attributions and secrecy in unemployed people with mental health problems. *Psychiatry Res.* 2019;272:447–449.

[182] Lebowitz MS, Ahn WK. Blue genes? Understanding and mitigating negative consequences of personalized information about genetic risk for depression. *J. Genet. Couns.* 2018;27:204–216.

[183] Corrigan PW, et al. Examining a progressive model of self-stigma and its impact on people with serious mental illness. *Psychiatry Res.* 2011;189:339–343.

[184] Rüsch N, et al. Self-stigma in women with borderline personality disorder and women with social phobia. *J. Nerv. Ment. Dis.* 2006;194:766–773.

[185] Deacon M. Personal experience: Being depressed is worse than having advanced cancer. *J. Psychiatr. Ment. Health Nurs.* 2015;22:457–459.

[186] Gallo KM. First person account: Self-stigmatization. *Schizophr. Bull.* 1994;20:407–410.

[187] Brohan E, et al. Self-stigma, empowerment and perceived discrimination among people with schizophrenia in 14 European countries: The GAMIAN-Europe study. *Schizophr. Res.* 2010;122:232–238.

[188] Brohan E, et al. Self-stigma, empowerment and perceived discrimination among people with bipolar disorder or depression in 13 European countries: The GAMIAN-Europe study. *J. Affect. Disord.* 2011;129:56–63.

[189] Corrigan PW, Watson AC. The paradox of self-stigma and mental illness. *Clin. Psychol. Sci. Pract.* 2002;9:35–53.

[190] Correll J, Park B. A model of the ingroup as a social resource. *Pers. Soc. Psychol. Rev.* 2005;9:341–359.

[191] Rüsch N, et al. Self-stigma, empowerment, and perceived legitimacy of discrimination among women with mental illness. *Psychiatr. Serv.* 2006;57:399–402.

[192] Rüsch N, et al. Ingroup perception and responses to stigma among persons with mental illness. *Acta Psychiatr. Scand.* 2009;120:320–328.

[193] Rogers ES, et al. Validating the empowerment scale with a multisite sample of consumers of mental health services. *Psychiatr. Serv.* 2010;61:933–936.

[194] Hansson L, Björkman T. Empowerment in people with a mental illness: Reliability and validity of the Swedish version of an empowerment scale. *Scand. J. Caring Sci.* 2005;19:32–38.

[195] WHO Regional Office for Europe. User Empowerment in Mental Health - A Statement by the WHO Regional Office for Europe. Copenhagen: WHO; 2010.

[196] Thoits PA. Resisting the stigma of mental illness. *Soc. Psychol. Q.* 2011;74:6–28.

[197] Firmin RL, et al. Stigma resistance is positively associated with psychiatric and psychosocial outcomes: A meta-analysis. *Schizophr. Res.* 2016;175:118–128.

[198] Dubreucq J, et al. Self-stigma in serious mental illness: A systematic review of frequency, correlates, and consequences. *Schizophr. Bull.* 2021;47:1261–1287.

[199] Xu Z, et al. Involuntary psychiatric hospitalisation, stigma stress, and recovery: A 2-year-study. *Epidemiol. Psychiatr. Sci.* 2019;28:458–465.

[200] Wang K, et al. Perceived provider stigma as a predictor of mental health service users' internalized stigma and disempowerment. *Psychiatry Res.* 2018;259:526–531.

[201] Lysaker PH, et al. Insight in schizophrenia spectrum disorders: Relationship with behavior, mood and perceived quality of life, underlying causes and emerging treatments. *World Psychiatry* 2018; 17:12–23.

[202] Lysaker PH, et al. Toward understanding the insight paradox: Internalized stigma moderates the association between insight and social functioning, hope, and self-esteem among people with schizophrenia spectrum disorders. *Schizophr. Bull.* 2007;33:192–199.

[203] Moritz S, et al. Embracing psychosis: A cognitive insight intervention improves personal narratives and meaning-making in patients with schizophrenia. *Schizophr. Bull.* 2018;44:307–316.

[204] Forgione FA. Diagnostic dissent: Experiences of perceived misdiagnosis and stigma in persons diagnosed with schizophrenia. *J. Humanist. Psychol.* 2019;59:69–98.

[205] Rüsch N, et al. Disclosure and quality of life among unemployed individuals with mental health problems: A longitudinal study. *J. Nerv. Ment. Dis.* 2019;207:137–139.

[206] Grice T, et al. Factors associated with mental health disclosure outside of the workplace: A systematic literature review. *Stigma Health* 2018;3:116–130.

[207] Pasek MH, et al. Identity concealment and social change: Balancing advocacy goals against individual needs. *J. Soc. Issues.* 2017;73:397–412.

[208] Garcia JA, Crocker J. Reasons for disclosing depression matter: The consequences of having egosystem and ecosystem goals. *Soc. Sci. Med.* 2008;67:453–462.

[209] Rüsch N, et al. A stress-coping model of mental illness stigma: I. Predictors of cognitive stress appraisal. *Schizophr. Res.* 2009;110:59–64.

[210] Rüsch N, et al. Stigma and disclosing one's mental illness to family and friends. *Soc. Psychiatry Psychiatr. Epidemiol.* 2014;49:1157–1160.

[211] Schibalski JV, et al. Stigma-related stress, shame and avoidant coping reactions among members of the general population with elevated symptom levels. *Compr. Psychiatry* 2017;74:224–230.

[212] Rüsch N, et al. Emotional reactions to involuntary psychiatric hospitalization and stigma as a stressor among people with mental illness. *Eur. Arch. Psychiatry Clin. Neurosci.* 2014;264:35–43.

[213] Rüsch N, et al. A stress-coping model of mental illness stigma: II. Emotional stress responses, coping behavior and outcome. *Schizophr. Res.* 2009;110:65–71.

[214] Rüsch N, et al. Stigma as a stressor and transition to schizophrenia after one year among young people at risk of psychosis. *Schizophr. Res.* 2015;166:43–48.

[215] Rüsch N, Kösters M. Honest, open, proud to support disclosure decisions and to decrease stigma's impact among people with mental illness: Conceptual review and meta-analysis of program efficacy. *Soc. Psychiatry Psychiatr. Epidemiol.* 2021;56:1513–1526.

[216] Scior K, et al. Supporting mental health disclosure decisions: The honest, open, proud programme. *Br. J. Psychiatry* 2020;216:243–245.

[217] Slade M. Personal Recovery and Mental Illness: A Guide for Mental Health Professionals. Cambridge: Cambridge University Press; 2009.

[218] Anthony WA. Recovery from mental illness: The guiding vision of the mental health service system in the 1990s. *Psychosoc. Rehabil. J.* 1993;16:11–23.

[219] Stein LI, Test MA. Alternative to mental hospital treatment. I. Conceptual model, treatment program, and clinical evaluation. *Arch. Gen. Psychiatry* 1980;37:392–397.

[220] Stratford AC, et al. The growth of peer support: An international charter. *J. Ment. Health* 2019;28:627–632.

[221] Rowe M, Davidson L. Recovering citizenship. *Isr. J. Psychiatry Relat. Sci.* 2016;53:14–20.

[222] Slade M. Everyday solutions for everyday problems: How mental health systems can support recovery. *Psychiatr. Serv.* 2012;63:702–704.

[223] Pincus HA, et al. A review of mental health recovery programs in selected industrialized countries. *Int. J. Ment. Health Syst.* 2016;10:73.

[224] Rose D. The mainstreaming of recovery. *J. Ment. Health* 2014;23:217–218.

[225] Thériault J, et al. Recovery colleges after a decade of research: A literature review. *Psychiatr. Serv.* 2020;71:928–940.

[226] Crowther A, et al. The impact of recovery colleges on mental health staff, services and society. *Epidemiol. Psychiatr. Sci.* 2019;28:481–488.

[227] Wood L, Alsawy S. Recovery in psychosis from a service user perspective: A systematic review and thematic synthesis of current qualitative evidence. *Community Ment. Health J.* 2018;54:793–804.

[228] Thornicroft G, et al. Undertreatment of people with major depressive disorder in 21 countries. *Br. J. Psychiatry* 2017;210:119–124.

[229] Degenhardt L, et al. Estimating treatment coverage for people with substance use disorders: An analysis of data from the World Mental Health Surveys. *World Psychiatry* 2017;16:299–307.

[230] Swift JK, et al. Treatment refusal and premature termination in psychotherapy, pharmacotherapy, and their combination: A meta-analysis of head-to-head comparisons. *Psychotherapy* 2017;54:47–57.

[231] Karyotaki E, et al. Predictors of treatment dropout in self-guided web-based interventions for depression: An 'individual patient data' meta-analysis. *Psychol. Med.* 2015;45:2717–2726.

[232] Ng JYY, et al. Self-determination theory applied to health contexts: A meta-analysis. *Perspect. Psychol. Sci.* 2012;7:325–340.

[233] Corrigan PW, et al. From adherence to self-determination: Evolution of a treatment paradigm for people with serious mental illnesses. *Psychiatr. Serv.* 2012;63:169–173.

[234] Priebe S, et al. Mental health care institutions in nine European countries, 2002 to 2006. *Psychiatr. Serv.* 2008;59:570–573.

[235] Angermeyer MC, et al. Attitudes of the German public to restrictions on persons with mental illness in 1993 and 2011. *Epidemiol. Psychiatr. Sci.* 2014;23:263–270.

[236] Burns T, Rugkåsa J. Hospitalisation and compulsion: The research agenda. *Br. J. Psychiatry* 2016; 209:97–98.

[237] de Jong MH, et al. Interventions to reduce compulsory psychiatric admissions: A systematic review and meta-analysis. *JAMA Psychiatry* 2016;73:657–664.

[238] Series L, Nilsson A. Article 12 CRPD: Equal recognition before the law. In: Bantekas I, Stein MA, Anastasiou D, eds. The UN ConVention on the Rights of Persons With Disabilities: A Commentary. Oxford: Oxford University Press; 2018. pp. 339–382.

[239] Borbé R, et al. Anwendung psychiatrischer Behandlungsvereinbarungen in Deutschland: Ergebnisse einer bundesweiten Befragung. *Nervenarzt.* 2012;83:638–643.

[240] Corrigan PW, et al. The impact of mental illness stigma on seeking and participating in mental health care. *Psychol. Sci. Public Interest* 2014;15:37–70.

[241] Clement S, et al. What is the impact of mental health-related stigma on help-seeking? A systematic review of quantitative and qualitative studies. *Psychol. Med.* 2015;45:11–27.

[242] Savage H, et al. Exploring professional help-seeking for mental disorders. *Qual. Health Res.* 2016; 26:1662–1673.

[243] Schomerus G, et al. Stigma as a barrier to recognizing personal mental illness and seeking help: A prospective study among untreated persons with mental illness. *Eur. Arch. Psychiatry Clin. Neurosci.* 2019;269:469–479.

[244] Rüsch N, et al. Shame, perceived knowledge and satisfaction with mental health as predictors of attitude patterns towards help-seeking. *Epidemiol. Psychiatr. Sci.* 2014;23:177–187.

[245] Schnyder N, et al. Association between mental health-related stigma and active help-seeking: Systematic review and meta-analysis. *Br. J. Psychiatry* 2017;210:261–268.

[246] Sirey JA, et al. Stigma as a barrier to recovery: Perceived stigma and patient-rated severity of illness as predictors of antidepressant drug adherence. *Psychiatr. Serv.* 2001;52:1615–1620.

[247] Rüsch N, et al. Predictors of dropout from inpatient dialectical behavior therapy among women with borderline personality disorder. *J. Behav. Ther. Exp. Psychiatry* 2008;39:497–503.

[248] Kovandžić M, et al. Access to primary mental health care for hard-to-reach groups: From 'silent suffering' to 'making it work'. *Soc. Sci. Med.* 2011;72:763–772.

[249] Wittchen HU, et al. Traumatic experiences and posttraumatic stress disorder in soldiers following deployment abroad: How big is the hidden problem? *Dtsch. Ärztebl. Int.* 2012;109:559–568.

[250] Hom MA, et al. A systematic review of help-seeking and mental health service utilization among military service members. *Clin. Psychol. Rev.* 2017;53:59–78.

[251] Coleman SJ, et al. Stigma-related barriers and facilitators to help seeking for mental health issues in the armed forces: A systematic review and thematic synthesis of qualitative literature. *Psychol. Med.* 2017;47:1880–1892.

[252] Haugen PT, et al. Mental health stigma and barriers to mental health care for first responders: A systematic review and meta-analysis. *J. Psychiatr. Res.* 2017;94:218–229.

[253] Rüsch N, et al. Attitudes towards disclosing a mental illness among German soldiers and their comrades. *Psychiatry Res.* 2017;258:200–206.

[254] Link B, Hatzenbuehler ML. Stigma as an unrecognized determinant of population health: Research and policy implications. *J. Health Polit. Policy Law* 2016;41:653–673.

[255] Schomerus G, et al. Preferences of the public regarding cutbacks in expenditure for patient care: Are there indications of discrimination against those with mental disorders? *Soc. Psychiatry Psychiatr. Epidemiol.* 2006;41:369–377.

[256] Hazo JB, et al. European Union investment and countries' involvement in mental health research between 2007 and 2013. *Acta Psychiatr. Scand.* 2016;134:138–149.

[257] Arseneault L. Mental Health Research Funding: We Are Still Not Getting Our Fair Share. 2019. Available at: www.nationalelfservice.net/mental-health/mental-health-research-funding/. Accessed 4 Jan 2020.

[258] Nicolini ME, et al. Should euthanasia and assisted suicide for psychiatric disorders be permitted? A systematic review of reasons. *Psychol. Med.* 2020;50:1241–1256.

[259] WHO. Preventing Suicide: A Global Imperative. Geneva: WHO; 2014.

[260] WHO. Suicide in the World: Global Health Estimates. 2019. Available at: apps.who.int/iris/bitstream/handle/10665/326948/WHO-MSD-MER-19.3-eng.pdf. Accessed 12 Feb 2020.

[261] Wray M, et al. The sociology of suicide. *Annu. Rev. Sociol.* 2011;37:505–528.

[262] Hofmann D. Suizid in der Spätantike: Seine Bewertung in der Lateinischen Literatur. Stuttgart: Steiner; 2007.

[263] Mayer L, et al. Anticipated suicide stigma, secrecy, and suicidality among suicide attempt survivors. *Suicide Life Threat. Behav.* 2020;50:706–713.

[264] Ludwig J, et al. Public stigma toward persons with suicidal thoughts: Do age, sex, and medical condition of affected persons matter? *Suicide Life Threat. Behav.* 2020;50:631–642.

[265] Sheehan L, et al. The self-stigma of suicide attempt survivors. *Arch. Suicide Res.* 2020;24:34–47.

[266] Sheehan L, et al. Benefits and risks of suicide disclosure. *Soc. Sci. Med.* 2019;223:16–23.

[267] Calear AL, Batterham PJ. Suicidal ideation disclosure: Patterns, correlates and outcome. *Psychiatry Res.* 2019;278:1–6.

[268] Oexle N, et al. Perceived suicide stigma, secrecy about suicide loss and mental health outcomes. *Death Studies* 2020;44:248–255.

[269] Bartone PT, et al. Peer support services for bereaved survivors: A systematic review. *Omega* 2019; 80:137–166.

[270] Chen JA, et al. The role of stigma and denormalization in suicide-prevention laws in East Asia: A sociocultural, historical, and ethical perspective. *Harv. Rev. Psychiatry* 2017;25:229–240.

[271] Rüsch N, et al. Self-contempt as a predictor of suicidality: A longitudinal study. *J. Nerv. Ment. Dis.* 2019;207:1056–1057.

[272] Christensen H, et al. Changing the direction of suicide prevention research: A necessity for true population impact. *JAMA Psychiatry* 2016;73:435–436.

[273] Oexle N, et al. Emerging trends in suicide prevention research. *Curr. Opin. Psychiatry* 2019;32:336–341.

[274] Bateson J. The Last and Greatest Battle: Finding the Will, Commitment, and Strategy to End Military Suicides. Oxford: Oxford University Press; 2015.

[275] Pourmand A, et al. Social media and suicide: A review of technology-based epidemiology and risk assessment. *Telemed. J. E. Health* 2019;25:880–888.

[276] Hofstra E, et al. Effectiveness of suicide prevention interventions: A systematic review and meta-analysis. *Gen. Hosp. Psychiatry* 2020;63:127–140.

[277] Hegerl U, et al. Prevention of suicidal behaviour: Results of a controlled community-based intervention study in four European countries. *PLoS One* 2019;14:e0224602.

[278] Wasserman D, et al. School-based suicide prevention programmes: The SEYLE cluster-randomised, controlled trial. *Lancet* 2015;385:1536–1544.

[279] Ahern S, et al. A cost-effectiveness analysis of school-based suicide prevention programmes. *Eur. Child Adolesc. Psychiatry* 2018;27:1295–1304.

[280] Bleuler E. Dementia Praecox or the Group of Schizophrenias [publ. in German 1913]. New York: Intern. Univ. Pr.; 1955.

[281] Bleuler E. Lehrbuch der Psychiatrie. 15th ed. Berlin, Heidelberg: Springer; 1983.

[282] Fusar-Poli P, et al. The psychosis high-risk state: A comprehensive state of the art review. *JAMA Psychiatry* 2013;70:107–120.

[283] Bosnjak Kuharic D, et al. Interventions for prodromal stage of psychosis. *Cochrane Database Syst. Rev.* 2019;2019:CD012236.

[284] Colizzi M, et al. Should we be concerned about stigma and discrimination in people at risk for psychosis? A systematic review. *Psychol. Med.* 2020;50:705–726.

[285] Selten JP, Cantor-Graae E. Hypothesis: Social defeat is a risk factor for schizophrenia? *Br. J. Psychiatry Suppl.* 2007;51:9–12.

[286] Pearce J, et al. Perceived discrimination and psychosis: A systematic review of the literature. *Soc. Psychiatry Psychiatr. Epidemiol.* 2019;54:1023–1044.

[287] Gronholm PC, et al. Mental health-related stigma and pathways to care for people at risk of psychotic disorders or experiencing first-episode psychosis: A systematic review. *Psychol. Med.* 2017;47:1867–1879.

[288] Rüsch N, et al. Attitudes towards help-seeking and stigma among young people at risk for psychosis. *Psychiatry Res.* 2013;210:1313–1315.

[289] Rüsch N, et al. Well-being among persons at risk of psychosis: The role of self-labeling, shame and stigma stress. *Psychiatr. Serv.* 2014;65:483–489.

[290] Xu Z, et al. Stigma and suicidal ideation among young people at risk of psychosis after one year. *Psychiatry Res.* 2016;243:219–224.

[291] Temesgen WA, et al. Conceptualizations of subjective recovery from recent onset psychosis and its associated factors: A systematic review. *Early Interv. Psychiatry* 2019;13:181–193.

[292] Mueser KT, et al. Clinical and demographic correlates of stigma in first-episode psychosis: The impact of duration of untreated psychosis. *Acta Psychiatr. Scand.* 2020;141:157–166.

[293] Lord C, et al. Autism spectrum disorder. *Lancet* 2018;392:508–520.

[294] Silberman S. NeuroTribes: The Legacy of Autism and the Future of Neurodiversity. New York: Avery; 2015.

[295] Baron-Cohen S. Neurodiversity - a revolutionary concept for autism and psychiatry. *J. Child Psychol. Psychiatry* 2017;58:744–747.

[296] O'Brolcháin F, Gordijn B. Risks of stigmatisation resulting from assistive technologies for people with autism spectrum disorder. *Stud. Health Technol. Inform.* 2017;242:265–268.

[297] Gilman SL. Madness as disability. *Hist. Psychiatry* 2014;25:441–449.

[298] Bonaventura. The Nightwatches of Bonaventura. Chicago: University of Chicago Press; 2014.

[299] Cage E, et al. Understanding, attitudes and dehumanisation towards autistic people. *Autism* 2019; 23:1373–1383.

[300] Botha M, Frost DM. Extending the minority stress model to understand mental health problems experienced by the autistic population. *Soc. Ment. Health* 2020;10:20–34.

[301] Reiff M, et al. "Set in Stone" or "Ray of Hope": Parents' beliefs about cause and prognosis after genomic testing of children diagnosed with ASD. *J. Autism Dev. Disord.* 2017;47:1453–1463.

[302] Austin JE, et al. Evaluating parental autism disclosure strategies. *J. Autism Dev. Disord.* 2018;48: 103–109.

[303] Sasson NJ, Morrison KE. First impressions of adults with autism improve with diagnostic disclosure and increased autism knowledge of peers. *Autism* 2019;23:50–59.

[304] Lindsay S, et al. Disclosure and workplace accommodations for people with autism: A systematic review. *Disabil. Rehabil.* 2021;43:597–610.

[305] Roleska M, et al. Autism and the right to education in the EU: Policy mapping and scoping review of the United Kingdom, France, Poland and Spain. *PLoS One* 2018;13:e0202336.

[306] Frank F, et al. Education and employment status of adults with autism spectrum disorders in Germany - a cross-sectional-survey. *BMC Psychiatry* 2018;18:75.

[307] Khalifa G, et al. Workplace accommodations for adults with autism spectrum disorder: A scoping review. *Disabil. Rehabil.* 2020;42:1316–1331.

[308] Price S, et al. Doctors with Asperger's: The impact of a diagnosis. *Clin. Teach.* 2019;16:19–22.

[309] Kinnear SH, et al. Understanding the experience of stigma for parents of children with autism spectrum disorder and the role stigma plays in families' lives. *J. Autism Dev. Disord.* 2016;46:942–953.

[310] Papadopoulos C, et al. Systematic review of the relationship between autism stigma and informal caregiver mental health. *J. Autism Dev. Disord.* 2019;49:1665–1685.

[311] Gillespie-Lynch K, et al. Changing college students' conceptions of autism: An online training to increase knowledge and decrease stigma. *J. Autism Dev. Disord.* 2015;45:2553–2566.

[312] Gillespie-Lynch K, et al. Whose expertise is it? Evidence for autistic adults as critical autism experts. *Front. Psychol.* 2017;8:438.

[313] Kras JF. The "Ransom Notes" affair: When the neurodiversity movement came of age. *Disabil. Stud. Q.* 2010;30:1065.

[314] Melle T. Die Welt im Rücken. 4th ed. Hamburg, Berlin: Rowohlt; 2019 (English translation by Biblioasis planned for Nov. 2022).

[315] Folstad S, Mansell W. 'The Button Question': A mixed-methods study of whether patients want to keep or remove bipolar disorder and the reasons for their decision. *J. Affect. Disord.* 2019;245: 708–715.

[316] Ellison N, et al. Bipolar disorder and stigma: A systematic review of the literature. *J. Affect. Disord.* 2013;151:805–820.

[317] Hawke LD, et al. Stigma and bipolar disorder: A review of the literature. *J. Affect. Disord.* 2013; 150:181–191.

[318] Perlick DA, et al. Stigma as a barrier to recovery: Adverse effects of perceived stigma on social adaptation of persons diagnosed with bipolar affective disorder. *Psychiatr. Serv.* 2001;52:1627–1632.

[319] Levy B, et al. Stigma, social anxiety, and illness severity in bipolar disorder: Implications for treatment. *Ann. Clin. Psychiatry* 2015;27:55–64.

[320] Howland M, et al. Mixed-methods analysis of internalized stigma correlates in poorly adherent individuals with bipolar disorder. *Compr. Psychiatry* 2016;70:174–180.
[321] Warwick H, et al. 'What people diagnosed with bipolar disorder experience as distressing': A meta-synthesis of qualitative research. *J. Affect. Disord.* 2019;248:108–130.
[322] Soo SA, et al. Randomized controlled trials of psychoeducation modalities in the management of bipolar disorder: A systematic review. *J. Clin. Psychiatry* 2018;79:17r11750.
[323] Ratheesh A, et al. Ethical considerations in preventive interventions for bipolar disorder. *Early Interv. Psychiatry* 2017;11:104–112.
[324] Lawrie SM, et al. Predicting major mental illness: Ethical and practical considerations. *BJPsych Open* 2019;5:e30.
[325] Gunderson JG, et al. Borderline personality disorder. *Nat. Rev. Dis. Primers* 2018;4:18029.
[326] Wetterborg D, et al. Borderline personality disorder: Prevalence and psychiatric comorbidity among male offenders on probation in Sweden. *Compr. Psychiatry* 2015;62:63–70.
[327] Temes CM, Zanarini MC. The longitudinal course of borderline personality disorder. *Psychiatr. Clin. North Am.* 2018;41:685–694.
[328] Rüsch N, et al. Shame and implicit self-concept in women with borderline personality disorder. *Am. J. Psychiatry* 2007;164:500–508.
[329] Curtis S, et al. Caring for young people who self-harm: A review of perspectives from families and young people. *Int. J. Environ. Res. Public Health* 2018;15:E950.
[330] de Marné D. Warum Normal Sein Gar Nicht so Normal Ist: ... Und Warum Reden Hilft. München: Scorpio Verlag; 2019.
[331] Ring D, Lawn S. Stigma perpetuation at the interface of mental health care: A review to compare patient and clinician perspectives of stigma and borderline personality disorder. *J. Ment. Health* 2022:1–21. doi:10.1080/09638237.2019.1581337.
[332] Lam DCK, et al. 'Judging a book by its cover': An experimental study of the negative impact of a diagnosis of borderline personality disorder on clinicians' judgements of uncomplicated panic disorder. *Br. J. Clin. Psychol.* 2016;55:253–268.
[333] Knaak S, et al. Stigma towards borderline personality disorder: Effectiveness and generalizability of an anti-stigma program for healthcare providers using a pre-post randomized design. *Borderline Personal. Disord. Emot. Dysregul.* 2015;2:9.
[334] Roehr S, et al. Is dementia incidence declining in high-income countries? A systematic review and meta-analysis. *Clin. Epidemiol.* 2018;10:1233–1247.
[335] WHO. Global Action Plan on the Public Health Response to Dementia 2017-2025. Geneva: WHO; 2017.
[336] Michalowsky B, et al. Ökonomische und gesellschaftliche Herausforderungen der Demenz in Deutschland – Eine Metaanalyse. *Bundesgesundheitsbl.* 2019;62:981–992.
[337] Ballenger JF. Framing confusion: Dementia, society, and history. *AMA J. Ethics* 2017;19:713–719.
[338] Johnston K, et al. Understandings of dementia in low and middle income countries and amongst indigenous peoples: A systematic review and qualitative meta-synthesis. *Aging Ment. Health* 2020; 24:1183–1195.
[339] Oscar N, et al. Machine learning, sentiment analysis, and tweets: An examination of Alzheimer's disease stigma on Twitter. *J. Gerontol. B Psychol. Sci. Soc. Sci.* 2017;72:742–751.
[340] Zeilig H. Dementia as a cultural metaphor. *Gerontologist* 2014;54:258–267.
[341] Behuniak SM. The living dead? The construction of people with Alzheimer's disease as zombies. *Ageing Soc.* 2011;31:70–92.
[342] von dem Knesebeck O, et al. Emotional reactions toward people with dementia: Results of a population survey from Germany. *Int. Psychogeriatr.* 2014;26:435–441.
[343] Alzheimer's Disease International. World Alzheimer Report 2019: Attitudes to dementia. 2019. Available at: www.alz.co.uk/research/WorldAlzheimerReport2019.pdf. Accessed 12 Feb 2020.
[344] Martin S, et al. Attitudes and preferences towards screening for dementia: A systematic review of the literature. *BMC Geriatr.* 2015;15:66.
[345] Draper B, et al. Early dementia diagnosis and the risk of suicide and euthanasia. *Alzheimers Dement.* 2010;6:75–82.
[346] Johnstone MJ. Metaphors, stigma and the 'Alzheimerization' of the euthanasia debate. *Dementia* 2013;12:377–393.

[347] Devlin K. Too much stigma attached to Alzheimer's, says author Terry Pratchett. *The Telegraph*, UK, 6 October 2008.

[348] O'Connor D, et al. Stigma, discrimination and agency: Diagnostic disclosure as an everyday practice shaping social citizenship. *J. Aging Stud.* 2018;44:45–51.

[349] Nguyen T, Li X. Understanding public-stigma and self-stigma in the context of dementia: A systematic review of the global literature. *Dementia* 2020;19:148–181.

[350] Werner P. Stigma and Alzheimer's disease: A systematic review of evidence, theory, and methods. In: Corrigan PW, ed. The Stigma of Disease and Disability: Understanding Causes and Overcoming Injustices. Washington: American Psychol. Association; 2014. pp. 223–244.

[351] Weetch J, et al. The involvement of people with dementia in advocacy: A systematic narrative review. *Aging Ment. Health* 2021;25:1595–1604.

[352] Zimmermann M. Poetics and Politics of Alzheimer's Disease Life-Writing. Cham: Palgrave Macmillan; 2017.

[353] Wolverson EL, et al. Living positively with dementia: A systematic review and synthesis of the qualitative literature. *Aging Ment. Health* 2016;20:676–699.

[354] Werner P, et al. Family stigma and caregiver burden in Alzheimer's disease. *Gerontologist* 2012; 52:89–97.

[355] Lopez RP, et al. Managing shame: A grounded theory of how stigma manifests in families living with dementia. *J. Am. Psychiatr. Nurses Assoc.* 2020;26:181–188.

[356] Low LF, et al. Communicating a diagnosis of dementia: A systematic mixed studies review of attitudes and practices of health practitioners. *Dementia* 2019;18:2856–2905.

[357] Werner P, Doron II. Alzheimer's disease and the law: Positive and negative consequences of structural stigma and labeling in the legal system. *Aging Ment. Health*. 2017;21:1206–1213.

[358] Cahill S. Dementia and Human Rights. Bristol: Policy Press; 2018.

[359] McDermott O, et al. Psychosocial interventions for people with dementia: A synthesis of systematic reviews. *Aging Ment. Health* 2019;23:393–403.

[360] Bienvenu B, Hanna G. Arts participation: Counterbalancing forces to the social stigma of a dementia diagnosis. *AMA J. Ethics* 2017;19:704–712.

[361] Krall R. Back to life: Art education for people living with dementia in the Kunsthistorisches Museum Vienna. In: Mateus-Berr R, Gruber V, eds. Arts & Dementia: Interdisciplinary Perspectives. Berlin: De Gruyter; 2021, pp. 354–365.

[362] Schicktanz S, et al. Patient representation and advocacy for Alzheimer disease in Germany and Israel. *J. Bioeth. Inq.* 2018;15:369–380.

[363] Chow S, et al. National dementia strategies: What should Canada learn? *Can. Geriatr. J.* 2018;21: 173–209.

[364] Bundesministerium für Familie, Senioren, Frauen und Jugend, Bundesministerium für Gesundheit. Gemeinsam für Menschen mit Demenz: Bericht zur Umsetzung der Agenda der Allianz für Menschen mit Demenz 2014–2018. Berlin; 2018.

[365] Laporte Uribe F, et al. Regional dementia care networks in Germany: Changes in caregiver burden at one-year follow-up and associated factors. *Int. Psychogeriatr.* 2017;29:991–1004.

[366] Jastreboff AM, et al. Obesity as a disease: The Obesity Society 2018 position statement. *Obesity* 2019;27:7–9.

[367] Vallgårda S, et al. Should Europe follow the US and declare obesity a disease? A discussion of the so-called utilitarian argument. *Eur. J. Clin. Nutr.* 2017;71:1263–1267.

[368] Arcelus J, et al. Mortality rates in patients with anorexia nervosa and other eating disorders: A meta-analysis of 36 studies. *Arch. Gen. Psychiatry* 2011;68:724–731.

[369] Reas DL. Public and healthcare professionals' knowledge and attitudes toward binge eating disorder: A narrative review. *Nutrients* 2017;9:E1267.

[370] Puhl R, Suh Y. Stigma and eating and weight disorders. *Curr. Psychiatry Rep.* 2015;17:10.

[371] O'Connor C, et al. How do people with eating disorders experience the stigma associated with their condition? A mixed-methods systematic review. *J. Ment. Health* 2021;30:454–469.

[372] Puhl R, Suh Y. Health consequences of weight stigma: Implications for obesity prevention and treatment. *Curr. Obes. Rep.* 2015;4:182–190.

[373] Blythin SPM, et al. Experiences of shame and guilt in anorexia and bulimia nervosa: A systematic review. *Psychol. Psychother.* 2020;93:134–159.

[374] Griffiths S, et al. How might eating disorders stigmatization worsen eating disorders symptom severity? Evaluation of a stigma internalization model. *Int. J. Eat. Disord.* 2018;51:1010–1014.

[375] Ali K, et al. Perceived barriers and facilitators towards help-seeking for eating disorders: A systematic review. *Int. J. Eat. Disord.* 2017;50:9–21.

[376] Watson HJ, et al. Genome-wide association study identifies eight risk loci and implicates metabo-psychiatric origins for anorexia nervosa. *Nat. Genet.* 2019;51:1207–1214.

[377] Angermeyer MC, et al. Biogenetic explanations and public acceptance of people with eating disorders. *Soc. Psychiatry Psychiatr. Epidemiol.* 2013;48:1667–1673.

[378] Easter MM. "Not all my fault": Genetics, stigma, and personal responsibility for women with eating disorders. *Soc. Sci. Med.* 2012;75:1408–1416.

[379] Culbert KM, et al. Research review: What we have learned about the causes of eating disorders - a synthesis of sociocultural, psychological, and biological research. *J. Child Psychol. Psychiatry* 2015; 56:1141–1164.

[380] Giordano S. Eating disorders and the media. *Curr. Opin. Psychiatry* 2015;28:478–482.

[381] Pirie I. Disordered eating and the contradictions of neoliberal governance. *Sociol. Health Illn.* 2016;38:839–853.

[382] Hausenblas HA, et al. Media effects of experimental presentation of the ideal physique on eating disorder symptoms: A meta-analysis of laboratory studies. *Clin. Psychol. Rev.* 2013;33: 168–181.

[383] Rodgers RF, et al. Longitudinal relationships among internalization of the media ideal, peer social comparison, and body dissatisfaction: Implications for the tripartite influence model. *Dev. Psychol.* 2015;51:706–713.

[384] Saul JS, Rodgers RF. Adolescent eating disorder risk and the online world. *Child Adolesc. Psychiatr. Clin. N. Am.* 2018;27:221–228.

[385] Chang PF, Bazarova NN. Managing stigma: Disclosure-response communication patterns in pro-anorexic websites. *Health Commun.* 2016;31:217–229.

[386] Rodgers RF, et al. A meta-analysis examining the influence of pro-eating disorder websites on body image and eating pathology. *Eur. Eat. Disord. Rev.* 2016;24:3–8.

[387] Aardoom JJ, et al. Internet and patient empowerment in individuals with symptoms of an eating disorder: A cross-sectional investigation of a pro-recovery focused e-community. *Eat. Behav.* 2014; 15:350–356.

[388] Oksanen A, et al. Pro-anorexia and anti-pro-anorexia videos on YouTube: Sentiment analysis of user responses. *J. Med. Internet Res.* 2015;17:e256.

[389] Rennick-Egglestone S, et al. Mental health recovery narratives and their impact on recipients: Systematic review and narrative synthesis. *Can. J. Psychiatry* 2019;64:669–679.

[390] Shaw LK, Homewood J. The effect of eating disorder memoirs in individuals with self-identified eating pathologies. *J. Nerv. Ment. Dis.* 2015;203:591–595.

[391] Iles IA, et al. Stigmatizing the other: An exploratory study of unintended consequences of eating disorder public service announcements. *J. Health Psychol.* 2017;22:120–131.

[392] Doley JR, et al. Interventions to reduce the stigma of eating disorders: A systematic review and meta-analysis. *Int. J. Eat. Disord.* 2017;50:210–230.

[393] Kelly AC, Waring SV. A feasibility study of a 2-week self-compassionate letter-writing intervention for nontreatment seeking individuals with typical and atypical anorexia nervosa. *Int. J. Eat. Disord.* 2018;51:1005–1009.

[394] Ruddock HK, et al. Obesity stigma: Is the 'food addiction' label feeding the problem? *Nutrients* 2019;11:E2100.

[395] Gilman SL. The Fat Person on the Edgware Road Omnibus: Fat, fashion, and public shaming in the British long eighteenth century. *Lit. Med.* 2017;35:431–447.

[396] Ringel MM, Ditto PH. The moralization of obesity. *Soc. Sci. Med.* 2019;237:112399.

[397] Kim TJ, et al. Obesity stigma in Germany and the United States - results of population surveys. *PLoS One* 2019;14:e0221214.

[398] Kersbergen I, Robinson E. Blatant dehumanization of people with obesity. *Obesity* 2019;27: 1005–1012.

[399] Lydecker JA, et al. Parents have both implicit and explicit biases against children with obesity. *J. Behav. Med.* 2018;41:784–791.

[400] Rand K, et al. "It is not the diet; it is the mental part we need help with." A multilevel analysis of psychological, emotional, and social well-being in obesity. *Int. J. Qual. Stud. Health Well-Being* 2017;12:1306421.

[401] Makowski AC, et al. Social deprivation, gender and obesity: Multiple stigma? Results of a population survey from Germany. *BMJ Open.* 2019;9:e023389.

[402] Nutter S, et al. Weight bias in educational settings: A systematic review. *Curr. Obes. Rep.* 2019;8: 185–200.

[403] Kim TJ, von dem Knesebeck O. Income and obesity: What is the direction of the relationship? A systematic review and meta-analysis. *BMJ Open* 2018;8:e019862.

[404] Tomiyama AJ. Stress and obesity. *Annu. Rev. Psychol.* 2019;70:703–718.

[405] Vartanian LR, Porter AM. Weight stigma and eating behavior: A review of the literature. *Appetite* 2016;102:3–14.

[406] Emmer C, et al. The association between weight stigma and mental health: A meta-analysis. *Obes. Rev.* 2020;21:e12935.

[407] Simone M, et al. Unhealthy weight control behaviors and substance use among adolescent girls: The harms of weight stigma. *Soc. Sci. Med.* 2019;233:64–70.

[408] Phelan SM, et al. Impact of weight bias and stigma on quality of care and outcomes for patients with obesity. *Obes. Rev.* 2015;16:319–326.

[409] Atanasova D, Koteyko N. Obesity frames and counter-frames in British and German online newspapers. *Health* 2017;21:650–669.

[410] Dickins M, et al. Social inclusion and the Fatosphere: The role of an online weblogging community in fostering social inclusion. *Sociol. Health Illn.* 2016;38:797–811.

[411] Hayward LE, Vartanian LR. Potential unintended consequences of graphic warning labels on sugary drinks: Do they promote obesity stigma? *Obes. Sci. Pract.* 2019;5:333–341.

[412] Ramos Salas X, et al. A critical analysis of obesity prevention policies and strategies. *Can. J. Public Health.* 2018;108:e598–e608.

[413] Brady J, Beausoleil N. A response to "A critical analysis of obesity prevention policies and strategies". *Can. J. Public Health.* 2018;108:e630–e632.

[414] Werner S, Roth D. Stigma in the field of intellectual disabilities: Impact and initiatives for change. In: Corrigan PW, ed. The Stigma of Disease and Disability: Understanding Causes and Overcoming Injustices. Washington: American Psychol. Association; 2014. pp. 73–91.

[415] Pelleboer-Gunnink HA, et al. Mainstream health professionals' stigmatising attitudes towards people with intellectual disabilities: A systematic review. *J. Intellect. Disabil. Res.* 2017;61:411–434.

[416] Clapton NE, et al. The role of shame in the development and maintenance of psychological distress in adults with intellectual disabilities: A narrative review and synthesis. *J. Appl. Res. Intellect Disabil.* 2018;31:343–359.

[417] Mitter N, et al. Stigma experienced by families of individuals with intellectual disabilities and autism: A systematic review. *Res. Dev. Disabil.* 2019;89:10–21.

[418] Friedman C. The relationship between disability prejudice and institutionalization of people with intellectual and developmental disabilities. *Intellect. Dev. Disabil.* 2019;57:263–273.

[419] Jahoda A, Markova I. Coping with social stigma: People with intellectual disabilities moving from institutions and family home. *J. Intellect. Disabil. Res.* 2004;48:719–729.

[420] Werner S, Scior K. Interventions aimed at tackling intellectual disability stigma: What works and what still needs to be done. In: Scior K, Werner S, eds. Intellectual Disability and Stigma: Stepping Out From the Margins. London: Palgrave Macmillan; 2016. pp. 129–147.

[421] Schomerus G, et al. The stigma of alcohol dependence compared with other mental disorders: A review of population studies. *Alcohol Alcohol.* 2011;46:105–112.

[422] Yang LH, et al. Stigma and substance use disorders: An international phenomenon. *Curr. Opin. Psychiatry* 2017;30:378–388.

[423] McGinty EE, et al. Portraying mental illness and drug addiction as treatable health conditions: Effects of a randomized experiment on stigma and discrimination. *Soc. Sci. Med.* 2015;126:73–85.

[424] Couto E Cruz C, et al. Mental and physical health correlates of discrimination against people who inject drugs: A systematic review. *J. Stud. Alcohol Drugs* 2018;79:350–360.

[425] Leach CW, Cidam A. When is shame linked to constructive approach orientation? A meta-analysis. *J. Pers. Soc. Psychol.* 2015;109:983–1002.

[426] Luoma JB, et al. Substance use and shame: A systematic and meta-analytic review. *Clin. Psychol. Rev.* 2019;70:1–12.

[427] Randles D, Tracy JL. Nonverbal displays of shame predict relapse and declining health in recovering alcoholics. *Clin. Psychol. Sci.* 2013;1:149–155.

[428] de Saint-Exupéry A. The Little Prince. London: Pan Books; 1974.

[429] Hammarlund R, et al. Review of the effects of self-stigma and perceived social stigma on the treatment-seeking decisions of individuals with drug- and alcohol-use disorders. *Subst. Abuse Rehabil.* 2018;9:115–136.

[430] Crapanzano KA, et al. The association between perceived stigma and substance use disorder treatment outcomes: A review. *Subst. Abuse Rehabil.* 2019;10:1–12.

[431] Burton CL, et al. Does getting stigma under the skin make it thinner? Emotion regulation as a stress-contingent mediator of stigma and mental health. *Clin. Psychol. Sci.* 2018;6:590–600.

[432] Zapolski TCB, et al. Less drinking, yet more problems: Understanding African American drinking and related problems. *Psychol. Bull.* 2014;140:188–223.

[433] van Boekel LC, et al. Stigma among health professionals towards patients with substance use disorders and its consequences for healthcare delivery: Systematic review. *Drug Alcohol Depend.* 2013;131:23–35.

[434] Livingston JD, et al. The effectiveness of interventions for reducing stigma related to substance use disorders: A systematic review. *Addiction* 2012;107:39–50.

[435] Bielenberg J, et al. A systematic review of stigma interventions for providers who treat patients with substance use disorders. *J. Subst. Abuse Treat.* 2021;131:108486.

[436] Luoma JB, et al. Slow and steady wins the race: A randomized clinical trial of acceptance and commitment therapy targeting shame in substance use disorders. *J. Consult. Clin. Psychol.* 2012;80:43–53.

[437] Corrigan PW, et al. Developing a research agenda for reducing the stigma of addictions, part II: Lessons from the mental health stigma literature. *Am. J. Addict.* 2017;26:67–74.

[438] McGinty E, et al. Communication strategies to counter stigma and improve mental illness and substance use disorder policy. *Psychiatr. Serv.* 2018;69:136–146.

[439] Schomerus G, et al. Das Stigma von Suchterkrankungen verstehen und überwinden. *Sucht* 2017; 63:253–259.

[440] Jackson-Best F, Edwards N. Stigma and intersectionality: A systematic review of systematic reviews across HIV/AIDS, mental illness, and physical disability. *BMC Public Health* 2018;18:919.

[441] Zerger S, et al. Differential experiences of discrimination among ethnoracially diverse persons experiencing mental illness and homelessness. *BMC Psychiatry* 2014;14:353.

[442] West ML, et al. The influence of mental illness and criminality self-stigmas and racial self-concept on outcomes in a forensic psychiatric sample. *Psychiatr. Rehabil. J.* 2015;38:150–157.

[443] Price M, et al. The intersectionality of identity-based victimization in adolescence: A person-centered examination of mental health and academic achievement in a U.S. high school. *J. Adolesc.* 2019;76: 185–196.

[444] Staiger T, et al. Intersections of discrimination due to unemployment and mental health problems: The role of double stigma for job- and help-seeking behaviors. *Soc. Psychiatry Psychiatr. Epidemiol.* 2018;53:1091–1098.

[445] Miler JA, et al. Provision of peer support at the intersection of homelessness and problem substance use services: A systematic 'state of the art' review. *BMC Publ. Health* 2020;20:641.

[446] Hatzenbuehler ML, et al. Stigma as a fundamental cause of population health inequalities. *Am. J. Public Health* 2013;103:813–821.

[447] Hinshaw SP. Another Kind of Madness: A Journey Through the Stigma and Hope of Mental Illness. New York: St. Martin's Press; 2017.

[448] Soklaridis S, et al. Where is the family voice? Examining the relational dimensions of the family-healthcare professional and its perceived impact on patient care outcomes in mental health and addictions. *PLoS One* 2019;14:e0215071.

[449] Corrigan PW, et al. Blame, shame, and contamination: The impact of mental illness and drug dependence stigma on family members. *J. Fam. Psychol.* 2006;20:239–246.

[450] Catthoor K, et al. Associative stigma in family members of psychotic patients in Flanders: An exploratory study. *World J. Psychiatry* 2015;5:118–125.

[451] Simpson-Adkins GJ, Daiches A. How do children make sense of their parent's mental health difficulties: A meta-synthesis. *J. Child Fam. Stud.* 2018;27:2705–2716.

[452] Moses T. Stigma and family. In: Corrigan PW, ed. The Stigma of Disease and Disability: Understanding Causes and Overcoming Injustices. Washington: American Psychol. Association; 2014. pp. 247–268.

[453] Riebschleger J, et al. Mental health literacy content for children of parents with a mental illness: Thematic analysis of a literature review. Brain Sci. 2017;7:E141.

[454] Wright A, et al. Evidence-based psychosocial treatment for individuals with early psychosis. Child Adolesc. Psychiatr. Clin. North Am. 2020;29:211–223.

[455] Gorrell S, et al. Family-based treatment of eating disorders: A narrative review. Psychiatr. Clin. North Am. 2019;42:193–204.

[456] Waid J, Kelly M. Supporting family engagement with child and adolescent mental health services: A scoping review. Health Soc. Care Community 2020;28:1333–1342.

[457] Sambrook Smith M, et al. Barriers to accessing mental health services for women with perinatal mental illness: Systematic review and meta-synthesis of qualitative studies in the UK. BMJ Open 2019;9:e024803.

[458] Song J, et al. Health of parents of individuals with developmental disorders or mental health problems: Impacts of stigma. Soc. Sci. Med. 2018;217:152–158.

[459] O'Shay-Wallace S. "We weren't raised that way": Using stigma management communication theory to understand how families manage the stigma of substance abuse. Health Commun. 2020;35:465–474.

[460] Amering M. Trialogue: An exercise in communication between users, carers, and professional mental health workers beyond role stereotypes. In: Gaebel W, Rössler W, Sartorius N, eds. The Stigma of Mental Illness - End of the Story? Cham: Springer; 2017. pp. 581–590.

[461] Barkmann C, Schulte-Markwort M. Prevalence of emotional and behavioural disorders in German children and adolescents: A meta-analysis. J. Epidemiol. Community Health 2012;66:194–203.

[462] Klipker K, et al. Mental health problems in children and adolescents in Germany: Results of the cross-sectional KiGGS Wave 2 study and trends. J. Health Monit. 2018;3:34–41.

[463] Perry BL, et al. Comparison of public attributions, attitudes, and stigma in regard to depression among children and adults. Psychiatr. Serv. 2007;58:632–635.

[464] Mulfinger N, et al. Secrecy versus disclosure of mental illness among adolescents: I. The perspective of adolescents with mental illness. J. Ment. Health. 2019;28:296–303.

[465] Kaushik A, et al. The stigma of mental illness in children and adolescents: A systematic review. Psychiatry Res. 2016;243:469–494.

[466] Moses T. Stigma apprehension among adolescents discharged from brief psychiatric hospitalization. J. Nerv. Ment. Dis. 2011;199:778–789.

[467] Mueller J, et al. Communications to children about mental illness and their role in stigma development: An integrative review. J. Ment. Health 2016;25:62–70.

[468] Ferrie J, et al. Psychosocial outcomes of mental illness stigma in children and adolescents: A mixed-methods systematic review. Child. Youth Serv. Rev. 2020;113:104961.

[469] Yamaguchi S, et al. Mental health literacy programs for school teachers: A systematic review and narrative synthesis. Early Interv. Psychiatry 2020;14:14–25.

[470] Gronholm PC, et al. Stigma related to targeted school-based mental health interventions: A systematic review of qualitative evidence. J. Affect. Disord. 2018;240:17–26.

[471] Hart LM, et al. teen Mental Health First Aid as a school-based intervention for improving peer support of adolescents at risk of suicide: Outcomes from a cluster randomised crossover trial. Aust. N. Z. J. Psychiatry 2020;54:382–392.

[472] Mulfinger N, et al. Honest, open, proud for adolescents with mental illness: Pilot randomized controlled trial. J. Child Psychol. Psychiatry 2018;59:684–691.

[473] Chen SP, et al. Contact in the classroom: Developing a program model for youth mental health contact-based anti-stigma education. Community Ment. Health J. 2016;52:281–293.

[474] International Organization for Migration. World Migration Report 2020. Geneva: IOM; 2019.

[475] UNHCR. The 1951 Convention Relating to the Status of Refugees and Its 1967 Protocol 2011. Available at: www.unhcr.org/about-us/background/4ec262df9/1951-convention-relating-status-refugees-its-1967-protocol.html. Accessed 12 May 2022.

[476] WHO Regional Office for Europe. Mental Health Promotion and Mental Health Care in Refugees and Migrants: Technical Guidance. Copenhagen: WHO; 2018.

[477] Morgan C, et al. Migration, ethnicity and psychoses: Evidence, models and future directions. World Psychiatry 2019;18:247–258.

[478] Bourque F, et al. A meta-analysis of the risk for psychotic disorders among first- and second-generation immigrants. *Psychol. Med.* 2011;41:897–910.

[479] Eylem O, et al. Stigma for common mental disorders in racial minorities and majorities: A systematic review and meta-analysis. *BMC Publ. Health* 2020;20:879.

[480] Satinsky E, et al. Mental health care utilisation and access among refugees and asylum seekers in Europe: A systematic review. *Health Policy* 2019;123:851–863.

[481] Byrow Y, et al. Perceptions of mental health and perceived barriers to mental health help-seeking amongst refugees: A systematic review. *Clin. Psychol. Rev.* 2020;75:101812.

[482] Grupp F, et al. 'Only God can promise healing': Help-seeking intentions and lay beliefs about cures for post-traumatic stress disorder among Sub-Saharan African asylum seekers in Germany. *Eur. J. Psychotraumatol.* 2019;10:1684225.

[483] Makowski AC, von dem Knesebeck O. Depression stigma and migration - results of a survey from Germany. *BMC Psychiatry* 2017;17:381.

[484] Nickerson A, et al. 'Tell Your Story': A randomized controlled trial of an online intervention to reduce mental health stigma and increase help-seeking in refugee men with posttraumatic stress. *Psychol. Med.* 2020;50:781–792.

[485] Ingleby D, et al. The MIPEX Health strand: A longitudinal, mixed-methods survey of policies on migrant health in 38 countries. *Eur. J. Public Health* 2019;29:458–462.

[486] International Organization for Migration. Summary Report on the MIPEX Health Strand and Country Reports. Geneva: IOM; 2016.

[487] Turrini G, et al. Efficacy and acceptability of psychosocial interventions in asylum seekers and refugees: Systematic review and meta-analysis. *Epidemiol. Psychiatr. Sci.* 2019;28:376–388.

[488] Salize HJ. Versorgungsrealität und Versorgungsgerechtigkeit in der Psychiatrie. *Archiv. Wiss. Prax. Soz. Arb.* 2017;4:2–12.

[489] Bennouna C, et al. School-based programs for supporting the mental health and psychosocial wellbeing of adolescent forced migrants in high-income countries: A scoping review. *Soc. Sci. Med.* 2019; 239:112558.

[490] Hynie M. The social determinants of refugee mental health in the post-migration context: A critical review. *Can. J. Psychiatry* 2018;63:297–303.

[491] Gühne U, Riedel-Heller SG. Die Arbeitssituation von Menschen Mit Schweren Psychischen Erkrankungen in Deutschland 2015. Available at: www.dgppn.de/_Resources/Persistent/6f086cca1fce87b992b2514621343930b0c398c5/Expertise_Arbeitssituation_2015-09-14_fin.pdf. Accessed 13 Feb 2020.

[492] Evans-Lacko S, et al. The mental health consequences of the recession: Economic hardship and employment of people with mental health problems in 27 European countries. *PLoS One* 2013;8:e69792.

[493] Techniker Krankenkasse. Gesundheitsreport 2019: Arbeitsunfähigkeiten 2019. Hamburg: TKK; 2019.

[494] Arends I, Baer N, et al. Mental Health and Work: Achieving Well-Integrated Policies and Service Delivery: OECD Social, Employment and Migration Working Papers, No. 161. Paris: OECD Publishing; 2014.

[495] Evans-Lacko S, Knapp M. Global patterns of workplace productivity for people with depression: Absenteeism and presenteeism costs across eight diverse countries. *Soc. Psychiatry Psychiatr. Epidemiol.* 2016;51:1525–1537.

[496] Angermeyer MC, et al. Public attitudes towards people with depression in times of uncertainty: Results from three population surveys in Germany. *Soc. Psychiatry Psychiatr. Epidemiol.* 2013;48:1513–1518.

[497] Mendel R, et al. Managers' reactions towards employees' disclosure of psychiatric or somatic diagnoses. *Epidemiol. Psychiatr. Sci.* 2015;24:146–149.

[498] Baer N. Was ist schwierig an "schwierigen" Mitarbeitern? Arbeitsprobleme und Potentiale bei Menschen mit psychischen Störungen. *Schw. Arch. Neur. Psychiatr.* 2013;164:123–131.

[499] Henderson C, et al. Mental health problems in the workplace: Changes in employers' knowledge, attitudes and practices in England 2006-2010. *Br. J. Psychiatry Suppl.* 2013;55:70–76.

[500] Yoshimura Y, et al. Psychiatric diagnosis and other predictors of experienced and anticipated workplace discrimination and concealment of mental illness among mental health service users in England. *Soc. Psychiatry Psychiatr. Epidemiol.* 2018;53:1099–1109.

[501] Brouwers EPM, et al. Discrimination in the workplace, reported by people with major depressive disorder: A cross-sectional study in 35 countries. *BMJ Open* 2016;6:e009961.

[502] Brohan E, et al. Systematic review of beliefs, behaviours and influencing factors associated with disclosure of a mental health problem in the workplace. *BMC Psychiatry* 2012;12:11.

[503] Hebl M, et al. Modern discrimination in organizations. *Annu. Rev. Organ. Psychol. Organ. Behav.* 2020;7:257–282.

[504] van Laar C, et al. Coping with stigma in the workplace: Understanding the role of threat regulation, supportive factors, and potential hidden costs. *Front. Psychol.* 2019;10:1879.

[505] McDowell C, Fossey E. Workplace accommodations for people with mental illness: A scoping review. *J. Occup. Rehabil.* 2015;25:197–206.

[506] European Commission. The Employment Equality Directive and Supporting People With Psychosocial Disabilities in the Workplace: A Legal Analysis of the Situation in the EU Member States. Luxembourg: Publications Office of the EU; 2016.

[507] Riechert I, Habib E. Betriebliches Eingliederungsmanagement bei Mitarbeitern mit Psychischen Störungen. Heidelberg: Springer; 2017.

[508] Gayed A, et al. Effectiveness of training workplace managers to understand and support the mental health needs of employees: A systematic review and meta-analysis. *Occup. Environ. Med.* 2018;75:462–470.

[509] Hanisch SE, et al. The effectiveness of interventions targeting the stigma of mental illness at the workplace: A systematic review. *BMC Psychiatry* 2016;16:1.

[510] Dobson KS, et al. The Working Mind: A meta-analysis of a workplace mental health and stigma reduction program. *Can. J. Psychiatry* 2019;64:39S–47S.

[511] Corrigan PW, et al. Key ingredients to contact-based stigma change: A cross-validation. *Psychiatr. Rehabil. J.* 2014;37:62–64.

[512] Oschmiansky F, Popp S, et al. Psychisch Kranke im SGB II: Situation und Betreuung (IAB-Forschungs-bericht, 14/2017). Nürnberg: Institut für Arbeitsmarkt- und Berufsforschung; 2017.

[513] Marmot M, Allen J, et al. Fair Society, Healthy Lives - The Marmot Review: Strategic Review of Health Inequalities in England Post-2010. London: The Marmot Review; 2010.

[514] Charette-Dussault É, Corbière M. An integrative review of the barriers to job acquisition for people with severe mental illnesses. *J. Nerv. Ment. Dis.* 2019;207:523–537.

[515] Henderson C, et al. Decision aid on disclosure of mental health status to an employer: Feasibility and outcomes of a randomised controlled trial. *Br. J. Psychiatry* 2013;203:350–357.

[516] Pinto AD, et al. Employment interventions in health settings: A systematic review and synthesis. *Ann. Fam. Med.* 2018;16:447–460.

[517] Rüsch N, et al. Efficacy of a peer-led group program for unemployed people with mental health problems: Pilot randomized controlled trial. *Int. J. Soc. Psychiatry* 2019;65:333–337.

[518] Richter D, Hoffmann H. Effectiveness of supported employment in non-trial routine implementation: Systematic review and meta-analysis. *Soc. Psychiatry Psychiatr. Epidemiol.* 2019;54:525–531.

[519] Nuechterlein KH, et al. Enhancing return to work or school after a first episode of schizophrenia: The UCLA RCT of individual placement and support and workplace fundamentals module training. *Psychol. Med.* 2020;50:20–28.

[520] Read H, et al. Early intervention in mental health for adolescents and young adults: A systematic review. *Am. J. Occup. Ther.* 2018;72:7205190040.

[521] Corrigan PW, et al. Strengths and challenges of peer coaches for supported education in colleges and universities. *Psychiatr. Rehabil. J.* 2020;43:175–178.

[522] Hoffmann H, et al. Long-term effectiveness of supported employment: 5-year follow-up of a randomized controlled trial. *Am. J. Psychiatry* 2014;171:1183–1190.

[523] Busch-Geertsema V, Henke J, Steffen A. Entstehung, Verlauf und Struktur von Wohnungslosigkeit und Strategien zu ihrer Vermeidung und Behebung: Ergebnisbericht. Berlin: Bundesministerium für Arbeit und Soziales; 2019.

[524] Busch-Geertsema V. Wohnungslosigkeit in Deutschland aus europäischer Perspektive. In: Bundeszentrale für Politische Bildung, ed. Aus Politik und Zeitgeschichte: Wohnungslosigkeit. Bonn; 2018. pp. 15–22.

[525] Fazel S, et al. The health of homeless people in high-income countries: Descriptive epidemiology, health consequences, and clinical and policy recommendations. *Lancet* 2014;384:1529–1540.

[526] Sundin EC, Baguley T. Prevalence of childhood abuse among people who are homeless in Western countries: A systematic review and meta-analysis. *Soc. Psychiatry Psychiatr. Epidemiol.* 2015;50:183–194.

[527] Ayano G, et al. Suicidal ideation and attempt among homeless people: A systematic review and meta-analysis. *Psychiatr. Q.* 2019;90:829–842.

[528] Tsai J, Huang M. Systematic review of psychosocial factors associated with evictions. *Health Soc. Care Community* 2019;27:e1–e9.

[529] Singh A, et al. Housing disadvantage and poor mental health: A systematic review. *Am. J. Prev. Med.* 2019;57:262–272.

[530] Petit J, et al. European public perceptions of homelessness: A knowledge, attitudes and practices survey. *PLoS One* 2019;14:e0221896.

[531] Heitmeyer W, ed. Deutsche Zustände: Folge 10. 4th ed. Berlin: Suhrkamp; 2016.

[532] Bhui K, et al. Homelessness and mental illness: A literature review and a qualitative study of perceptions of the adequacy of care. *Int. J. Soc. Psychiatry* 2006;52:152–165.

[533] Manning RM, Greenwood RM. Recovery in homelessness: The influence of choice and mastery on physical health, psychiatric symptoms, alcohol and drug use, and community integration. *Psychiatr. Rehabil. J.* 2019;42:147–157.

[534] Hwang SW, Burns T. Health interventions for people who are homeless. *Lancet* 2014;384:1541–1547.

[535] Omerov P, et al. Homeless persons' experiences of health- and social care: A systematic integrative review. *Health Soc. Care Community* 2020;28:1–11.

[536] Canavan R, et al. Service provision and barriers to care for homeless people with mental health problems across 14 European capital cities. *BMC Health Serv. Res.* 2012;12:222.

[537] Pahwa R, et al. The ties that bind and unbound ties: Experiences of formerly homeless individuals in recovery from serious mental illness and substance use. *Qual. Health Res.* 2019;29:1313–1323.

[538] Corrigan PW, et al. Using peer navigators to address the integrated health care needs of homeless African Americans with serious mental illness. *Psychiatr. Serv.* 2017;68:264–270.

[539] Montgomery AE, et al. Rethinking homelessness prevention among persons with serious mental illness. *Soc. Issues Policy Rev.* 2013;7:58–82.

[540] Salize HJ, et al. Verbesserung der psychiatrischen Behandlungsprävalenz bei Risikopersonen vor dem Abrutschen in die Wohnungslosigkeit. *Psychiatr. Prax.* 2017;44:21–28.

[541] Bhugra D, ed. Urban Mental Health. Oxford: Oxford University Press; 2019.

[542] Stewart JL. The ghettoization of persons with severe mental illnesses. *Ment. Health Soc. Incl.* 2019;23:53–57.

[543] Richter D, Hoffmann H. Preference for independent housing of persons with mental disorders: Systematic review and meta-analysis. *Adm. Policy Ment. Health* 2017;44:817–823.

[544] Richter D, Hoffmann H. Independent housing and support for people with severe mental illness: Systematic review. *Acta Psychiatr. Scand.* 2017;136:269–279.

[545] Stergiopoulos V, et al. Long-term effects of rent supplements and mental health support services on housing and health outcomes of homeless adults with mental illness: Extension study of the At Home/Chez Soi randomised controlled trial. *Lancet Psychiatry* 2019;6:915–925.

[546] Baxter AJ, et al. Effects of housing first approaches on health and well-being of adults who are homeless or at risk of homelessness: Systematic review and meta-analysis of randomised controlled trials. *J. Epidemiol. Community Health* 2019;73:379–387.

[547] Becker T, Hoffmann H, et al. Versorgungsmodelle in Psychiatrie und Psychotherapie. Stuttgart: Kohlhammer; 2008.

[548] Hinshaw SP, Stier A. Stigma as related to mental disorders. *Annu. Rev. Clin. Psychol.* 2008;4:367–393.

[549] Liu NH, et al. Excess mortality in persons with severe mental disorders: A multilevel intervention framework and priorities for clinical practice, policy and research agendas. *World Psychiatry* 2017;16:30–40.

[550] Lancet. The health crisis of mental health stigma. *Lancet* 2016;387:1027.

[551] Perry A, et al. Stigmatisation of those with mental health conditions in the acute general hospital setting. A qualitative framework synthesis. *Soc. Sci. Med.* 2020;255:112974.

[552] Vistorte AOR, et al. Stigmatizing attitudes of primary care professionals towards people with mental disorders: A systematic review. *Int. J. Psychiatry Med.* 2018;53:317–338.

[553] Stone EM, et al. General medical clinicians' attitudes toward people with serious mental illness: A scoping review. *J. Behav. Health Serv. Res.* 2019;46:656–679.

[554] Druss BG, et al. Mental disorders and use of cardiovascular procedures after myocardial infarction. *JAMA* 2000;283:506–511.

[555] van Nieuwenhuizen A, et al. Emergency department staff views and experiences on diagnostic overshadowing related to people with mental illness. *Epidemiol. Psychiatr. Sci.* 2013;22:255–262.

[556] Henderson C, et al. Mental health-related stigma in health care and mental health-care settings. *Lancet Psychiatry* 2014;1:467–482.

[557] Nordt C, et al. Attitudes of mental health professionals toward people with schizophrenia and major depression. *Schizophr. Bull.* 2006;32:709–714.

[558] Valery KM, Prouteau A. Schizophrenia stigma in mental health professionals and associated factors: A systematic review. *Psychiatry Res.* 2020;290:113068.

[559] Sweeney A, et al. The role of fear in mental health service users' experiences: A qualitative exploration. *Soc. Psychiatry Psychiatr. Epidemiol.* 2015;50:1079–1087.

[560] Harangozo J, et al. Stigma and discrimination against people with schizophrenia related to medical services. *Int. J. Soc. Psychiatry* 2014;60:359–366.

[561] Stovell D, et al. Shared treatment decision-making and empowerment-related outcomes in psychosis: Systematic review and meta-analysis. *Br. J. Psychiatry* 2016;209:23–28.

[562] Hamann J, et al. Self-stigma and consumer participation in shared decision making in mental health services. *Psychiatr. Serv.* 2017;68:783–788.

[563] Schmidbauer W. Hilflose Helfer: Über die Seelische Problematik der Helfenden Berufe. 21st ed. Reinbek: Rowohlt; 2018.

[564] Riley R, et al. 'Treading water but drowning slowly': What are GPs' experiences of living and working with mental illness and distress in England? A qualitative study. *BMJ Open* 2018;8:e018620.

[565] Fink-Miller EL, Nestler LM. Suicide in physicians and veterinarians: Risk factors and theories. *Curr. Opin. Psychol.* 2018;22:23–26.

[566] Ventriglio A, et al. Suicide among doctors: A narrative review. *Indian J. Psychiatr.* 2020;62:114–120.

[567] Tay S, et al. Mental health problems among clinical psychologists: Stigma and its impact on disclosure and help-seeking. *J. Clin. Psychol.* 2018;74:1545–1555.

[568] Adams EFM, et al. What stops us from healing the healers: A survey of help-seeking behaviour, stigmatisation and depression within the medical profession. *Int. J. Soc. Psychiatry* 2010;56:359–370.

[569] Vayr F, et al. Barriers to seeking help for physicians with substance use disorder: A review. *Drug Alcohol Depend.* 2019;199:116–121.

[570] Bhugra D, et al. EPA guidance on how to improve the image of psychiatry and of the psychiatrist. *Eur. Psychiatry* 2015;30:423–430.

[571] Angermeyer MC, et al. Public attitudes towards psychiatry and psychiatric treatment at the beginning of the 21st century: A systematic review and meta-analysis of population surveys. *World Psychiatry* 2017;16:50–61.

[572] Knaak S, Patten S. A grounded theory model for reducing stigma in health professionals in Canada. *Acta Psychiatr. Scand.* 2016;134:53–62.

[573] Winkler P, et al. Short video interventions to reduce mental health stigma: A multi-centre randomised controlled trial in nursing high schools. *Soc Psychiatry Psychiatr. Epidemiol.* 2017;52:1549–1557.

[574] Deb T, et al. Responding to experienced and anticipated discrimination (READ): Anti-stigma training for medical students towards patients with mental illness - study protocol for an international multisite non-randomised controlled study. *BMC Med. Educ.* 2019;19:41.

[575] Lebowitz MS, Ahn WK. Using personification and agency reorientation to reduce mental-health clinicians' stigmatizing attitudes toward patients. *Stigma Health* 2016;1:176–184.

[576] Helmus K, et al. Decreasing stigmatization: Reducing the discrepancy between "us" and "them" - an intervention for mental health care professionals. *Front. Psychiatry* 2019;10:243.

[577] Mutschler C, et al. Transition experiences following psychiatric hospitalization: A systematic review of the literature. *Community Ment. Health J.* 2019;55:1255–1274.

[578] Steinhart I, Wienberg G, eds. Rundum ambulant: Funktionales Basismodell psychiatrischer Versorgung in der Gemeinde. Köln: Psychiatrie Verlag; 2017.

[579] Rössler W, Melchinger H. Die ambulante Soziotherapie nach § 37a SGB V ist gescheitert. *Psychiatr. Prax.* 2012;39:106–107.

[580] Gaebel W, Hasan A, Falkai P. (DGPPN) S3-Leitlinie Schizophrenie. Berlin: Springer; 2019.

[581] McGinty EE, et al. Quality of medical care for persons with serious mental illness: A comprehensive review. *Schizophr. Res.* 2015;165:227–235.

[582] Bongiorno DM, et al. Comorbid psychiatric disease is associated with lower rates of thrombolysis in ischemic stroke. *Stroke* 2018;49:738–740.

[583] Hoffmann-Donner H. Auf heiteren Pfaden: Gesammelte Gedichte. 2nd ed. Frankfurt: Literarische Anstalt Rütten & Löning; 1873.

[584] Chrysikou E. Psychiatric institutions and the physical environment: Combining medical architecture methodologies and architectural morphology to increase our understanding. *J. Healthc. Eng.* 2019; 2019:4076259.

[585] Jovanović N, et al. How to design psychiatric facilities to foster positive social interaction: A systematic review. *Eur. Psychiatry* 2019;60:49–62.

[586] Liddicoat S. Designing a supportive emergency department environment for people with self harm and suicidal ideation: A scoping review. *Australas. Emerg. Care* 2019;22:139–148.

[587] Friedrich-Ebert-Stiftung. Es ist Zeit für einen neuen Aufbruch! Handlungsbedarfe zur Reform der psychosozialen Versorgung 44 Jahre nach der Psychiatrie-Enquete. Bonn: Friedrich-Ebert-Stiftung; 2019.

[588] Firth J, et al. The Lancet Psychiatry Commission: A blueprint for protecting physical health in people with mental illness. *Lancet Psychiatry* 2019;6:675–712.

[589] Deister A, Wilms B. Regionale Verantwortung übernehmen: Modellprojekte in Psychiatrie und Psychotherapie nach §64b SGB V. Köln: Psychiatrie Verlag; 2014.

[590] Ebert DD, Cuijpers P. It is time to invest in the prevention of depression. *JAMA Netw. Open* 2018;1:e180335.

[591] Rüsch N, Thornicroft G. Does stigma impair prevention of mental disorders? *Br J Psychiatry* 2014;204:249–251.

[592] Embry DD. Behavioral vaccines and evidence-based kernels: Nonpharmaceutical approaches for the prevention of mental, emotional, and behavioral disorders. *Psychiatr. Clin. North Am.* 2011;34:1–34.

[593] Prinz RJ, et al. Population-based prevention of child maltreatment: The U.S. Triple P System Population Trial. *Prev. Sci.* 2009;10:1–12.

[594] Gilbert R, et al. Burden and consequences of child maltreatment in high-income countries. *Lancet* 2009;373:68–81.

[595] Furlong M, et al. Cochrane review: Behavioural and cognitive-behavioural group-based parenting programmes for early-onset conduct problems in children aged 3 to 12 years. *Evid. Based Child Health* 2013;8:318–692.

[596] Ormel J, et al. Prevention of depression will only succeed when it is structurally embedded and targets big determinants. *World Psychiatry* 2019;18:111–112.

[597] Buck-Zerchin DS. Auf der Spur des Morgensterns: Psychose als Selbstfindung. Neumünster, Norderstedt: Paranus Verlag, Anne Fischer Verlag; 2005.

[598] Utschakowski J, Sielaff G, Bock T, Winter A, eds. Experten aus Erfahrung: Peerarbeit in der Psychiatrie. Köln: Psychiatrie Verlag; 2016.

[599] Shalaby RAH, Agyapong VIO. Peer support in mental health: Literature review. *JMIR Ment. Health* 2020;7:e15572.

[600] Burke E, et al. The effects of peer support on empowerment, self-efficacy, and internalized stigma: A narrative synthesis and meta-analysis. *Stigma Health* 2019;4:337–356.

[601] Johnson S, et al. Peer-supported self-management for people discharged from a mental health crisis team: A randomised controlled trial. *Lancet* 2018;392:409–418.

[602] Chien WT, et al. Peer support for people with schizophrenia or other serious mental illness. *Cochrane Database Syst. Rev.* 2019;4:CD010880.

[603] Cabassa LJ, et al. Peer-based health interventions for people with serious mental illness: A systematic literature review. *J. Psychiatr. Res.* 2017;84:80–89.

[604] Ibrahim N, et al. A systematic review of influences on implementation of peer support work for adults with mental health problems. *Soc Psychiatry Psychiatr. Epidemiol.* 2020;55:285–293.

[605] Gillard S. Peer support in mental health services: Where is the research taking us, and do we want to go there? *J. Ment. Health* 2019;28:341–344.

[606] Gerlinger G, et al. Nach der Reform ist vor der Reform: Ergebnisse der Novellierungsprozesse der Psychisch-Kranken-Hilfe-Gesetze der Bundesländer. *Nervenarzt* 2019;90:45–57.

[607] Priebe S. Involuntary hospitalization of suicidal patients: Time for new answers to basic questions? *Am. J. Bioeth.* 2019;19:90–92.

[608] Sheridan Rains L, et al. Variations in patterns of involuntary hospitalisation and in legal frameworks: An international comparative study. *Lancet Psychiatry* 2019;6:403–417.

[609] Wahl OF. Media Madness: Public Images of Mental Illness. New Brunswick: Rutgers University Press; 1995.

[610] Morris G. Mental Health Issues and the Media: An Introduction for Health Professionals. London: Routledge; 2006.

[611] Signorielli N. The stigma of mental illness on television. *J. Broadcast. Electron. Media* 1989;33:325–331.

[612] Fahmüller E-M. Geniale Psychopathen - labile Kommissare: Figuren mit psychischen Störungen im aktuellen deutschen Krimi. Berlin: Master School Drehbuch Edition; 2018.

[613] Goodwin J. The horror of stigma: Psychosis and mental health care environments in twenty-first-century horror film (part II). *Perspect. Psychiatr. Care* 2014;50:224–234.

[614] Stollfuß S. Zwischen Stigmatisierung und Differenzierung: Krankheit in Filmen und Fernsehserien. In: Bundeszentrale für Politische Bildung, ed. Aus Politik und Zeitgeschichte: Krankheit und Gesellschaft. Bonn; 2018. pp. 36–40.

[615] Angermeyer MC, et al. Media consumption and desire for social distance towards people with schizophrenia. *Eur. Psychiatry* 2005;20:246–250.

[616] Hoffmann-Richter U. Psychiatrie in der Zeitung: Urteile und Vorurteile. Bonn: Ed. Das Narrenschiff; 2000.

[617] Kroll M, et al. Die Darstellung der Depression in deutschen Tageszeitungen - Eine Trendanalyse. *Psychiatr. Prax.* 2003;30:367–371.

[618] Whitley R, Wang J. Good news? A longitudinal analysis of newspaper portrayals of mental illness in Canada 2005 to 2015. *Can. J. Psychiatry* 2017;62:278–285.

[619] Anderson C, et al. Changes in newspaper coverage of mental illness from 2008 to 2016 in England. *Epidemiol. Psychiatr. Sci.* 2020;29:e9.

[620] Dietrich S, et al. Influence of newspaper reporting on adolescents' attitudes toward people with mental illness. *Soc. Psychiatry Psychiatr. Epidemiol.* 2006;41:318–322.

[621] Schomerus G, et al. Impact of the Germanwings plane crash on mental illness stigma: Results from two population surveys in Germany before and after the incident. *World Psychiatry* 2015;14:362–363.

[622] von dem Knesebeck O, et al. Changes in depression stigma after the Germanwings crash - findings from German population surveys. *J. Affect. Disord.* 2015;186:261–265.

[623] Alvarez-Mon MA, et al. Areas of interest and stigmatic attitudes of the general public in five relevant medical conditions: Thematic and quantitative analysis using Twitter. *J. Med. Internet Res.* 2019;21:e14110.

[624] Miller BJ, et al. How connected are people with schizophrenia? Cell phone, computer, email, and social media use. *Psychiatry Res.* 2015;225:458–463.

[625] Robinson P, et al. Measuring attitudes towards mental health using social media: Investigating stigma and trivialisation. *Soc. Psychiatry Psychiatr. Epidemiol.* 2019;54:51–58.

[626] Naslund JA, et al. Naturally occurring peer support through social media: The experiences of individuals with severe mental illness using YouTube. *PLoS One* 2014;9:e110171.

[627] Smith-Merry J, et al. Social connection and online engagement: Insights from interviews with users of a mental health online forum. *JMIR Ment. Health* 2019;6:e11084.

[628] Sangeorzan I, et al. Exploring the experiences of people vlogging about severe mental illness on YouTube: An interpretative phenomenological analysis. *J. Affect. Disord.* 2019;246:422–428.

[629] Jakubowska A, et al. Internet use for social interaction by people with psychosis: A systematic review. *Cyberpsychol. Behav. Soc. Netw.* 2019;22:336–343.

[630] Naslund JA, et al. The future of mental health care: Peer-to-peer support and social media. *Epidemiol. Psychiatr. Sci.* 2016;25:113–122.

[631] Naslund JA, Aschbrenner KA. Risks to privacy with use of social media: Understanding the views of social media users with serious mental illness. *Psychiatr. Serv.* 2019;70:561–568.

[632] de Choudhury M, De S. Mental health discourse on reddit: Self-disclosure, social support, and anonymity. In: AAAI Press, ed. Proceedings of the Eighth International AAAI Conference on Weblogs and Social Media. Palo Alto; 2014. pp. 71–80.

[633] Royal Society for Public Health. #StatusOfMind: Social media and young people's mental health and wellbeing 2017. Available at: www.rsph.org.uk/our-work/campaigns/status-of-mind.html. Accessed 17 Feb 2020.

[634] Pagoto S, et al. A call for a public health agenda for social media research. *J. Med. Internet Res.* 2019;21:e16661.

[635] Ferrari M, et al. Gaming with stigma: Analysis of messages about mental illnesses in video games. *JMIR Ment. Health* 2019;6:e12418.

[636] Baumann A, et al. Das Bild psychisch Kranker im Spielfilm: Auswirkungen auf Wissen, Einstellungen und soziale Distanz am Beispiel des Films "Das weisse Rauschen". *Psychiatr. Prax.* 2003;30:372–378.

[637] Ritterfeld U, Jin SA. Addressing media stigma for people experiencing mental illness using an entertainment-education strategy. *J. Health Psychol.* 2006;11:247–267.

[638] Eder J. Depressionsdarstellung und Zuschauergefühle im Film. In: Poppe S, ed. Emotionen in Literatur und Film. Würzburg: Königshausen & Neumann; 2012. pp. 219–245.

[639] Fuchs T. Temporality and psychopathology. *Phenomenol. Cogn. Sci.* 2013;12:75–104.

[640] Corrigan PW, et al. The effects of news stories on the stigma of mental illness. *J. Nerv. Ment. Dis.* 2013;201:179–182.

[641] Happer C, Philo G. The role of the media in the construction of public belief and social change. *J. Soc. Polit. Psychol.* 2013;1:321–336.

[642] Corrigan PW, et al. Newspaper stories as measures of structural stigma. *Psychiatr. Serv.* 2005;56: 551–556.

[643] Goepfert NC, et al. Effects of stigmatizing media coverage on stigma measures, self-esteem, and affectivity in persons with depression - an experimental controlled trial. *BMC Psychiatry* 2019;19:138.

[644] Maier JA, et al. Media influences on self-stigma of seeking psychological services: The importance of media portrayals and person perception. *Psychol. Pop. Media Cult.* 2014;3:239–256.

[645] Ross AM, et al. A systematic review of the impact of media reports of severe mental illness on stigma and discrimination, and interventions that aim to mitigate any adverse impact. *Soc. Psychiatry Psychiatr. Epidemiol.* 2019;54:11–31.

[646] Till B, et al. Associations of tabloid newspaper use with endorsement of suicide myths, suicide-related knowledge, and stigmatizing attitudes toward suicidal individuals. *Crisis* 2018;39:428–437.

[647] Lutter M, et al. Anomie or imitation? The Werther effect of celebrity suicides on suicide rates in 34 OECD countries, 1960-2014. *Soc. Sci. Med.* 2020;246:112755.

[648] Whitley R, et al. Suicide mortality in Canada after the death of Robin Williams, in the context of high-fidelity to suicide reporting guidelines in the Canadian media. *Can. J. Psychiatry* 2019;64:805–812.

[649] Schäfer M, Quiring O. Gibt es Hinweise auf einen "Enke-Effekt"? Die Presseberichterstattung über den Suizid von Robert Enke und die Entwicklung der Suizidzahlen in Deutschland. *Publizistik* 2013;58:141–160.

[650] Niederkrotenthaler T, et al. Association of increased youth suicides in the United States with the release of 13 Reasons Why. *JAMA Psychiatry* 2019;76:933–940.

[651] Till B, et al. Determining the effects of films with suicidal content: A laboratory experiment. *Br. J. Psychiatry* 2015;207:72–78.

[652] Niederkrotenthaler T, Till B. Effects of suicide awareness materials on individuals with recent suicidal ideation or attempt: Online randomised controlled trial. *Br. J. Psychiatry* 2020;217:693–700.

[653] Pirkis J, et al. Suicide prevention media campaigns: A systematic literature review. *Health Commun.* 2019;34:402–414.

[654] Niederkrotenthaler T, et al. Celebrity suicide on Twitter: Activity, content and network analysis related to the death of Swedish DJ Tim Bergling alias Avicii. *J. Affect. Disord.* 2019;245:848–855.

[655] Shanahan N, et al. Self-harm and social media: Thematic analysis of images posted on three social media sites. *BMJ Open* 2019;9:e027006.

[656] Brown RC, et al. #cutting: Non-suicidal self-injury (NSSI) on Instagram. *Psychol. Med.* 2018;48: 337–346.

[657] Lavis A, Winter R. #Online harms or benefits? An ethnographic analysis of the positives and negatives of peer-support around self-harm on social media. *J. Child Psychol. Psychiatry* 2020;61:842–854.

[658] Paul E, et al. Has information on suicide methods provided via the Internet negatively impacted suicide rates? *PLoS One* 2017;12:e0190136.

[659] Till B, Niederkrotenthaler T. Surfing for suicide methods and help: Content analysis of websites retrieved with search engines in Austria and the United States. *J. Clin. Psychiatry* 2014;75:886–892.

[660] Henderson L. Selling suffering: Mental illness and media values. In: Philo G, ed. Media and Mental Distress. London/New York: Longman; 1996. pp. 18–36.

[661] Mueller AS. Does the media matter to suicide? Examining the social dynamics surrounding media reporting on suicide in a suicide-prone community. *Soc. Sci. Med.* 2017;180:152–159.

[662] Gilman SL. Seeing the Insane. Lincoln and London: University of Nebraska Press; 1996.

[663] Merke F. History and Iconography of Endemic Goitre and Cretinism. Lancaster: MTP; 1984.

[664] Gilman SL. Disease and Representation: Images of Illness From Madness to AIDS. Ithaca: Cornell University Press; 1988.

[665] WHO, Dept. of Mental Health and Substance Abuse, International Association for Suicide Prevention (IASP). Preventing Suicide: A Resource for Media Professionals. Geneva: WHO; 2008.

[666] Maiorano A, et al. Reducing stigma in media professionals: Is there room for improvement? Results from a systematic review. *Can. J. Psychiatry* 2017;62:702–715.

[667] Carmichael V, et al. Media coverage of mental illness: A comparison of citizen journalism vs. professional journalism portrayals. *J. Ment. Health* 2019;28:520–526.

[668] Rawls J. A Theory of Justice. Cambridge, Mass: Harvard Univ. Press; 1999.

[669] Sen A. Commodities and Capabilities. New Delhi: Oxford University Press; 2018.

[670] Davidson L, et al. A capabilities approach to mental health transformation: A conceptual framework for the recovery era. *Can. J. Commun. Ment. Health* 2009;28:35–46.

[671] Höffe O. Democracy in An Age of Globalisation. Berlin, Heidelberg: Springer; 2007.

[672] Corrigan PW, Al-Khouja MA. Reactions to solidarity versus normalcy messages for antistigma campaigns. *J. Nerv. Ment. Dis.* 2019;207:1001–1004.

[673] Aichele V, Althoff N. Nicht-Diskriminierung und angemessene Vorkehrungen in der UN-Behindertenrechtskonvention. In: Welke A, ed. UN-Behindertenrechtskonvention mit rechtlichen Erläuterungen. Berlin: Dt. Verein für öffentliche u. private Fürsorge; 2012. pp. 104–118.

[674] WHO Regional Office for Europe. Mental Health, Human Rights and Standards of Care: Assessment of the Quality of Institutional Care for Adults With Psychosocial and Intellectual Disabilities in the WHO European Region. Copenhagen: WHO; 2018.

[675] von Boetticher A. Das neue Teilhaberecht. 2nd ed. Baden-Baden: Nomos; 2020.

[676] BMAS. Studie zum aktiven und passiven Wahlrecht von Menschen mit Behinderung: Forschungsbericht 470. Berlin: Bundesministerium für Arbeit und Soziales; 2016.

[677] Bhugra D, et al. Mental illness and the right to vote: A review of legislation across the world. *Int. Rev. Psychiatry* 2016;28:395–399.

[678] Corrigan PW. Where is the evidence supporting public service announcements to eliminate mental illness stigma? *Psychiatr. Serv.* 2012;63:79–82.

[679] Klerings I, et al. Information overload in healthcare: Too much of a good thing? *Z. Evid. Fortbild. Qual. Gesundhwes.* 2015;109:285–290.

[680] Khaleel I, et al. Health information overload among health consumers: A scoping review. *Patient Educ. Couns.* 2020;103:15–32.

[681] Nyhan B, et al. Effective messages in vaccine promotion: A randomized trial. *Pediatrics* 2014;133:e835–e842.

[682] Schomerus G, et al. An online intervention using information on the mental health-mental illness continuum to reduce stigma. *Eur. Psychiatry* 2016;32:21–27.

[683] Violeau L, et al. How continuum beliefs can reduce stigma of schizophrenia: The role of perceived similarities. *Schizophr. Res.* 2020;220:46–53.

[684] Romme M. Living With Voices: 50 Stories of Recovery. Ross on Wye: PCCS Books/Birmingham City Univ.; 2009.

[685] Paluck EL, Green DP. Prejudice reduction: What works? A review and assessment of research and practice. *Annu Rev Psychol.* 2009;60:339–367.

[686] Nous Group. Independent Evaluation of Beyondblue 2014. Available at: www.beyondblue.org.au/docs/default-source/research-project-files/bw0265.pdf. Accessed 10 Jan 2020.

[687] Corrigan PW, et al. Examining the impact of public service announcements on help seeking and stigma: Results of a randomized controlled trial. *J. Nerv. Ment. Dis.* 2015;203:836–842.

[688] Evans-Lacko S, et al. Influence of time to change's social marketing interventions on stigma in England 2009-2011. *Br. J. Psychiatry Suppl.* 2013;55:S77–S88.

[689] Henderson C, et al. Relationships between anti-stigma programme awareness, disclosure comfort and intended help-seeking regarding a mental health problem. *Br. J. Psychiatry* 2017;211:316–322.

[690] Collins RL, et al. Social marketing of mental health treatment: California's mental illness stigma reduction campaign. *Am. J. Public Health* 2019;109:S228–S235.

[691] Makowski AC, et al. Changes in beliefs and attitudes toward people with depression and schizophrenia: Results of a public campaign in Germany. *Psychiatry Res.* 2016;237:271–278.

[692] Kohls E, et al. Public attitudes toward depression and help-seeking: Impact of the OSPI-Europe depression awareness campaign in four European regions. *J. Affect. Disord.* 2017;217:252–259.

[693] Morgan AJ, et al. Systematic review and meta-analysis of Mental Health First aid training: Effects on knowledge, stigma, and helping behaviour. *PLoS One* 2018;13:e0197102.

[694] Forthal S, et al. Mental Health First Aid: A systematic review of trainee behavior and recipient mental health outcomes. *Psychiatr. Serv.* 2022;73:439–446.

[695] Brijnath B, et al. Do web-based mental health literacy interventions improve the mental health literacy of adult consumers? Results from a systematic review. *J. Med. Internet Res.* 2016;18:e165.

[696] Corrigan PW, et al. Challenging the public stigma of mental illness: A meta-analysis of outcome studies. *Psychiatr. Serv.* 2012;63:963–973.

[697] Morgan AJ, et al. Interventions to reduce stigma towards people with severe mental illness: Systematic review and meta-analysis. *J. Psychiatr. Res.* 2018;103:120–133.

[698] Link BG, et al. A school-based intervention for mental illness stigma: A cluster randomized trial. *Pediatrics* 2020;145:e20190780.

[699] Koike S, et al. Effect of name change of schizophrenia on mass media between 1985 and 2013 in Japan: A text data mining analysis. *Schizophr. Bull.* 2016;42:552–559.

[700] Chen HC, et al. Renaming schizophrenia alone has not altered negative wording in newspaper articles: A text-mining finding in Taiwan. *Psychiatry Clin. Neurosci.* 2019;73:594–595.

[701] Corrigan PW, et al. Three strategies for changing attributions about severe mental illness. *Schizophr. Bull.* 2001;27:187–195.

[702] Pettigrew TF, et al. Recent advances in intergroup contact theory. *Int. J. Intercult. Relat.* 2011;35:271–280.

[703] Turner RN, et al. Reducing explicit and implicit outgroup prejudice via direct and extended contact: The mediating role of self-disclosure and intergroup anxiety. *J. Pers. Soc. Psychol.* 2007;93:369–388.

[704] Maunder RD, White FA. Intergroup contact and mental health stigma: A comparative effectiveness meta-analysis. *Clin. Psychol. Rev.* 2019;72:101749.

[705] Jorm AF. Effect of contact-based interventions on stigma and discrimination: A critical examination of the evidence. *Psychiatr. Serv.* 2020;71:735–737.

[706] Miles E, Crisp RJ. A meta-analytic test of the imagined contact hypothesis. *Group Process Intergroup Relat.* 2014;17:3–26.

[707] West K, et al. Enhancing imagined contact to reduce prejudice against people with schizophrenia. *Group Process Intergroup Relat.* 2011;14:407–428.

[708] Janoušková M, et al. Can video interventions be used to effectively destigmatize mental illness among young people? A systematic review. *Eur. Psychiatry* 2017;41:1–9.

[709] Martínez-Hidalgo MN, et al. Social contact as a strategy for self-stigma reduction in young adults and adolescents with mental health problems. *Psychiatry Res.* 2018;260:443–450.

[710] Reimer NK, et al. Intergroup contact and social change: Implications of negative and positive contact for collective action in advantaged and disadvantaged groups. *Pers. Soc. Psychol. Bull.* 2017;43:121–136.

[711] Corrigan PW, et al. The California schedule of key ingredients for contact-based antistigma programs. *Psychiatr. Rehabil. J.* 2013;36:173–179.

[712] Corrigan PW. Strategic Stigma Change (SSC): Five principles for social marketing campaigns meant to erase the prejudice and discrimination of mental illness. *Psychiatr. Serv.* 2011;62:824–826.

[713] Conrad I, et al. Präventiv und stigmareduzierend? Evaluation des Schulprojekts "Verrückt? Na und!". *Z. Psychiatr. Psychol. Psychother.* 2010;58:257–264.

[714] Wechsler D, et al. Effects of contact-based, short term anti-stigma training for medical students: Results from a randomized controlled trial. *Neuropsychiatr.* 2020;34:66–73.

[715] Bock T, et al. Was macht die Seele im Knast? Trialogische Fortbildung zum Thema psychischer Gesundheit/Krankheit für werdende Justizvollzugsbeamte. *Recht. Psychiatrie.* 2019;37:20–25.

[716] Gaebel W, et al. Promoting stigma coping and empowerment in patients with schizophrenia and depression: Results of a cluster-RCT. *Eur. Arch. Psychiatry Clin. Neurosci.* 2020;270:501–511.

[717] Lucksted A, et al. Outcomes of a psychoeducational intervention to reduce internalized stigma among psychosocial rehabilitation clients. *Psychiatr. Serv.* 2017;68:360–367.

[718] Alonso M, et al. Interventions to reduce internalized stigma in individuals with mental illness: A systematic review. *Span. J. Psychol.* 2019;22:e27.

[719] Yanos PT, et al. A randomized-controlled trial of treatment for self-stigma among persons diagnosed with schizophrenia-spectrum disorders. *Soc. Psychiatry Psychiatr. Epidemiol.* 2019;54:1363–1378.

[720] Han CS, Oliffe JL. Photovoice in mental illness research: A review and recommendations. *Health* 2016;20:110–126.

[721] Fleming J, et al. An ethnographic approach to interpreting a mental illness photovoice exhibit. *Arch. Psychiatr. Nurs.* 2009;23:16–24.

[722] Molloy JK. Photovoice as a tool for social justice workers. *J. Progress Hum. Serv.* 2007;18:39–55.

[723] Russinova Z, et al. A randomized controlled trial of a peer-run antistigma photovoice intervention. *Psychiatr. Serv.* 2014;65:242–246.

[724] Mills H, et al. Self-help interventions to reduce self-stigma in people with mental health problems: A systematic literature review. *Psychiatry Res.* 2020;284:112702.

[725] Thoits PA. "I'm not mentally ill": Identity deflection as a form of stigma resistance. *J. Health Soc. Behav.* 2016;57:135–151.

[726] Quinn DM. When stigma is concealable: The costs and benefits for health. In: Major B, Dovidio JF, Link BG, eds. The Oxford Handbook of Stigma, Discrimination, and Health. Oxford: Oxford University Press; 2018. pp. 287–299.

[727] Corrigan PW, et al. Reducing self-stigma by coming out proud. *Am. J. Public Health* 2013;103:794–800.

[728] Corrigan PW, et al. Adapting disclosure programs to reduce the stigma of mental illness. *Psychiatr. Serv.* 2018;69:826–828.

[729] Rüsch N, et al. Efficacy of Coming Out Proud to reduce stigma's impact among people with mental illness: Pilot randomised controlled trial. *Br. J. Psychiatry* 2014;204:391–397.

[730] Corrigan PW, et al. Diminishing the self-stigma of mental illness by Coming Out Proud. *Psychiatry Res.* 2015;229:148–154.

[731] Conley CS, et al. Honest, Open, Proud–college: Effectiveness of a peer-led small-group intervention for reducing the stigma of mental illness. *Stigma Health* 2020;5:168–178.

[732] Xu Z, et al. Effectiveness of interventions to promote help-seeking for mental health problems: Systematic review and meta-analysis. *Psychol. Med.* 2018;48:2658–2667.

[733] Klawiter M. Breast cancer in two regimes: The impact of social movements on illness experience. *Sociol. Health Illn.* 2004;26:845–874.

[734] Bailey ZD, et al. Structural racism and health inequities in the USA: Evidence and interventions. *Lancet* 2017;389:1453–1463.

[735] Sprague L, et al. Participatory praxis as an imperative for health-related stigma research. *BMC Med.* 2019;17:32.

[736] Henderson C, et al. The Time to Change Programme to reduce stigma and discrimination in England and its wider context. In: Gaebel W, Rössler W, Sartorius N, eds. The Stigma of Mental Illness - End of the Story? Cham: Springer; 2017. pp. 339–356.

[737] Henderson C, et al. Mental illness stigma after a decade of Time to Change England: Inequalities as targets for further improvement. *Eur. J. Public Health* 2020;30:526–532.

[738] Robinson EJ, Henderson C. Public knowledge, attitudes, social distance and reporting contact with people with mental illness 2009-2017. *Psychol. Med.* 2019;49:2717–2726.

[739] Robertson J. See Me: Scotland case study. In: Gaebel W, Rössler W, Sartorius N, eds. The Stigma of Mental Illness - End of the Story? Cham: Springer; 2017. pp. 379–403.

[740] Quinn N, et al. The impact of a national mental health arts and film festival on stigma and recovery. *Acta Psychiatr. Scand.* 2011;123:71–81.

[741] Chen SP, et al. Fighting stigma in Canada: Opening minds anti-stigma initiative. In: Gaebel W, Rössler W, Sartorius N, eds. The Stigma of Mental Illness - End of the Story? Cham: Springer; 2017. pp. 237–261.

[742] Stuart H. Reducing the stigma of mental illness. *Glob. Ment. Health* 2016;3:e17.

[743] Ramge A, Becker H. The German mental health alliance. In: Gaebel W, Rössler W, Sartorius N, eds. The Stigma of Mental Illness - End of the Story? Cham: Springer; 2017. pp. 405–416.

[744] Evans-Lacko S, et al. How much does mental health discrimination cost: Valuing experienced discrimination in relation to healthcare care costs and community participation. *Epidemiol. Psychiatr. Sci.* 2015;24:423–434.

[745] McCrone P, et al. The economic impact of initiatives to reduce stigma: Demonstration of a modelling approach. *Epidemiol. Psichiatr. Soc.* 2010;19:131–139.

[746] Corrigan PW. Lessons learned from unintended consequences about erasing the stigma of mental illness. *World Psychiatry* 2016;15:67–73.

[747] Jacob KS, et al. Mental health systems in countries: Where are we now? *Lancet* 2007;370:1061–1077.

[748] WHO. The Global Burden of Disease: 2004 Update. Geneva; 2008.

[749] Thyloth M, et al. Increasing burden of mental illnesses across the globe: Current status. *Indian J. Soc. Psychiatry* 2016;32:254–256.

[750] Yatham S, et al. Depression, anxiety, and post-traumatic stress disorder among youth in low and middle income countries: A review of prevalence and treatment interventions. *Asian J. Psychiatr.* 2018;38:78–91.

[751] Wang PS, et al. Use of mental health services for anxiety, mood, and substance disorders in 17 countries in the WHO world mental health surveys. *Lancet* 2007;370:841–850.

[752] Horton R. Launching a new movement for mental health. *Lancet* 2007;370:806.

[753] Saxena S, et al. Resources for mental health: Scarcity, inequity, and inefficiency. *Lancet* 2007;370:878–889.

[754] Patel V, et al. Scaling up services for mental and neurological disorders in low-resource settings. *Intern. Health* 2009;1:37–44.

[755] Sweetland AC, et al. Closing the mental health gap in low-income settings by building research capacity: Perspectives from Mozambique. *Ann. Glob. Health* 2014;80:126–133.

[756] WHO, Dept of Mental Health and Substance Abuse. mhGAP Intervention Guide for Mental, Neurological and Substance-Use Disorders in Non-Specialized Health Settings: Version 2.0. Geneva: WHO; 2016.

[757] Lora A, et al. Service availability and utilization and treatment gap for schizophrenic disorders: A survey in 50 low- and middle-income countries. *Bull. World Health Organ.* 2012;90:47–54, 54A–54B.

[758] Alloh FT, et al. Mental Health in low-and middle income countries (LMICs): Going beyond the need for funding. *Health Prospect* 2018;17:12–17.

[759] Petersen I, et al. Optimizing mental health services in low-income and middle-income countries. *Curr. Opin. Psychiatry* 2011;24:318–323.

[760] National Institute of Mental Health and Neuro Sciences. National Mental Health Survey of India, 2015-16: Summary 2016. Available at: www.indianmhs.nimhans.ac.in/Docs/Summary.pdf. Accessed 18 Mar 2021.

[761] Arvind BA, et al. Prevalence and socioeconomic impact of depressive disorders in India: Multisite population-based cross-sectional study. *BMJ Open* 2019;9:e027250.

[762] Gopalkrishnan N. Cultural diversity and mental health: Considerations for policy and practice. *Front. Public Health* 2018;6:179.

[763] Gater R, et al. The pathways to psychiatric care: A cross-cultural study. *Psychol. Med.* 1991;21:761–774.

[764] James S, et al. Demand for, access to and use of community mental health care: Lessons from a demonstration project in India and Pakistan. *Intern. J. Soc. Psychiatry* 2002;48:163–176.

[765] Hanlon C. Next steps for meeting the needs of people with severe mental illness in low- and middle-income countries. *Epidemiol. Psychiatr. Sci.* 2017;26:348–354.

[766] Rathod S, et al. Mental health service provision in low- and middle-income countries. *Health Serv. Ins.* 2017;10:1178632917694350.

[767] van der Watt ASJ, et al. The perceived effectiveness of traditional and faith healing in the treatment of mental illness: A systematic review of qualitative studies. *Soc. Psychiatry Psychiatr. Epidem.* 2018; 53:555–566.

[768] Saraceno B, et al. Barriers to improvement of mental health services in low-income and middle-income countries. *Lancet* 2007;370:1164–1174.

[769] Hanlon C, et al. Challenges and opportunities for implementing integrated mental health care: A district level situation analysis from five low- and middle-income countries. *PLoS One* 2014;9:e88437.

[770] Jacob KS. Mental health services in low-income and middle-income countries. *Lancet Psychiatr.* 2017;4:87–89.

[771] Angdembe M, et al. Situational analysis to inform development of primary care and community-based mental health services for severe mental disorders in Nepal. *Int. J. Ment. Health Syst.* 2017;11:69.

[772] Gómez-Dantés O, Frenk J. Neither myth nor stigma: Mainstreaming mental health in developing countries. *Salud Publica de Mex.* 2018;60:212–217.

[773] Thornicroft G, et al. Stigma: Ignorance, prejudice or discrimination? *Br. J. Psychiatry* 2007;190:192–193.

[774] Koschorke M, et al. Experiences of stigma and discrimination faced by family caregivers of people with schizophrenia in India. *Soc. Sci. Med.* 2017;178:66–77.

[775] Ubaka CM, et al. Health professionals' stigma towards the psychiatric ill in Nigeria. *Ethiop. J. Health Sci.* 2018;28:483–494.

[776] Nyblade L, et al. Stigma in health facilities: Why it matters and how we can change it. *BMC Med.* 2019;17:25.

[777] Pryor J, Reeder G. HIV-related stigma. In: Hall JC, Hall BJ, Cockerell CJ, eds. HIV/AIDS in the Post-HAART Era: Manifestations, Treatment, and Epidemiology. Shelton: People's Medical Pub House; 2011. pp. 790–806.

[778] Mascayano F, et al. Addressing stigma relating to mental illness in low- and middle-income countries. *Front. Psychiatry* 2015;6:38.

[779] Semrau M, et al. Strengthening mental health systems in low- and middle-income countries: The Emerald programme. *BMC Med.* 2015;13:79.

[780] Mehta N, et al. Evidence for effective interventions to reduce mental health-related stigma and discrimination in the medium and long term: Systematic review. *Br. J. Psychiatry* 2015;207:377–384.

[781] Thornicroft G, et al. Evidence for effective interventions to reduce mental health related stigma and discrimination. *Lancet* 2016;387:1123–1132.

[782] Heim E, et al. Reducing mental health-related stigma among medical and nursing students in low- and middle-income countries: A systematic review. *Epidemiol. Psychiatr. Sci.* 2019;29:e28.

[783] Kleinman A. Clinical relevance of anthropological and cross-cultural research: Concepts and strategies. *Am. J. Psychiatry* 1978;135:427–431.

[784] Raguram R. The ache of exile: Travails of stigma and social exclusion among the mentally ill in India. *Psychol. Dev. Soc. J.* 2015;27:254–269.

[785] Mascayano F, et al. Including culture in programs to reduce stigma toward people with mental disorders in low- and middle-income countries. *Transcult. Psychiatry* 2020;57:140–160.

[786] Weiss MG, et al. Psychiatric stigma across cultures: Local validation in Bangalore and London. *Anthropol. Med.* 2001;8:71–87.

[787] Thara R, Srinivasan TN. How stigmatising is schizophrenia in India? *Int. J. Soc. Psychiatry* 2000; 46:135–141.

[788] Charles H, et al. Stigma and explanatory models among people with schizophrenia and their relatives in Vellore, south India. *Int. J. Soc. Psychiatry* 2007;53:325–332.

[789] Raguram R, et al. Schizophrenia and the cultural epidemiology of stigma in Bangalore, India. *J. Nerv. Ment. Dis.* 2004;192:734–744.

[790] Loganathan S, Murthy SR. Experiences of stigma and discrimination endured by people suffering from schizophrenia. *Indian J. Psychiatry* 2008;50:39–46.

[791] Loganathan S, Murthy RS. Living with schizophrenia in India: Gender perspectives. *Transcult. Psychiatry* 2011;48:569–584.

[792] Thara R, et al. Women with schizophrenia and broken marriages—doubly disadvantaged? Part I: Patient perspective. *Intern. J. Soc. Psychiatry* 2003;49:225–232.

[793] Rao D, et al. Gender inequality and structural violence among depressed women in South India. *Soc. Psychiatry Psychiatr. Epidem.* 2012;47:1967–1975.

[794] Kleinman A. Experience and its moral modes: Culture, human conditions, and disorder. In: Peterson GB, ed. Tanner Lectures on Human Values. Salt Lake City: Univ Utah Press; 1999. pp. 357–420.

[795] Hernandez M, et al. Cultural competence: A literature review and conceptual model for mental health services. *Psychiatr. Serv.* 2009;60:1046–1050.

[796] Kim BSK, et al. The Asian Values Scale: Development, factor analysis, validation, and reliability. *J. Couns. Psychol.* 1999;46:342–352.

[797] Abdullah T, Brown TL. Mental illness stigma and ethnocultural beliefs, values, and norms: An integrative review. *Clin. Psychol. Rev.* 2011;31:934–948.

[798] Thara R, et al. Beliefs about mental illness: A study of a rural South-Indian community. *Int. J. Ment. Health.* 1998;27:70–85.

[799] Pereira B, et al. The explanatory models of depression in low income countries: Listening to women in India. *J. Affect. Disord.* 2007;102:209–218.

[800] Mathews M, et al. Explanatory models of mental illness among family caregivers of persons in psychiatric rehabilitation services: A pilot study. *Int. J. Soc. Psychiatry* 2019;65:589–602.

[801] Shankar BR, et al. Explanatory models of common mental disorders among traditional healers and their patients in rural south India. *Int. J. Soc. Psychiatry* 2006;52:221–233.

[802] Raguram R, et al. Traditional community resources for mental health: A report of temple healing from India. *BMJ* 2002;325:38–40.

[803] Johnson S, et al. Insight, psychopathology, explanatory models and outcome of schizophrenia in India: A prospective 5-year cohort study. *BMC Psychiatry* 2012;12:159.

[804] Kohrt BA, Hruschka DJ. Nepali concepts of psychological trauma: The role of idioms of distress, ethnopsychology and ethnophysiology in alleviating suffering and preventing stigma. *Cult. Med. Psychiatry* 2010;34:322–352.

[805] Neupane D, et al. Caregivers' attitude towards people with mental illness and perceived stigma: A cross-sectional study in a tertiary hospital in Nepal. *PLoS One* 2016;11:e0158113.

[806] Clarke K, et al. Understanding psychological distress among mothers in rural Nepal: A qualitative grounded theory exploration. *BMC Psychiatry* 2014;14:60.

[807] Chase LE, et al. Culture and mental health in Nepal: An interdisciplinary scoping review. *Glob. Ment. Health* 2018;5:e36.

[808] Shah I, et al. Impact of conventional beliefs and social stigma on attitude towards access to mental health services in Pakistan. *Comm. Ment. Health J.* 2019;55:527–533.

[809] Dein S, et al. Jinn, psychiatry and contested notions of misfortune among east London Bangladeshis. *Transcult. Psychiatry* 2008;45:31–55.

[810] Nuri NN, et al. Pathways to care of patients with mental health problems in Bangladesh. *Int. J. Ment. Health Syst.* 2018;12:39.

[811] Hossain MD, et al. Mental disorders in Bangladesh: A systematic review. *BMC Psychiatry* 2014;14:216.

[812] Islam A. Mental health and the health system in Bangladesh: Situation analysis of a neglected domain. *AJPN* 2015;3:57–62.

[813] Kudva KG, et al. Stigma in mental illness: Perspective from eight Asian nations. *Asia Pac. Psychiatry* 2020;12:e12380.

[814] Phillips MR, et al. Stigma and expressed emotion: A study of people with schizophrenia and their family members in China. *Br. J. Psychiatry* 2002;181:488–493.

[815] Yang LH, et al. Culture and stigma: Adding moral experience to stigma theory. *Soc. Sci. Med.* 2007;64:1524–1535.

[816] Farmer PE, et al. Structural violence and clinical medicine. *PLoS Med* 2006;3:e449.

[817] Burnard P, et al. Views of mental illness and mental health care in Thailand: A report of an ethnographic study. *J. Psychiatr. Ment. Health Nurs.* 2006;13:742–749.

[818] Hamdan-Mansour AM, Wardam LA. Attitudes of Jordanian mental health nurses toward mental illness and patients with mental illness. *Issues Ment. Health Nurs.* 2009;30:705–711.

[819] Bener A, Ghuloum S. Gender difference on patients' satisfaction and expectation towards mental health care. *Nig. J. Clin. Pract.* 2013;16:285–291.

[820] Alzayani S. Effect of Cultural Background and Training on Stigmatized Attitudes Among Healthcare Professionals: A Randomized Study of Medical Students' Attitude and Behaviors Toward Alcohol Dependent Individuals in the Middle East [Doctoral Diss.]: University of Connecticut; 2015.

[821] Koura M, et al. Qualitative research: Stigma associated with psychiatric diseases. *Middle East J. Fam. Med.* 2012;10:44–47.

[822] Alosaimi FD, et al. The prevalence of psychiatric disorders among visitors to faith healers in Saudi Arabia. *Pak. J. Med. Sci.* 2014;30:1077–1082.

[823] Alosaimi FD, et al. Public awareness, beliefs, and attitudes toward bipolar disorder in Saudi Arabia. *Neuropsychiatr. Dis. Treat.* 2019;15:2809–2818.

[824] Alsughayir MA. Public view of the "Evil Eye" and its role in psychiatry. A Study in Saudi society. *Arab. J. Psychiatry* 1996;7:152–160.

[825] Khalil AI. Stigma versus mental health literacy: Saudi public knowledge and attitudes towards mental disorders. *IJIER* 2017;5:59–76.

[826] Abolfotouh MA, et al. Attitudes toward mental illness, mentally ill persons, and help-seeking among the Saudi public and sociodemographic correlates. *Psychol. Res. Behav. Manag.* 2019;12:45–54.

[827] Alahmed S, et al. Perceptions of mental illness etiology and treatment in Saudi Arabian healthcare students: A cross-sectional study. *SAGE Open Med.* 2018;6:2050312118788095.

[828] Tayeb H, et al. Supernatural explanations of neurological and psychiatric disorders among health care professionals at an academic tertiary care hospital in Saudi Arabia. *J. Nerv. Ment. Dis.* 2018;206:589–592.

[829] Alqahtani MM, Salmon P. Cultural influences in the aetiological beliefs of saudi arabian primary care patients about their symptoms: The association of religious and psychological beliefs. *J. Religion Health* 2008;47:302–313.

[830] AlAteeq D, et al. The experience and impact of stigma in Saudi people with a mood disorder. *Ann. Gen. Psychiatry* 2018;17:51.

[831] Alamri Y. Mental illness in Saudi Arabia: Stigma and acceptability. *Int. J. Soc. Psychiatry* 2016;62: 306–307.

[832] Dalky HF. Mental illness stigma reduction interventions: Review of intervention trials. *West. J. Nurs. Res.* 2012;34:520–547.

[833] Dalky HF, et al. Quality of life, stigma and burden perception among family caregivers and patients with psychiatric illnesses in Jordan. *Comm. Ment. Health J.* 2017;53:266–274.

[834] Dalky HF, et al. Assessment of mental health stigma components of mental health knowledge, attitudes and behaviors among Jordanian healthcare providers. *Comm. Ment. Health J.* 2020;56:524–531.

[835] Al Ali NM, et al. Factors affecting help-seeking attitudes regarding mental health services among attendance of primary health care centers in Jordan. *Int. J. Ment. Health* 2017;46:38–51.

[836] Taghva A, et al. Stigma barriers of mental health in Iran: A qualitative study by stakeholders of mental health. *Iran. J. Psychiatry* 2017;12:163–171.

[837] Shamsaei F, et al. Meaning of health from the perspective of family member caregiving to patients with bipolar disorder. *J. Mazand. Univ. Med. Sci.* 2012;22:51–65.

[838] Akbari M, et al. Challenges of family caregivers of patients with mental disorders in Iran: A narrative review. *Iran. J. Nurs. Midwifery Res.* 2018;23:329–337.

[839] Abi Doumit C, et al. Knowledge, attitude and behaviors towards patients with mental illness: Results from a national Lebanese study. *PLoS One* 2019;14:e0222172.

[840] Rayan A, Fawaz M. Cultural misconceptions and public stigma against mental illness among Lebanese university students. *Perspect. Psychiatr. Care* 2018;54:258–265.

[841] Aramouny C, et al. Knowledge, attitudes, and beliefs of Catholic clerics' regarding mental health in Lebanon. *J. Relig. Health* 2020;59:257–276.

[842] Weissbecker I, Fitzgerald C. IMC Libya Mental Health and Psychosocial Support Assessment Report 2011. Available at: https://internationalmedicalcorps.org/wp-content/uploads/2017/07/International-Medical-Corps-Libya-MHPSS-Assessment-Report-Nov-2011.pdf. Accessed 24 Mar 2021.

[843] Spagnolo J, et al. Mental health knowledge, attitudes, and self-efficacy among primary care physicians working in the Greater Tunis area of Tunisia. *Int. J. Ment. Health Syst.* 2018;12:63.

[844] Okello E, Musisi S. The role of traditional healers in mental health care in Africa. In: Hill AG, Kleinman A, Akyeampong EK, eds. The Culture of Mental Illness and Psychiatric Practice in Africa. Bloomington: Indiana Univ Press; 2015. pp. 249–261.

[845] Amuyunzu-Nyamongo M. The Social and Cultural Aspects of Mental Health in African Societies. Commonwealth Health Partnerships. 2013; pp. 59–63. Available at: www.commonwealthhealth.org/wp-content/uploads/2013/07/The-social-and-cultural-aspects-of-mental-health-in-African-societies_CHP13.pdf. Accessed 3 Mar 2021.

[846] Ventevogel P, et al. Madness or sadness? Local concepts of mental illness in four conflict-affected African communities. *Confl. Health* 2013;7:3.

[847] van Duijl M, et al. Unravelling the spirits' message: A study of help-seeking steps and explanatory models among patients suffering from spirit possession in Uganda. *Int. J. Ment. Health Syst.* 2014;8:24.

[848] Kpobi L, Swartz L. Explanatory models of mental disorders among traditional and faith healers in Ghana. *Int. J. Cult. Ment. Health* 2018;11:605–615.

[849] Dako-Gyeke M, Asumang ES. Stigmatization and discrimination experiences of persons with mental illness: Insights from a qualitative study in southern Ghana. *Soc. Work Soc.* 2013;11.

[850] Read UM, et al. Local suffering and the global discourse of mental health and human rights: An ethnographic study of responses to mental illness in rural Ghana. *Global. Health* 2009;5:13.

[851] Yaro PB, et al. Stakeholders' perspectives about the impact of training and sensitization of traditional and spiritual healers on mental health and illness: A qualitative evaluation in Ghana. *Int. J. Soc. Psychiatry* 2020;66:476–484.

[852] Sorsdahl KR, Stein DJ. Knowledge of and stigma associated with mental disorders in a South African community sample. *J. Nerv. Ment. Dis.* 2010;198:742–747.

[853] Girma E, et al. Public stigma against people with mental illness in the Gilgel Gibe Field Research Center (GGFRC) in Southwest Ethiopia. *PLoS One* 2013;8:e82116.

[854] Hatzenbuehler ML, Link BG. Introduction to the special issue on structural stigma and health. *Soc. Sci. Med.* 2014;103:1–6.

[855] Böge K, et al. Perceived stigmatization and discrimination of people with mental illness: A survey-based study of the general population in five metropolitan cities in India. *Ind. J. Psychiatry* 2018; 60:24–31.

[856] Bhugra D, et al. Legislative provisions related to marriage and divorce of persons with mental health problems: A global review. *Int. Rev. Psychiatry* 2016;28:386–392.

[857] Ministry of Health and Family Welfare Government of India. The Mental Healthcare Act: An Act to Provide for Mental Healthcare and Services for Persons with Mental Illness and to Protect, Promote and Fulfil the Rights of Such Persons During Delivery of Mental Healthcare and Services and for Matters Connected Therewith or Incidental Thereto. 2017. Available at: www.prsindia.org/uploads/media/Mental%20Health/Mental%20Healthcare%20Act,%202017.pdf. Accessed 18 Mar 2021.

[858] Bhugra D, et al. Right to property, inheritance, and contract and persons with mental illness. *Int. Rev. Psychiatry* 2016;28:402–408.

[859] Rosenthal E, Sundram CJ. The Role of International Human Rights in National Mental Health Legislation 2004. Available at: www.who.int/mental_health/policy/international_hr_in_national_mhlegislation.pdf. Accessed 23 Mar 2021.

[860] Petersen I, et al. Strengthening mental health system governance in six low- and middle-income countries in Africa and South Asia: Challenges, needs and potential strategies. *Health Policy Plan.* 2017;32:699–709.

[861] Evans-Lacko S, et al. Evaluation of capacity-building strategies for mental health system strengthening in low- and middle-income countries for service users and caregivers, policymakers and planners, and researchers. *BJPsych Open* 2019;5:e67.

[862] Sharan P, et al. Mental health policies in South-East Asia and the public health role of screening instruments for depression. *WHO South-East Asia J. Publ. Health* 2017;6:5–11.

[863] Okasha A, Okasha T. Religion, spirituality and the concept of mental illness. *Actas Esp. Psiquiatr.* 2012;40:73–79.

[864] Sankoh O, et al. Mental health in Africa. *Lancet Glob. Health* 2018;6:e954–e955.

[865] Bruckner TA, et al. The mental health workforce gap in low- and middle-income countries: A needs-based approach. *Bull. WHO* 2011;89:184–194.

[866] National Academies of Sciences, Engineering, and Medicine. Ending Discrimination Against People With Mental and Substance Use Disorders: The Evidence for Stigma Change. Washington DC; 2016.

[867] Xu Z, et al. Challenging mental health related stigma in China: Systematic review and meta-analysis. I. Interventions among the general public. *Psychiatry Res.* 2017;255:449–456.

[868] Yang LH, et al. Recent advances in cross-cultural measurement in psychiatric epidemiology: Utilizing 'what matters most' to identify culture-specific aspects of stigma. *Int. J. Epidemiol.* 2014;43:494–510.

[869] Fung KM, et al. Randomized controlled trial of the self-stigma reduction program among individuals with schizophrenia. *Psychiatry Res.* 2011;189:208–214.

[870] Ahuja KK, et al. Breaking barriers: An education and contact intervention to reduce mental illness stigma among Indian college students. *Psychosocl. Intervention* 2017;26:103–109.

[871] Fernandez A, et al. Effects of brief psychoeducational program on stigma in Malaysian pre-clinical medical students: A randomized controlled trial. *Acad. Psychiatry* 2016;40:905–911.

[872] Maulik PK, et al. Longitudinal assessment of an anti-stigma campaign related to common mental disorders in rural India. *Br. J. Psychiatry* 2019;214:90–95.

[873] Loganathan S, Kreuter M. Audience segmentation: Identifying key stakeholders for mental health literacy interventions in India. *J. Public Ment. Health* 2014;13:159–170.

[874] Chatterjee S, et al. Effectiveness of a community-based intervention for people with schizophrenia and their caregivers in India (COPSI): A randomised controlled trial. *Lancet* 2014;383:1385–1394.

[875] Gutiérrez-Maldonado J, et al. Effects of a psychoeducational intervention program on the attitudes and health perceptions of relatives of patients with schizophrenia. *Soc. Psychiatry Psychiatr. Epidemiol.* 2009;44:343–348.

[876] John S, et al. Addressing stigma and discrimination towards mental illness: A community based intervention programme from India. *J. Psychosoc. Rehab. Ment. Health* 2015;2:79–85.

[877] Shamsaei F, et al. The effect of training interventions of stigma associated with mental illness on family caregivers: A quasi-experimental study. *Ann. Gen. Psychiatry* 2018;17:48.

[878] Worakul P, et al. Effects of psycho-educational program on knowledge and attitude upon schizophrenia of schizophrenic patients' caregivers. *J. Med. Assoc. Thai.* 2007;90:1199–1204.

REFERENCES

263

[879] Balaji M, et al. The development of a lay health worker delivered collaborative community based intervention for people with schizophrenia in India. *BMC Health Serv. Res.* 2012;12:42.
[880] Li J, et al. Effectiveness of an anti-stigma training on improving attitudes and decreasing discrimination towards people with mental disorders among care assistant workers in Guangzhou, China. *Int. J. Ment. Health Syst.* 2019;13:1.
[881] Armstrong G, et al. A mental health training program for community health workers in India: Impact on knowledge and attitudes. *Int. J. Ment. Health Syst.* 2011;5:17.
[882] Makanjuola V, et al. Impact of a one-week intensive 'training of trainers' workshop for community health workers in south-west Nigeria. *Ment. Health Fam. Med.* 2012;9:33–38.
[883] Chinnayya HP, et al. Training primary care health workers in mental health care: Evaluation of attitudes towards mental illness before and after training. *Intern. J. Soc. Psychiatry* 1990;36:300–307.
[884] Ng YP, et al. Determining the effectiveness of a video-based contact intervention in improving attitudes of Penang primary care nurses towards people with mental illness. *PLoS One* 2017;12: e0187861.
[885] Bayar MR, et al. Reducing mental illness stigma in mental health professionals using a web-based approach. *Isr. J. Psychiatry Relat. Sci.* 2009;46:226–230.
[886] Rong Y, et al. Improving knowledge and attitudes towards depression: A controlled trial among Chinese medical students. *BMC Psychiatry* 2011;11:36.
[887] Reddy JP, et al. The effect of a clinical posting in psychiatry on the attitudes of medical students towards psychiatry and mental illness in a Malaysian medical school. *Ann. Acad. Med. Singap.* 2005; 34:505–510.
[888] Arkar H, Eker D. Influence of a 3-week psychiatric training programme on attitudes toward mental illness in medical students. *Soc. Psychiatry Psychiatr. Epidemiol.* 1997;32:171–176.
[889] Altindag A, et al. Effects of an antistigma program on medical students' attitudes towards people with schizophrenia. *Psychiatry Clin. Neurosci.* 2006;60:283–288.
[890] Vargas D de. The impact of clinical experience with alcoholics on Brazilian nursing students' attitudes toward alcoholism and associated problems. *J. Addict. Nurs.* 2013;24:180–186.
[891] Kakuma R, et al. Mental health stigma: What is being done to raise awareness and reduce stigma in South Africa? *Afr. J. Psychiatry* 2010;13:116–124.
[892] Petersen I, et al. Lessons from case studies of integrating mental health into primary health care in South Africa and Uganda. *Int. J. Ment. Health Syst.* 2011;5:8.
[893] Pejović-Milovancević M, et al. Changing attitudes of high school students towards peers with mental health problems. *Psychiatr. Danub.* 2009;21:213–219.
[894] Chan JYN, et al. Combining education and video-based contact to reduce stigma of mental illness: "The Same or Not the Same" anti-stigma program for secondary schools in Hong Kong. *Soc. Sci. Med.* 2009;68:1521–1526.
[895] Kutcher S, et al. Improving Malawian teachers' mental health knowledge and attitudes: An integrated school mental health literacy approach. *Glob. Ment. Health* 2015;2:e1.
[896] Khairy N, et al. Impact of the first national campaign against the stigma of mental illness. *Egypt. J. Psychiatr.* 2012;33:35–39.
[897] Maulik PK, et al. Evaluation of an anti-stigma campaign related to common mental disorders in rural India: A mixed methods approach. *Psychol. Med.* 2017;47:565–575.
[898] Dharitri R, et al. Stigma of mental illness: An interventional study to reduce its impact in the community. *Ind. J. Psychiatry* 2015;57:165–173.
[899] Knaak S, et al. Mental illness-related stigma in healthcare: Barriers to access and care and evidence-based solutions. *Healthc. Manage. Forum* 2017;30:111–116.
[900] Uys L, et al. Evaluation of a health setting-based stigma intervention in five African countries. *AIDS Patient Care STDS* 2009;23:1059–1066.
[901] Grandón P, et al. An integrative program to reduce stigma in primary healthcare workers toward people with diagnosis of severe mental disorders: A protocol for a randomized controlled trial. *Front. Psychiatry* 2019;10:110.
[902] Corrigan PW, Watson AC. Understanding the impact of stigma on people with mental illness. *World Psychiatry* 2002;1:16–20.
[903] Loganathan S, Varghese M. Formative research on devising a street play to create awareness about mental illness: Cultural adaptation and targeted approach. *Int. J. Soc. Psychiatry* 2019;65:279–288.

[904] Park S, Park KS. Family stigma: A concept analysis. *Asian Nurs. Res.* 2014;8:165–171.
[905] Yu BCL et al. Internalization process of stigma of people with mental illness across cultures: A meta-analytic structural equation modeling approach. *Clin. Psychol. Rev.* 2021;87:102029.
[906] Mittal D, et al. Empirical studies of self-stigma reduction strategies: A critical review of the literature. *Psychiatr. Serv.* 2012;63:974–981.
[907] Xu Z, et al. Challenging mental health related stigma in China: Systematic review and meta-analysis. II. Interventions among people with mental illness. *Psychiatry Res.* 2017;255:457–464.
[908] Medical Research Council. The MRC Funds £2m Study to Address Global Mental Health Stigma - News and Features - Medical Research Council 2018. Available at: webarchive.nationalarchives.gov. uk/20200923122015/https://mrc.ukri.org/news/browse/mrc-funds-2m-study-to-address-global-mental-health-stigma/. Accessed 18 Mar 2021.
[909] Thornicroft G, et al. Key lessons learned from the INDIGO global network on mental health related stigma and discrimination. *World Psychiatry* 2019;18:229–230.
[910] O'Reilly CL, et al. Consumer-led mental health education for pharmacy students. *Am. J. Pharm. Educ.* 2010;74:167.
[911] Friedrich B, et al. Anti-stigma training for medical students: The education not discrimination project. *Br. J. Psychiatry Suppl.* 2013;55:s89–s94.
[912] Thornicroft G. Physical health disparities and mental illness: The scandal of premature mortality. *Br. J. Psychiatry* 2011;199:441–442.
[913] Thornicroft G. Premature death among people with mental illness. *BMJ* 2013;346:f2969.
[914] WHO, Dept. of Mental Health and Substance Abuse. mhGAP Intervention Guide for Mental, Neurological and Substance-Use Disorders in Non-Specialized Health Settings: Version 1.0. Geneva: WHO; 2010.
[915] Kohrt BA, et al. Reducing mental illness stigma in healthcare settings: Proof of concept for a social contact intervention to address what matters most for primary care providers. *Soc. Sci. Med.* 2020; 250:112852.
[916] Lewin S, et al. Supporting the delivery of cost-effective interventions in primary health-care systems in low-income and middle-income countries: An overview of systematic reviews. *Lancet* 2008;372: 928–939.
[917] Druetz T. Integrated primary health care in low- and middle-income countries: A double challenge. *BMC Med. Ethics* 2018;19:48.
[918] Lund C, et al. PRIME: A programme to reduce the treatment gap for mental disorders in five low- and middle-income countries. *PLoS Med.* 2012;9:e1001359.
[919] Keynejad RC, et al. WHO Mental Health Gap Action Programme (mhGAP) Intervention Guide: A systematic review of evidence from low and middle-income countries. *Evid. Based Ment. Health* 2018; 21:30–34.
[920] Singh OP. District Mental Health Program - need to look into strategies in the era of Mental Health Care Act, 2017 and moving beyond Bellary Model. *Indian J. Psychiatry* 2018;60:163–164.
[921] Acharya B, et al. Partnerships in mental healthcare service delivery in low-resource settings: Developing an innovative network in rural Nepal. *Global. Health* 2017;13:2.
[922] Hall T, et al. Social inclusion and exclusion of people with mental illness in Timor-Leste: A qualitative investigation with multiple stakeholders. *BMC Publ. Health* 2019;19:702.
[923] Maitra S, et al. An approach to mental health in low and middle income countries: A case example from urban India. *Int. J. Ment. Health* 2015;44:215–230.
[924] Amenta E, Polletta F. The cultural impacts of social movements. *Annu. Rev. Sociol.* 2019;45:279–299.
[925] Clair M, et al. Destigmatization and health: Cultural constructions and the long-term reduction of stigma. *Soc. Sci. Med.* 2016;165:223–232.
[926] Tokmic F, et al. Development of a behavioral health stigma measure and application of machine learning for classification. *Innov. Clin. Neurosci.* 2018;15:34–42.
[927] Brannan C, et al. Preventing discrimination based on psychiatric risk biomarkers. *Am. J. Med. Genet. B Neuropsychiatr. Genet.* 2019;180:159–171.
[928] Mullor D, et al. Effect of a serious game (Stigma-Stop) on reducing stigma among psychology students: A controlled study. *Cyberpsychol. Behav. Soc. Netw.* 2019;22:205–211.
[929] Zhang J, Centola D. Social networks and health: New developments in diffusion, online and offline. *Annu. Rev. Sociol.* 2019;45:91–109.

INTERNET ADDRESSES

The internet addresses listed here in alphabetical order (as of February 2022) are listed in the text. More information can be found in the text sections mentioned.

https://alz.co.uk/everythreeseconds	Sect. 5.4.4
https://alzheimerfest.it	Sect. 5.4.4
https://alzpoetry.com	Sect. 5.4.4
https://bagw.de	Sect. 7.2.1
https://bastagegenstigma.de	Sect. 8.4.7
https://bergundmental.de	Sect. 5.4.3
https://bibb.de/en	Sect. 7.2.1
https://blaupause-gesundheit.de	Sect. 7.3.2
https://bzga.de/home/bzga/	Sect. 5.2.3
https://cartercenter.org	Sect. 7.4.7
https://cochrane.org	Sect. 1.5
https://deutsche-depressionshilfe.de	Sect. 5.2.3
https://dgbs.de	Sects. 5.4.2, 7.3.2
https://empowerment-college.com	Sect. 5.1.6
https://ex-in.de	Sects. 7.3.4, 9.1.5
https://ex-in.eu	Sect. 9.1.5
https://feantsa.org	Sect. 7.2.1
https://frnd.de	Sects. 5.2.3, 7.4.5
https://gedenkort-t4.eu	Sect. 2.1.2
https://hearing-voices.org	Sect. 8.1.4
https://hopprogram.org	Sect. 9.2.5
https://indigo-group.org	Sect. 1.5
https://institut-fuer-menschenrechte.de/en	Sect. 7.5.2
https://iom.int	Sect. 5.8
https://irremenschlich.de	Sect. 8.4.6
https://irrsinnig-menschlich.de	Sect. 8.4.5
https://itgetsbetter.org	Sect. 4.3.4
https://konfetti-im-kopf.de	Sect. 5.4.4
https://mentalhealthcrowd.de	Sect. 5.4.3
https://muenchen-depression.de	Sect. 8.1.6
https://mutmachleute.de	Sect. 8.4.3
https://neunerhaus.at	Sect. 7.2.3
https://ohrenkuss.de	Sect. 5.4.6
https://projekt-yam.at	Sect. 5.2.3
https://promenz.at	Sect. 5.4.4
https://psychenet.de	Sect. 8.1.6
https://recoverycollegeberlin.de	Sect. 5.1.6
https://refukey.org	Sect. 5.8
https://robert-enke-stiftung.de	Sect. 5.2.3
https://scope.org.uk/campaigns/end-the-awkward	Sect. 5.4.6
https://seelischegesundheit.net	Sect. 12.2
https://seemescotland.org	Sect. 12.1
https://suizidpraevention.de	Sect. 5.2.3

INDEX

Page numbers followed by 'f', indicate figure; 't', tables; 'b', boxes.

Healthcare system
  adequate staffing levels, 157–158
  antistigma interventions, 139
  antistigma interventions for professionals, 142–143
  architecture, 147–148
  attitudes of professionals, 139–140
  avoidance of coercion and violence, 155–157
  experiences of patients, 140
  fragmentation, 144–145
  at individual level, 139–142
  inequality and stigma, 138
  initiatives against structural discrimination in, 148–158
  integrated care and regional budget, 150–151
  interfaces, 144–145
  lack of psychosocial interventions, 145–146
  levels of, 139
  patients *vs.* professionals, 140–141
  peer support, 153–155
  prejudice and discrimination, 138
  prevention, 151–153
  professionals with mental illness, 141
  psychiatrists, 141–142
  shared decision-making, 141
  somatic care, 146–147
  strengthening outpatient care, 148–150, 149f
  structural discrimination, 143–148, 200
  trialogue, 153–155
  wrong incentives, 144–145
Health consequences of secrecy, 58b
Help-seeking, 75–79, 109, 198–199, 206. *See also* Treatment and stigma
Henderson, Claire, 131, 180, 202
Henryism, John, 56
Heracles, 13, 15
Herodotus, 29
Hinshaw, Stephen, 105
Hippocrates, 15
Hoche, Alfred, 16–17
Hölderlin, Friedrich, 227
Homelessness
  discrimination, 135–136
  and health, 134–135
  media coverage of, 135
  public opinion on, 135
  support and treatment for, 136–137
Homer, 1, 85
Home Treatment, 148
Honest, Open, Proud (HOP) programme, 194–197
  approach of, 194–195
  for different target groups, 196
  format and content, 195–196
  group facilitators and participants, 196
  identity as mentally ill and disclosure, 194
Hope, 3

Housing, 134–138
Housing First, 137–138

I
Ignorance
  media, 166–167
  and negative attitudes, 108–109
Illness
  and impairments, 4
  prevention, 50
  in work environment, disclosure of, 128
Incentives, wrong, 144–145
India, mental illness in, 208
INDIGO Partnership Research Programme, 221–222
Individual discrimination, 32
Individual Placement and Support (IPS). *See* Supported employment
Individual studies, 7
Inequality and stigma, 138
Insecurity, fear and, 52
Integrated care and regional budget, 150–151
Intellectual disability, 100–102
Interfaces, 144–145
Intersectionality, 104
Intervention studies, 5–6
In Würde zu sich stehen. *See* Honest, Open, Proud
Iran, mental illness in, 210
Irre Menschlich Hamburg, 189–190
Irrsinnig Menschlich (Madly Human), 189

J
Jaadu-tona, 209
Jaspers, Karl, 27
Jesus, 29, 64
Jinn, 209, 210
Job search, disclosure in, 131
Jordan, mental illness in, 210
Jorm, Tony, 179
Just world belief, 46–47

K
Kafka, Franz, 11, 157
Kalanka, 209
karma, 208
Khoutweh Khoutweh, 212
Kissling, Werner, 190
Klee, Ernst, 17–18
Kleitias, 14f
Knaak, Stephanie, 93
Knapp, Martin, 22
Kwan, 209